Microbiology Theory for MLT

Microbiology Theory for MLT

(Medical Laboratory Technology)

Second Edition

Namita Jaggi
MBBS MD
Consultant Microbiologist
Director
Department of Laboratory and Infection Control
Artemis Health Institute
Gurgaon, Haryana, India

JAYPEE

JAYPEE BROTHERS MEDICAL PUBLISHERS (P) LTD

New Delhi • London • Philadelphia • Panama

Jaypee Brothers Medical Publishers (P) Ltd

Headquarters
Jaypee Brothers Medical Publishers (P) Ltd
4838/24, Ansari Road, Daryaganj
New Delhi 110 002, India
Phone: +91-11-43574357
Fax: +91-11-43574314
Email: jaypee@jaypeebrothers.com

Overseas Offices

J.P. Medical Ltd
83 Victoria Street, London
SW1H 0HW (UK)
Phone: +44-2031708910
Fax: +02-03-0086180
Email: info@jpmedpub.com

Jaypee Medical Inc
The Bourse
111 South Independence Mall East
Suite 835, Philadelphia, PA 19106, USA
Mobile: +267-519-9789
Email: joe.rusko@jaypeebrothers.com

Jaypee Brothers Medical Publishers (P) Ltd
Shorakhute, Kathmandu
Nepal
Phone: +00977-9841528578
Email: jaypee.nepal@gmail.com

Jaypee-Highlights Medical Publishers Inc
City of Knowledge, Bld. 237, Clayton
Panama City, Panama
Phone: +507-301-0496
Fax: +507-301-0499
Email: cservice@jphmedical.com

Jaypee Brothers Medical Publishers (P) Ltd
17/1-B Babar Road, Block-B, Shaymali
Mohammadpur, Dhaka-1207
Bangladesh
Mobile: +08801912003485
Email: jaypeedhaka@gmail.com

Website: www.jaypeebrothers.com
Website: www.jaypeedigital.com

Inquiries for bulk sales may be solicited at: jaypee@jaypeebrothers.com

Microbiology Theory for MLT

First Edition: 2003
Reprint: 2005, 2008
Second Edition: 2013, **Reprint: 2025**

ISBN 978-93-5090-646-0

Printed in India

Dedicated to

Vikram,

Karan, Raghav, Shagun

... the joy of my life

Preface to the Second Edition

In the years that have elapsed since the first edition of this book was released, a lot of new developments have taken place in the expanding field of microbiology.

Automation in microbiology is one of them. As of now, automation exists in bacterial identification and sensitivity, *Mycobacterium tuberculosis* cultures, urine analysis, blood cultures and serological and molecular tests. They have definitely led to an ease in diagnosis in terms of a rapid turn-around time, and increased accuracy. This is due to incorporation of many automated steps such as pipetting, which excludes variation because of different staff members performing the test. These machines operate on the basis of stringent quality control measures and increase the level of confidence in the laboratory reports. While automation in the field of microbiology cannot completely replace manual methods as in the field of biochemistry and hematology, it is being successfully used in high volume larger laboratories today and is gradually being considered as an option in medium-sized laboratories also. It is important to realize, however, that basic microbiological techniques and knowledge and a sound clinical judgment cannot replace automation. Basic bench work such as plate reading, Gram's stain and bacterial identification on the basis of colony morphology or biochemical tests should be continued. Having a good mix of manual and automated tests would prove useful as well as cost effective.

The last few years have exposed us to the pandemic caused by the novel H1N1 influenza virus. This edition has a chapter dedicated to that. As microbiology technicians, we must be well versed with the way the samples are collected as also the various diagnostic techniques that are available for the diagnosis of this virus. At the same time, one should be aware of the infection control measures, that have to be adopted to prevent transmission of this virus to others. This would include hand hygiene and observance of contact precautions.

The last couple of years have also seen the rise of the field of clinical microbiology, which is the future direction microbiology is taking. It is now moving beyond the laboratory benches into the wards or the intensive care units (ICUs). With the indiscriminate use of antibiotics, antibiotic resistance is on the rise and there is a fear that we may enter the post-antibiotic era very soon, which would be similar to the pre-antibiotic era when we had no antibiotics to treat patients. Microbiologists and clinicians are struggling with extended-spectrum beta-lactamases (ESBLs) in gram-negative bacteria, methicillin-resistant *Staphylococcus aureus* (MRSA), vancomycin-resistant enterococci and PAN-resistant *Acinetobacter* and *Pseudomonas* in the hospital setting. More of the resistant bacteria are causing hospital-acquired infections. The role of the microbiology laboratory is increasing and the antibiotic sensitivities and resistance patterns that it supplies are being used to help clinicians select the appropriate antibiotic for the patients. The microbiology laboratory and the infection control department also partner in setting up the antibiotic policy, which then should be followed to encourage the judicious use of antibiotics. As a result of this change, there has to be a shift in our training perspective from a theoretical to a clinically-oriented approach in which the diagnosis has to be given in conjunction with the clinical history of the patient. It is *as important* to report the organism isolated with its antibiotic sensitivities *as it is not* to report organisms, which are thought to be colonizers. Here lies the importance of correlating the microbiology report with the clinical history. We would be saving the patient from the unnecessary intake of antibiotics and also helping in stopping the march of antibiotic resistance. In today's age, the microbiologists' opinion is being sought on ICU rounds when decisions about the antibiotic sensitivity patterns of the patients are discussed to be able to decide the treatment of patients. So, they have a very critical role as advisors to the clinicians.

Molecular methods and serological techniques are being increasingly used as methods of diagnosis especially in those organisms, which take a long time to grow on conventional media or are very fastidious such as *Mycobacterium tuberculosis*, *Haemophilus* species, *Chlamydia*, gonorrhea, anaerobic organisms and viruses. These methodologies are known to give some false-positive reactions and should be interpreted carefully in conjunction with the clinical history. Also, stringent quality control measures need to be instituted in these tests to be able to benefit from the newer technologies.

Fungus as a cause of infections especially in the hospital ICUs is raising. This is the result of the fungus being selected out because of the wiping out of the bacterial flora by heavy antibiotic intake in hospitals. It is important to be well versed with fungal diagnostic techniques as also antifungal-sensitivities and resistance patterns.

Quality control in microbiology is becoming an integral part of the functioning of a good laboratory. There are two types of quality control procedures, that we adopt in the laboratory—external and internal. External quality control is required to validate our results and test processes from an external authorized agency and internal quality control takes care of the day-to-day accuracy of our results. This involves running of all our controls in the morning daily before the start of the day's work. Whether we are working at larger hospital laboratories or smaller diagnostic centers, we need to formulate an effective internal quality control program, get it validated from our senior doctors and follow it religiously in the laboratories.

Infection control is also falling under the purview of medical microbiologists in hospitals. As one-third of the hospital-acquired infections can be prevented, we need to adopt an infection control plan at our hospitals, which can lead to a decrease in the hospital-acquired infections. This involves a thorough understanding of the microbiology of the bacterial organisms and, their antibiotic sensitivities and the methods to stop transmission.

I would also like to make a special mention of Pushpa Kumari Nirwan, MSc (Microbiology), who has helped me with the formulation of the second edition of this book and has added valuable insights.

Namita Jaggi

Preface to the First Edition

Medical microbiology is the vital link between the clinicians and the patients for the effective diagnosis and treatment of infectious diseases.

An accurate microbiological diagnosis requires the joint effort of a medical microbiologist and the laboratory technician.

The role of the medical laboratory technologist is vital in the effective running of any laboratory. It is he/she who actually runs the tests whether it is performing routine diagnostic tests or working on *molecular diagnostic and genetic techniques*. His/her training, expertise and knowledge in the field of medical microbiology has to be appropriate for him/her to do justice to the subject.

Medical laboratory technology (MLT) as a field is making rapid advances and is becoming a specialty in its own right.

Having been involved in teaching medical microbiology to MLT students (Diploma and BSc), I have realized that there is a paucity of comprehensive and reader-friendly books in microbiology for them. It is with this view in mind, I felt inspired to write a textbook which would help them to understand the basics of medical microbiology and then gently guide them into details wherever required.

Keeping in mind the MLT syllabus, a greater stress has been laid on General Bacteriology, Systemic Bacteriology and Parasitology, which form the backbone of routine microbiological diagnosis. Outlines have been provided on Virology, Mycology, Immunology and Applied Microbiology to give an insight into these upcoming fields.

It has been my sincere effort to stress upon topics relevant to MLT students such as laboratory diagnosis of diseases and basic culture techniques; whereas, at the same time, outlining facts on the antigenic structure of bacteria, that may be required by those who go into research fields. The subject matter in each chapter has been broken down into smaller segments in the form of a lesson plan to aid understanding.

It has been my sincere endeavor to put down on paper my experiences in the field of teaching Medical Microbiology and running a Medical Diagnostic Laboratory for the past decade. I hope students will be benefitted from this book. I welcome suggestions for the improvement of the same.

Namita Jaggi

Acknowledgments

Writing this book has been a satisfying and enjoyable experience. I wish to acknowledge all those who were with me in this endeavor.

I wish to thank my father-in-law, Professor (Dr) OP Jaggi, who provided me with the inspiration and encouragement for writing this book. A renowned author, he has over 50 medical books to his credit including an eighteen volume treatise on the History and Science of Medicine. His guidance, wisdom and expertise have helped me at every stage. I also wish to thank my mother-in-law, Mrs Sudershan Jaggi, for her constant cooperation and sharing of my responsibilities, whereas I devoted myself to this project.

I am grateful as always to my parents, Rear Adm (Retd) KL Malhan and Sushma Malhan, for their unconditional love, encouragement and support. Their affectionate prodding spurred me on to successfully finish this book.

I also thank Dr Manu, Ritu, Sumedha, Madhu, Niten and Neha, for their good wishes and support.

I am indebted to my husband, Dr Vikram Jaggi, for being an anchor of love and strength for me and letting me involve myself in this mammoth task.

I am especially grateful to my children, Karan, Raghav and Shagun, for the time that I snatched away from them to be able to do justice to the book. They patiently accepted my involvement and actively cooperated towards the project.

Thanks are also due to my teachers at Maulana Azad Medical College, my guide Dr UK Baveja, Dr VK Sharma, Dr Krishna Prakash and the faculty at MAMC, for instilling in me sound basic knowledge of the subject.

I would be failing in my duty if I do not thank my MLT students, who provided me with the necessary feedback and the stimulus for writing this book.

Finally, I would like to acknowledge the staff at my clinic—Poonam, Renu, Dhananjay and Rajeev and also Meena my house-help, for holding the fort and enabling me to find time for writing.

I am thankful to Shri Jitendar P Vij (Group Chairman), Mr Ankit Vij (Managing Director) and Mr Tarun Duneja (Director-Publishing) of M/s Jaypee Brothers Medical Publishers (P) Ltd, New Delhi, India, for having provided an ideal environment for the writing up of this book.

I am grateful to Ms Samina Khan, for effective coordination and help at various stages of publication of this book. Thanks are also due to Ms Sunita Katla, Mr KK Raman, Mr Gopal Singh, Ms Seema Dogra, Mr Laxmidhar Padhiary and others at the Jaypee Publishing Department, for their competent professional help.

Contents

Section 1: General Bacteriology

Section 2: Immunology

Section 3: Systemic Bacteriology

Section 4: Virology

Section 5: Parasitology

Section 6: Mycology

Section 7: Applied Microbiology

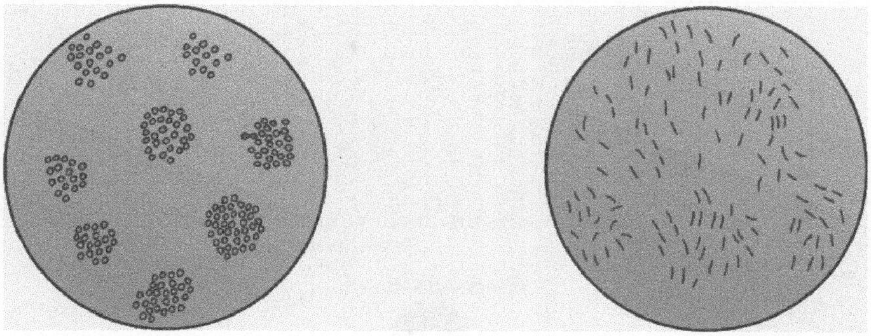

Gram-positive cocci in clusters *Staphylococcus aureus* Gram-negative rods *Escherichia coli*

Fig. 3.1: Gram-positive and gram-negative organisms

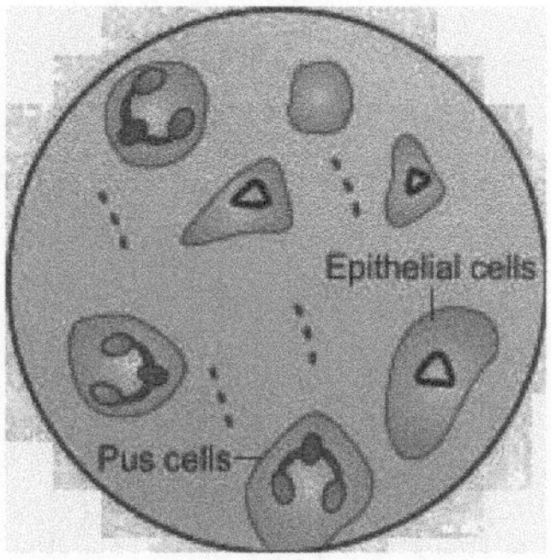

Fig. 3.2: Acid fast bacteria (*Mycobacterium tuberculosis*)

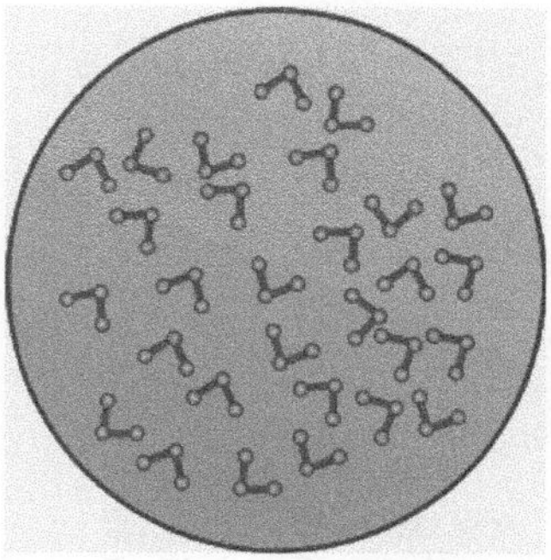

Fig. 3.3: *Corynebacterium diphtheriae* (Albert staining)

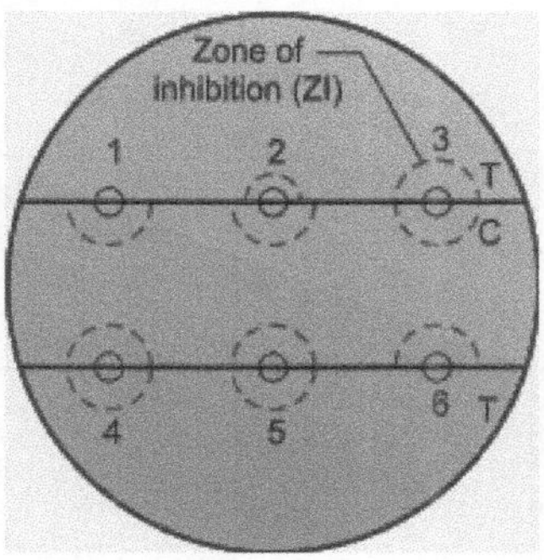

Fig. 12.1: Diagram showing interpretation of Stokes method

C = Control; T = Test; ZI = Zone of inhibition; 1 = Resistant; 2 = Intermediate resistant; 3 = Sensitive; 4 = Sensitive; 5 = Sensitive; 6 = Resistant

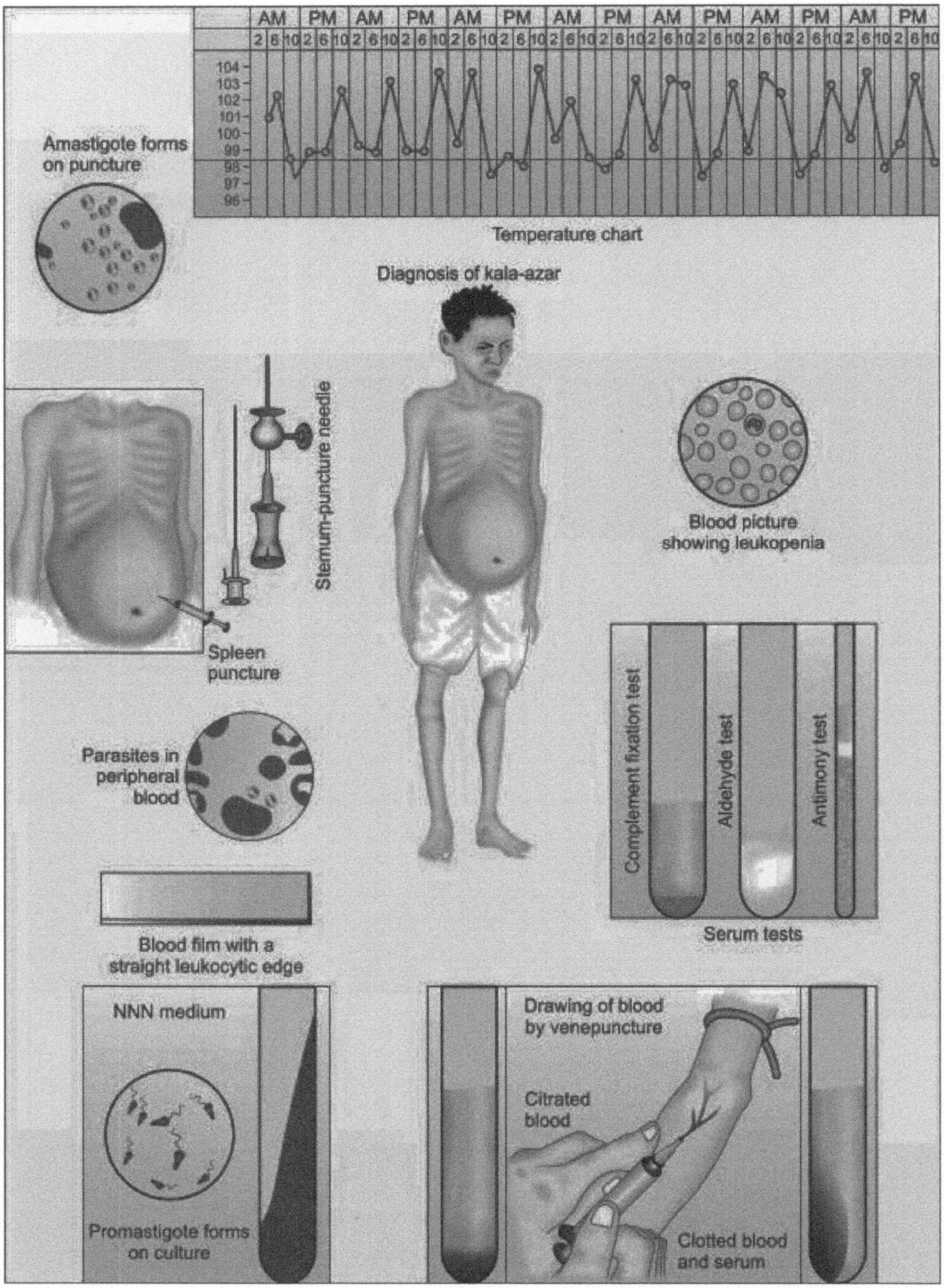

Fig. 38.10: Diagram showing the methods of diagnosis of kala-azar

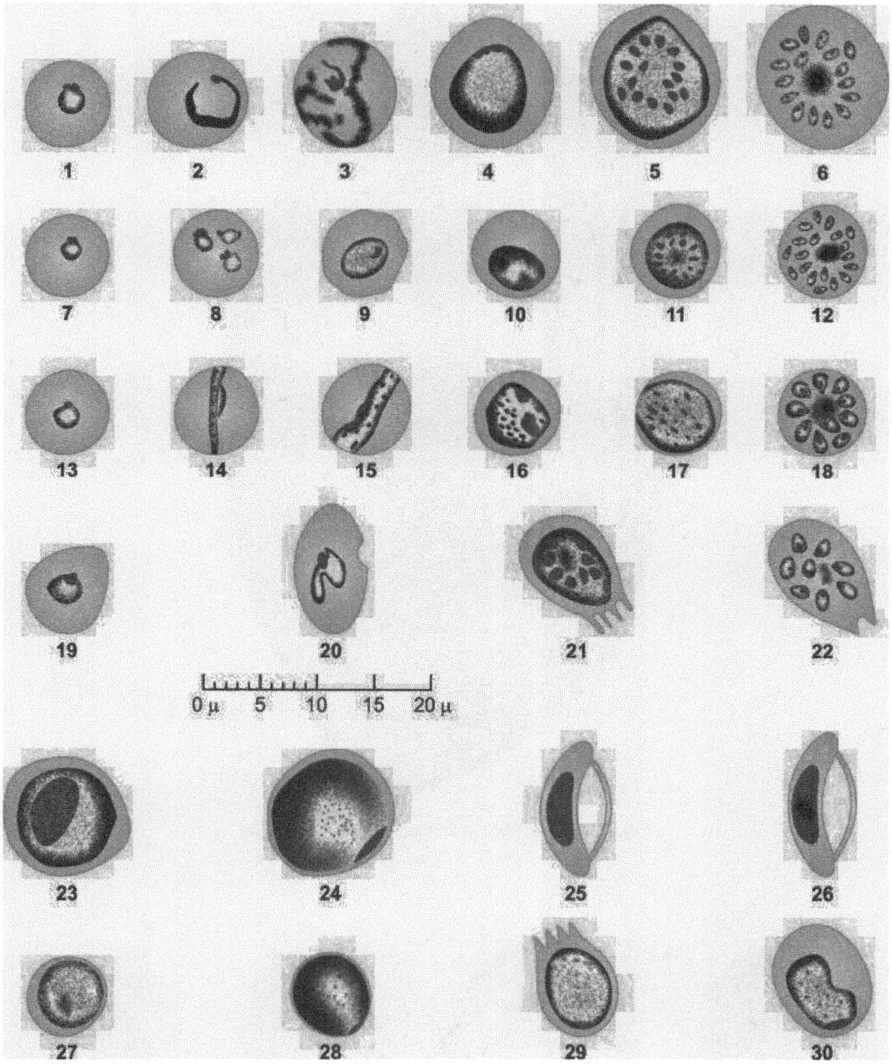

Fig. 38.12: Malarial parasites of man: Differential characters of erythrocytic phases (color):

1,6, *P. vivax*, 1,2,3, trophozoites (1 early ring-form, 2 &3 larger ring-forms with Schüffiner's dots, 3 amoeboid form); 4,5,6, schizonts—early to mature (rosette) stage.

7 to 12, *P. falciparum*. 7,8,9, trophozoites; 10,11,12, growth of a schizont (inside the capillary of internal organ); 8, showing multiple infections with form "accole"; 9 & 10, showing Maurer's dots in the host-cell. Note the normal size of the infected cell.

13 to 18, *P. malariae*. 13, ring-form; 14,15, band-form; 16,17,18, growth of a schizont. Note the normal size of the host-cell and undotted erythrocytes.

19 to 22, *P. ovale*. 19, 20, trophozoites; 21,22, developing schizonts. Note Jame's dots in all the stages as also the irregular and oval shape of the enlarged host-cell.

23 to 30, mature gametocytes *P. vivax* (23 male, 24 female), *P. falciparum* (25 male, 26 female), *P. malariae* (27 male, 28 female) and *P. ovale* (29 male, 30 female).

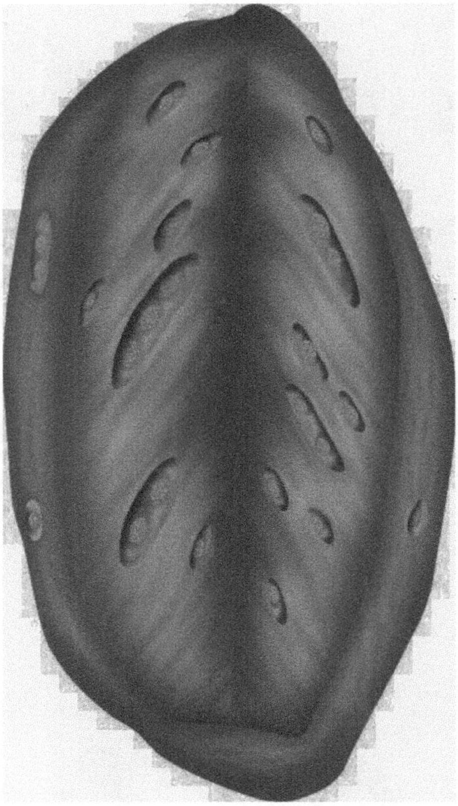

Fig. 39.5: Cysticercus cellulosae in pig's muscle

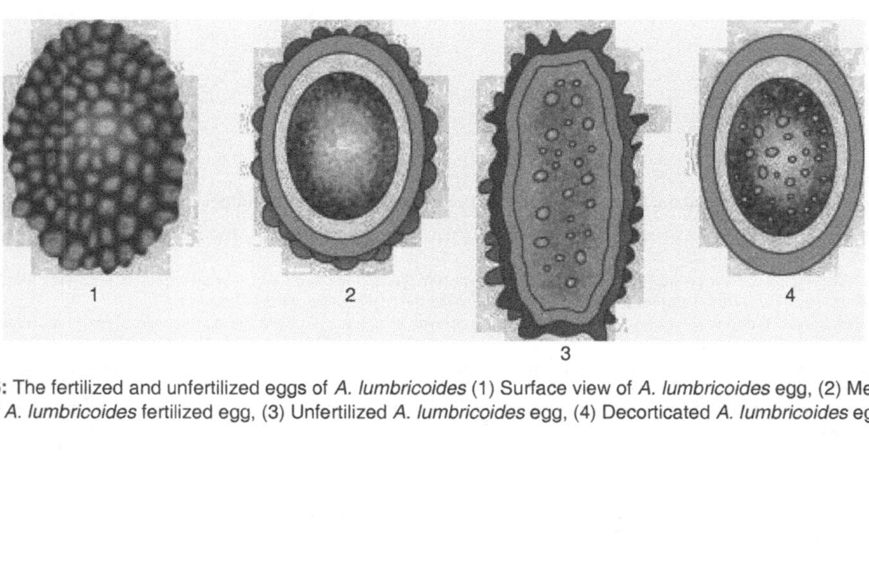

Fig. 39.16: The fertilized and unfertilized eggs of *A. lumbricoides* (1) Surface view of *A. lumbricoides* egg, (2) Median view of *A. lumbricoides* fertilized egg, (3) Unfertilized *A. lumbricoides* egg, (4) Decorticated *A. lumbricoides* egg

Section 1

General Bacteriology

- Introduction and History of Microbiology
- Microscopy
- Staining
- Morphology of Bacteria
- Growth and Nutrition of Bacteria
- Sterilization and Disinfection
- Cultivation of Microorganisms-I: Culture Medium
- Cultivation of Microorganisms-II: Inoculation Techniques
- Classification of Microorganisms
- Bacterial Identification
- Infection
- Antibiotic Sensitivity Test
- Bacterial Genetics

General Bacteriology

Introduction

This section deals with the basics of microbiology. The principles and techniques learnt in these chapters will help you to understand the other sections of the book better.

The studies of bacterial morphology, growth, nutrition and culture as discussed in this section are very important to arrive at an accurate bacteriological diagnosis in clinical laboratory practice.

The chapters on Classification and Identification of Bacteria help us to identify and classify bacteria. Antibiotic sensitivity testing is an essential prerequisite for the treatment of bacterial diseases and has been discussed in detail in the chapter devoted to it. Lastly, a chapter on Bacterial Genetics has been included to give an insight into the bacterial mechanisms of resistance and into the field of genomics.

Mastering this section before going on to others would help MLT students to have a strong foundation in Medical Microbiology.

CHAPTER 1

Introduction and History of Microbiology

LESSON PLAN

- What is Microbiology?
- History of Microbiology
  - Antony Van Leeuwenhoek
  - Louis Pasteur
  - Robert Koch
- Microorganisms and Diseases
  - Free Living Orgenisms
  - Saprophytes
  - Parasites—Commensal, Pathogenic
  - Epidemiology of Diseases
- Branches of Microbiology
- Uses of Studying Medical Microbiology

WHAT IS MICROBIOLOGY?

Definition

Microbiology is a branch of science that deals with the study of microbes which are living organisms of microscopic size.

- This term was introduced by a French chemist named **Louis Pasteur** who demonstrated that breakdown of sugar solutions (fermentation) was caused by microbes.
- All microorganisms are smaller than 0.1 to 0.2 mm (200 microns) in diameter. One micron is 10^{-6} of a meter. With the naked eye we cannot see objects smaller than 200 microns. So we require a microscope for their study.
- Microbes are present everywhere (air, water, soil, etc.). Only some of these microorganisms are disease producing or pathogenic. The majority do not cause disease and are non-pathogenic. Medical microbiology is concerned with the causation of disease by the pathogenic microorganisms, their diagnosis and cure.

HISTORY OF MICROBIOLOGY

Antony Van Leeuwenhoek

Microorganisms were first seen by Antony Van Leeuwenhoek (pronounced as Layvenhook) who was from Holland. He was a cloth merchant but his hobby was to grind lenses and observe things through them. His microscope was a single biconvex lens that magnified 200 times. He found many microorganisms in materials like water, mud, saliva and the stools. He recognized them as living because they swam about actively. He called them animalcules. He made various drawings which we now recognize as bacterial cocci and rods and stated that their size was 1/6 of the blood cell. He sent his findings to the Royal Society of London in 1683 but it was only two centuries later that their importance came to be understood.

Louis Pasteur (1822–1895)

He is known as the **Father of Microbiology.** He has many contributions in the field of microbiology.

a. He was a French chemist but was greatly interested in fermentation. His studies on fermentation established the presence and activity of different kinds of microorganisms.
b. He established the basic principles and techniques of bacteriology.
   i. He proved that all forms of life arose from life and not de novo (by itself)
   ii. He introduced techniques of sterilization and developed hot air oven and autoclave
   iii. Pasteurization (a process which slows microbial growth in food by subjecting it to temperature below boiling point) was named after its creator Louis Pasteur. This process was originally conceived as a way of preventing wine and beer and is now used for heat labile liquids
   iv. He said that different bacteria need different conditions for growth.
c. He discovered the process of attenuation and development of live vaccines.
   Attenuation: It is the process of making a bacteria lose its ability to cause disease but retaining its ability to cause production of protective antibodies. This is a way of making a live vaccine and this when introduced into the body protects the body, from further attack by the bacteria. He attenuated cultures of anthrax bacillus by heating to high temperatures (42–43°C). This, when introduced into animals protected them from infection with anthrax.
d. He first used the term vaccine for Rabies. Subsequently, the preparation of cow pox used by Edward Jenner for protection against smallpox, was also called vaccine. Pasteur Institute, Paris is named after him.

Robert Koch (1843–1910)

a. He is known as the Father of bacteriology. He established bacteriological techniques in Germany, during his studies on anthrax bacteria just as Louis Pasteur had done in France.
b. He first used solid media for growing bacteria in pure culture.
c. He introduced staining techniques.
d. He discovered the bacteria of tuberculosis and cholera in 1882 and 1883, respectively and said that different microorganisms cause different kinds of diseases.
e. Robert Koch is known for the **Koch's postulates.** According to this a microorganism can be accepted as a causative agent of an infectious disease only if the following conditions are satisfied. These were first indicated by Henle and later enunciated by Koch and are known as **Koch's postulates:**
   - The bacteria should always be present with the lesions of the disease.
   - It should be possible to isolate the bacterium in pure culture from the lesion.
   - When we inoculate the above culture into lab animals it should reproduce the lesions of the disease.
   - It should be possible to reisolate the bacterium in pure culture from the lesions produced in experimental animals.
f. Koch in 1890 observed that when tubercle bacillus or its protein was injected in guinea pig already infected with the bacteria, an exaggerated response took place which was named as a hypersensitivity reaction known as **Koch's phenomenon**. This forms the basis of what we now call Mantoux skin test for tuberculosis.

Table 1.1 shows the achievements of other great scientists during that period.

MICROORGANISMS AND DISEASES

Microorganisms are of three types:

a. *Free living*: Most microorganisms are free living in soil, water and air, and are not found on the human body. Some of these organisms obtain their energy from daylight and some from oxidation of inorganic matter.

Table 1.1: Achievements of other great scientists

Name	*Achievements*
Ivanovsky (1892)	He was the first to report a viral disease (Tobacco mosaic disease) in plants
Walter Reed (1902)	He proved that yellow fever had a viral etiology. It was the first human viral disease discovered
Goodpasture (1930)	He developed the technique of growing viruses on chick embryo
Edward Jenner (1796)	Vaccination against smallpox
Metchnikoff (1883)	Observed the phenomenon of phagocytosis and established that it is a defence mechanism against microbial invasion
Alexander Fleming (1929)	Discovered Penicillin in 1929 and used it in the 2nd World War
Ehrlich, Burnet (1908)	Contributed towards immunology
Behring, Kitasato (1890)	Discovered antibodies
Neisser (1979)	Discovered gonococcus
Ogston (1881)	Discovered staphylococcus
Loeffler (1884)	Discovered diphtheria bacillus
Hansen (1874)	Discovered leprosy bacillus
Landsteiner (1900)	Discovered blood groups
Joseph lister (1854)	– Father of antiseptic surgery – Techniques of antiseptic and aseptic surgery for prevention of wound sepsis
Watson and Crick (1961)	Genetic code, structure of DNA
Ruska (1934)	Discovered electron microscope
Twort (1915) and d'Herelle (1917)	Discovered bacteriophage

b. *Saprophytes*: These grow on dead decaying matter to obtain energy.

c. *Parasites*: These are microorganisms that live in or on a living host and obtain their nourishment from them. They are divided into:

   i. Commensal

   ii. Pathogenic

Commensal

These are normally found on the skin and mucous membranes of the upper respiratory tract, intestine and vagina and obtain nourishment from the body secretions and food remains. These microorganisms are called normal flora. They are normally harmless because they do not enter the human body. In certain conditions, however when the body's defence mechanisms are weak, they can enter the tissues and cause disease. Thus, they act as ***opportunistic pathogens*** that is pathogenic only when the opportunity arises.

Pathogenic

Pathogenic microorganisms are disease causing microorganisms. They can overcome the normal defences of the body, produce toxins and damage the tissues causing signs and symptoms of the disease.

The process of microbial invasion and multiplication in the body is called infection. It may or may not lead to disease (appearance of signs and symptoms) depending on the fighting capacity of the body.

Those infective diseases that are readily spread from person to person are called infectious diseases or communicable diseases.

Epidemiology of Diseases

It is a study of the factors that influence the prevalence and distribution of diseases of the community. It includes the study of the source of infection, the mode of transmission from one person to another and the prevention of diseases. The source of infection is where the pathogenic organisms grow and multiply. Sources can be a clinical patient or a carrier. A carrier is a person who does not suffer from the disease himself but carries the pathogen in his body and so can transmit the disease to others.

BRANCHES OF MICROBIOLOGY

Microbiology is very important in modern society. It has great use in various fields such as industry, food and agriculture. The various branches of microbiology are:

a. Medical microbiology
b. Industrial microbiology
c. Food microbiology
d. Soil microbiology
e. Plant microbiology.

Here we are concerned with medical microbiology. We will study it under the following heads:

1. *Bacteriology*: It is the branch of medical microbiology that deals with the study of bacteria.
2. *Virology*: It is the branch of medical microbiology that deals with the study of viruses.
3. *Parasitology*: It is the branch of medical microbiology that deals with the study of parasites.
4. *Mycology*: It is the branch of medical microbiology that deals with the study of fungi.
5. *Immunology*: It is the branch of medical microbiology that deals with the study of antigens, antibodies and immunity in the body.
6. *Serology*: It is the branch of medical microbiology that deals with the study of the presence of antibodies in the serum, their levels and significance.
7. *Molecular biology and genetics*: It is the branch of medical microbiology that deals with genetic material (DNA and RNA) and its detection for diagnosis. This branch is also utilized in research on genes in microorganisms.

USES OF STUDYING MEDICAL MICROBIOLOGY

1. The knowledge of medical microbiology helps us to find out the causative agents of diseases, their diagnosis, prevention and treatment.
2. Microorganisms are the smallest forms of living beings and serve as models for studies on genetics and biochemistry.

CHAPTER

2

Microscopy

LESSON PLAN

- Introduction
- Principle of an Ordinary Light Microscope
- Parts of Microscope
  - Mechanical Parts
  - Magnifying Parts
  - Illuminating Parts
- Magnification
- Resolution
- Method of Use of Light Microscope
- Care of the Microscope
- Types of Microscopes
  - Simple
  - Compound
  - Dark Ground
  - Phase Contrast
  - Fluorescence Microscope
  - Electron Microscope

INTRODUCTION

What is a Microscope?

A microscope is an optical instrument consisting of a combination of lenses which magnifies the image of the object seen through it. It is used for the morphological study of very small organisms which are not visible to the naked eye. Micro means small and scope means to view.

PRINCIPLE OF AN ORDINARY LIGHT MICROSCOPE

It is important to understand the optical principles and construction of the microscope to obtain the best performance from the instrument.

The specimen/sample is kept on a glass slide. Light from an external/internal source falls on the mirror and is focussed on the specimen. The specimen throws a shadow in the beam of light which is magnified in two stages as it passes up the microscope into the eye. The objective lens starts the magnifying process. It operates at a distance that is roughly equivalent to its focal length and a real, inverted and enlarged primary image is formed in the upper part of the tube. Here, the field lens collects the diverging rays of the primary image. These rays then pass through the eyepiece lens which magnifies it still further. When the rays leave the eyepiece lens to reach the lens of the observor's eye they are divergent and the image seen by the retina is virtual and enlarged.

PARTS OF MICROSCOPE

1. **Mechanical parts** — Stand, Stage, Limb
2. **Magnifying parts** — Optical lens system
Objectives
Eyepieces

3. **Illuminating parts** — Substage condensor
Iris diaphragm
Filter holder
Mirror

A microscope can be monocular which has a single eyepiece or binocular with two eyepieces.

Monocular

- This microscope is for beginners who have difficulty in fusing images.
- Used for photography.
- No adjustment of interocular distance.

Binocular

- No tilting required as the body, is inclined.
- Inclined body may increase overall magnification.
- No eye strain.
- Stage is horizontal, so there is no running-off of solution on the slide.

Mechanical Parts

See Figure 2.1 for binocular microscope.

Stand

It forms the base of the microscope. It has a horse-shoe shaped foot to give stability in case of a monocular microscope or a rectangular base in case of a binocular microscope.

Limb

It is attached to the foot by a hinge joint so that it can be set at a comfortable angle for the observer. To the limb are attached the illuminating parts and the optical tube. In case of binocular microscope, the body itself is inclined and the limb is immovable.

Stage

This is a horizontal platform which has a hole in it. On this, the slide with the specimen is held with clips. It can be fixed or mobile. The latter is preferable when a large area is to be examined. The mechanical stage adjustments move the slide in two directions.

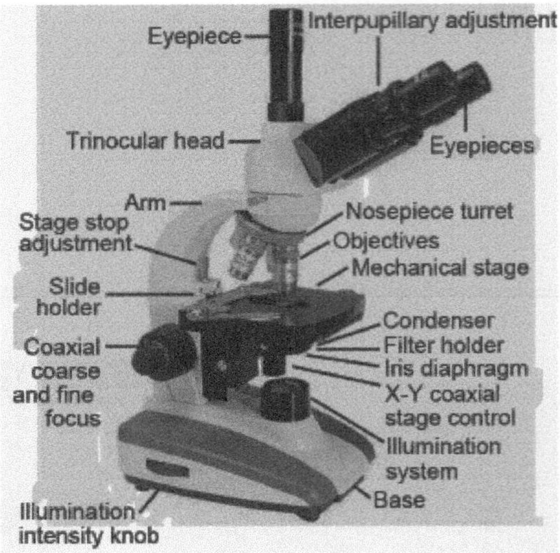

Fig. 2.1: Binocular microscope

Magnifying Parts

This consists of the eye-pieces and objectives attached to either end of the optical tube. The tube can be moved up and down by means of coarse and fine adjustment screws. Alternatively, the stage can be racked up or down.

Eyepieces

The optical tube bears on its upper end an inclined binocular head with two eyepieces or one eyepiece in a monocular microscope. They have a magnification of 5X, 6X, 10X, or 15X.

Objectives

The three objectives are screwed on to the revolving nose-piece which is attached to the lower end of the tube. They are:

1. Low power objective 10X
2. High power objective 40X
3. Oil immersion objective 100X.

Illuminating Parts

Mirror

Either the light source is inbuilt inside the microscope or an external mirror is given. It forms the lowermost of the illuminating parts. It is planoconcave. It can reflect the light of the sun or a lamp on to the condensor. Flat surface is used when oil immersion lens is used and concave surface is used with low and high power objectives. In case of an inbuilt source of light, the light is reflected up through a mirror on to the condensor.

Filter Holder

Above the mirror is a ring shaped filter holder which holds a circular coloured blue glass. It absorbs the red/yellow component of the light and reduces glare.

Iris Diaphragm

Just like the ciliary muscles contract the iris in the eye to control the size of the pupil in bright and dark so as to allow the right amount of light to pass in, the iris diaphragm controls the amount of light reaching the sub-stage condensor. The iris diaphragm has a small lever which controls the amount of light reaching the object. The oil immersion lens requires maximum light and hence the iris diaphragm is kept open. The low power lens requires minimum light and the iris diaphragm is kept partially closed. In high power it is open to a medium extent.

Substage Condensor

It is made up of a system of convex lenses which focus light from the illuminating source on to the plane of the object. The height of the condensor can be changed with the help of a condensor adjustment. Lowering the condensor decreases the light whereas raising it increases the illumination. While using oil immersion objective the condensor is kept at the highest position and at low power the condensor is kept at the lowest position. In 40X it is kept in between the above two.

MAGNIFICATION

Magnification means the **degree of enlargement** that is the number of times the length, breadth or diameter is multiplied.

There are two types of magnification:

Empty magnification: The image is magnified but the sharpness of the image is lost. Larger images are blurred. No details are observed. This is of no use.

Useful magnification: The image is magnified up to a limit where the details are clearly observed.

Since we know that magnification is carried out in two stages, the overall magnification of the microscope can be calculated by multiplying the magnifying power of the objective by the magnifying power of the eyepiece. If the microscope has an inclined binocular head, then the product should be further multiplied by this factor.

To calculate the magnifying power of the objective. We see that:

$$\text{Magnification} = \frac{\text{Size of image}}{\text{Size of object}}$$

$$= \frac{\text{Distance of image from objective}}{\text{Distance of object from objective}}$$

$$= \frac{\text{Mechanical tube length}}{\text{Focal length of objective}}$$

Mechanical tube length = Optical tube length = 160 mm.

Focal length of 10X objective = 16 mm.

∴ Magnification of low power

$$\Rightarrow \frac{160}{16} = 10X$$

Likewise, the 40X objective has a focal length of 4 mm and a magnification of 40X and the oil immersion has a focal length < 2 mm and a magnification of 100.

When these objectives are used the overall magnifications of the microscope become 10 × 10 = 100X, 40 × 10 = 400X and 10 × 100 = 1000X, respectively for low, high and oil immersion lens. (This is assuming the magnifying power of the eyepiece is 10X).

RESOLUTION

Limit of useful magnification of a microscope is set by its resolving power, i.e. its ability to show closely adjacent structural details as separate and distinct. The **limit** of **resolution** is the minimum distance between two visible bodies at which they are seen as separate and not in contact with one another. The limit of resolution of the naked eye is 0.2 mm or 200 microns. The limit of resolution of light microscope is 0.2 micron. The limit of resolution of electron microscope is 1 A° or 1/10 of a nanometer.

METHOD OF USE OF LIGHT MICROSCOPE

1. Place the microscope at a convenient position. Adjust the height and position of the observors chair. Adjust eyepieces in a binocular microscope. Spectacles may be used or removed.
2. Check that the objectives and eyepieces are free from dust and oil.
3. Oil immersion objective should be cleaned after use each day with a well-washed fine cotton cloth or lens cleaning tissue paper soaked in a lens cleaning solution. This is made by mixing Isopropyl alcohol and Ether in the ratio of 70:30.
4. Likewise, eyepieces, objectives, condensor lenses and mirror surfaces should be wiped free from dust with a soft cotton cloth or lens cleaning paper.
5. Check that the condensor can be racked up fully and that the substage iris is open fully. Place the slide with the object on the stage. For viewing in low power:
   - Bring the dry objective into view.
   - Use coarse focussing and fine adjustment only to obtain and maintain exact focus.

   For viewing in high power: The condensor is brought to a medium position. The iris diaphragm is opened to a medium degree. The 40X objective is brought into view and focussed with the help of coarse and fine adjustments.

   For viewing in oil-immersion: First rack down the stage to get adequate clearance. Place a moderately large drop of oil on the slide. Rotate the nose-piece until the oil immersion lens is in place. Use the coarse focussing adjustment slowly to raise the stage until the oil on the slide makes contact with the objective and the oil lights up. Then, with coarse adjustment raise the stage a little further to bring the surface of the slide as close as possible to the objective lens without actually touching it. Apply the eyes to the eye-pieces and while watching slowly focus the objective away from the slide by lowering the stage with coarse focussing. Stop as soon as focus is reached and specimen is seen. Obtain exact focus by use of fine adjustment. Condenser should be at the highest position and the diaphragm should be fully opened.
6. After use, wipe the oil.

We use 10X or 40X for examination of urine, stool or fungal preparation. 100X is reserved for examination of the slide for malarial parasite, bacteria or blood cell morphology.

CARE OF THE MICROSCOPE

- The objectives, eyepieces, mirrors, etc. should be cleaned with lens cleaning solution and lens cleaning tissue.
- When not in use, the microscope should be protected with a wooden or plastic cover.

TYPES OF MICROSCOPES

Simple Microscope

Consists of a single magnifying lens.

Compound Microscope

Compound microscopes include the monocular and the binocular microscopes which we have discussed.

Dark Ground Microscope

Introduction

The dark ground microscope allows us to view objects brightly lit against a dark background. The surfaces and internal bodies of the bacteria are shown brightly lit and in contrast to a dark background. This is especially used for unstained preparations.

Principle

The basic *principle* of a dark ground microscope is that the specimen is illuminated only by rays of light so oblique, that unless they are scattered by the specimen they fail to enter the objective and reach the eye. Some of the scattered rays from the objects enter the objective and reach the eye, so that they appear gleaming brightly against a dark background. The oil immersion lens is used in this microscope.

Use

It is used to view delicate organisms like spirochetes and vibrio which become clearer due to increased contrast. The film of fluid and the coverslip should be thin and the number of bacteria should not be excessive because too many bacteria will scatter light.

Phase Contrast Microscope

Introduction

Phase contrast microscope provides greater contrast in the internal structure of bacteria, so that we can see it better.

Principle

Unstained bacteria and cells consist of alternate strips of material of slightly different refractive indices which act as a diffraction grating. The diffracted and undiffracted rays of light acquire small phase differences. These differences are maximized in the microscope and then allowed to recombine in such a way that they interfere with each other and so reduce light intensity in the area of image corresponding to the object. It helps us to view unstained living organisms with good contrast and high resolution.

Use

It is used to study flagellar movement, living blood cells, internal structure of bacteria, the cytopathic effect of viruses on tissue cell cultures and the growth and subdivision of bacteria.

Fluorescence Microscope

Introduction and Principle

When certain materials, e.g. oil or fat droplets or certain dyes are exposed to ultraviolet radiation, they convert the invisible short wave radiation into longer wave length of visible light and so become luminous and are said to fluoresce. So if microorganisms or tissue cells are stained with a fluorescent dye and are examined under the microscope with UV radiation (instead of ordinary visible light), they are seen as bright objects against a dark background.

Wave length of
UV light ⇒ 280–500 nm
Visible light → 500 nm

Use

Some of these fluorescent dyes have a special affinity for microorganisms or cell components and can be used to directly stain them and so make them easily visible with ultraviolet light, i.e.:

Auramine O—Stains tubercle bacilli with yellow fluorescence.

Acridine orange-R—It has affinity for nucleic acids. It fluoresces orange red with RNA and yellow green with DNA. It can be used to stain viral nucleic acids in infected cells and tissues.

Other are: *Thiazo yellow and Thioflavin.*

Immunofluorescence

Principle

Certain fluorescent dyes can be used to label immunoglobulins or anti-immunoglobulins. Dyes used are:

- Fluorescein isothiocyanate which gives yellow green fluorescence.
- Lissamine rhodamine which gives orange fluorescence. Fluorescent antiserum is applied like a stain to a film of microorganisms and the fluorescent antibody is allowed to combine firmly with the corresponding antigen in the film.

After washing the slide is examined under a fluorescent microscope.

Use

Fluorescence is used to study tubercle bacilli, rickettsia, viruses and distribution of bacterial antigen. Immunofluorescence is used in diagnostic immunology.

Electron Microscope

Introduction

As we have learnt earlier electron microscope has a limit of resolution of 1 A° and can be used to study very small organisms. Electron microscope is used to observe very small microorganisms like viruses or to see structural details within cells.

Principle

The object is scanned with a high speed beam of electrons instead of visible light. To allow the passage of electrons, the column or the tube of the microscope is evacuated to make it completely devoid of air and gas (vacuum). It is focussed with electromagnetic lenses. High resolving power of the instrument is due to the electron beam having a small wavelength of about 0.005 nm which is 100,000 times shorter than the wavelength of light. The atoms of the object scatter electrons and form a shadow in the electron beam. If the material in small organisms or particles is not dense enough it may help to outline them with a layer of heavy metal called shadowing or shadow casting.

Working

The specimen to be examined under the electron microscope is fixed, dried and then mounted onto a thin membrane made from collodion. Electron microscope consists of a tubular column at the top of which is mounted the source of electrons which is the electron gun which emits electrons from a hot tungsten filament which serves as a cathode. Beneath this filament is placed a cathode shield and then an anode with a small hole in its centre. A high voltage is applied which may be 50 kV or 100 kV to accelerate the emitted electrons.

The narrow beam of electrons passes at high speed through the hole and down the column of the microscope. Focussing and magnification is achieved by a series of electromagnetic lenses. The final magnification is 100,000. The final image is formed on a fluorescent screen at the lower end of the column and is viewed through a glass window. It can be photographed also. A binocular microscope is used to view the fluorescent screen.

Disadvantage of electron microscope is that it cannot be used to observe organisms in the wet living state.

CHAPTER

3

Staining

LESSON PLAN

- Introduction
- Why is Staining Required?
- What are Stains?
  - Types of Stains
  - Basic Stains
- Fixation
  - Use of Fixation
  - Methods of Fixation
  - Effects of Fixation
- Stains Used in Microbiology
  - Simple Stains
  - Differential Stains
  - Gram's Stain
  - Acid Fast Stain or the Ziehl-Neelsen Stain
  - Fluorescent Stains
  - Albert Staining
  - Negative Staining—Capsular Staining

INTRODUCTION

Staining means to add color contrast to a microscopic preparation for better visibility under the microscope.

WHY IS STAINING REQUIRED?

1. It is difficult to observe the bacteria in unstained state as bacteria are semi-transparent and consist of a clear protoplasmic matter
2. Staining helps us to observe better structural details of bacteria.
3. It helps us to differentiate between bacteria.
4. Easy identification of bacteria is possible especially if bacteria are small in size and less in number, e.g. acid fast bacteria in sputum are identified by an acid fast stain.
5. It also helps us to observe the chemical nature of cellular contents, e.g. fats and enzymes.

WHAT ARE STAINS?

Stains are aqueous preparations of a dye or group of dyes and are used for providing color to biological material. Dyes are coloring agents that are derivatives of coal tar usually having one or more rings connected by well-defined chemical bonds called chromophores.

The term stain and dye are not the same. A coloring agent that is used for general purposes is called a dye. The one that is used for biological purposes is called a stain.

Types of Stains

Based on their chemical behavior, the dyes are classified as acidic, basic and neutral. Stains can be: basic, acidic or neutral (Table 3.1).

Basic Stains

The basic radical is a positively charged cat ion and it is colored. The acidic radical is colorless.

Table 3.1: Types of stains

Acidic	*Basic*	*Neutral*
	Methylene blue	Giemsa
Picric acid	Crystal violet	Leishman's
Nigrosin	Basic fuchsin	Wright's
Acid fuchsin	Hematoxylin	
Eosin	Methyl green	
	Auramine	
	Thionin	
	Neutral red	
	Safranines	

The bacterial protoplasm especially the phosphate groups in the abundant nucleic acids are negatively charged and have an affinity for basic dyes which have a positively charged cat ion.

Acidic Stains

Negatively charged anion is colored and basic radical is colorless. These do not stain bacteria strongly except at a very acidic pH and thus are used for negative staining.

Neutral Stains

The coloring matter is contained in both acidic and basic components.

Staining can be:
- Supravital
- Vital/intravital

Supravital staining: This is a technique of staining in which the cell is killed by the stain itself and not by fixation, e.g. Janus green stain.

Vital/intravital staining: This is a method of staining in which the viability of the bacteria is maintained. This type of staining is used to stain structures within living cells which are normally poorly visible, e.g. Chlorazol Black E is a vital stain.

Before we learn further about staining we must know about a step we use before staining—fixation.

FIXATION

Definition

Any process either physical or chemical which kills and immobilizes the organisms is called fixation. Before the bacterial cell is stained, it is fixed.

Uses of Fixation

- Causes the bacteria to stick to the slide, so that it is not washed away.
- Preserves the internal structure and increases its visibility.
- It helps in the increase in affinity towards dyes.
- It kills the bacteria and therefore safer to work with.

Fixation procedures should avoid shrinkage and swelling of parts of the cell or autolysis.

Methods of Fixation

- Physical-heat
- Chemical

Heat fixation is commonly employed in the staining reactions performed in microbiology. It is done by passing the prepared smear over the flame two or three times.

Chemical fixation: The chemical fixatives are:
- Formalin
- Mercuric chloride
- Methyl alcohol
- Ethyl alcohol
- Osmic acid.

Effects of Fixation

It causes:
1. Denaturation of proteins
2. Solidification of cell structure.

Fixation alters the chemistry of the cell but a fair amount of information can still be obtained about its structure.

STAINS USED IN MICROBIOLOGY

Simple Stains

These are basic dyes, e.g. Loeffler's methylene blue or dilute carbol fuchsin which stains all bacteria of the same color. There is no differentiation between bacteria.

Differential Stains

- These stains are used for differentiating different types of organisms in the same film.
- More than one stain is used and the background and the organisms may be of different colors.

For example, Gram's stain and AFB stain (Ziehl-Neelsen).

Gram's Stain

Introduction

- It is the most widely used stain in Microbiology.
- It was introduced by Christian Gram in 1884.
- It differentiates between Gram-positive and Gram-negative organisms.

Basic Steps

- Make a smear on a slide. Dry and heat fix.
- Cover the smear with crystal violet or gentian violet or methyl violet for one minute (Gentian violet = Methyl violet + Crystal violet).
- Tip off the crystal violet. Hold the slide at a steep slope and wash off the residual stain with an excess of iodine solution. Begin by pouring the iodine from the upper end of the slide and rapidly work downwards. It is important to use enough iodine solution to wash away all the crystalline deposit that forms when the stain and iodine mix. Iodine acts as a mordant (One which fixes and enhances the color. We shall discuss mordants later). Let the iodine solution stay on the slide and act for one minute. The dye iodine complex or lake is insoluble in water but moderately soluble in acetone or alcohol which is used as decolorizer in the next step.
- Decolorize with 100 percent acetone solution. First tip off the iodine and hold the slide at a steep slope. Then pour acetone on the slide from its upper end so as to cover the whole surface. De colorization is very rapid and is usually complete in 2 to 3 seconds. After this period, the acetone must first be removed by washing thoroughly under running tap water.
- Counter stain with safranine or neutral red or carbol fuchsin for one minute.
- Wash.
- Blot dry.

Principle of Gram's Stain

When bacteria are stained, some organisms retain the primary dye and when treated with decolorizing agent do not lose their original color. They are termed as 'Gram-positive' and they appear violet because of crystal violet dye.

Other bacteria lose their primary color on decolorization and take up the second stain or counter stain. Counter stain is usually pink in color and the 'Gram-negative' organisms appear pink.

The Gram-positive organisms and fibrin appear dark violet in color, and Gram-negative organisms, nuclei, protoplasm of pus cells and tissue cells appear pink.

The reason for this phenomenon is explained in the theories given below:

Theories of Gram's Stain

1. The Gram-positive bacteria have more acidic protoplasm. So the dye iodine complex binds more firmly as the dye is a basic dye. Hence, on decolorization, it does not easily flow out. Gram-positive organisms have 1000 times' greater affinity for the dye.
2. Magnesium ribonucleoprotein esters are present in Gram-positive bacteria which help in binding of basic dye.
3. The dye iodine complex flows out in case of Gram-negative and does not flow out in Gram-positive because:
   a. The *lipopolysaccharide present (LPS)* in Gram-negative cell walls dissolves in acetone creating holes through which the dye can go outside.

b. The cell wall and the cyloplasmic membrane are more permeable in Gram-negative bacteria.
c. Techoic acid and mucopeptide (peptidoglycan) in cell wall of Gram-positive makes it very thick causing more osmotic pressure inside. So, when it is decolorized, the stain does not go out.
d. Pores of Gram-positive bacteria are small; hence the out flow of the stain is inhibited.

Mordant

These are chemical substances which have the power of fixing and enhancing the color of the dye. They have a strong affinity for both, the substrate and the dye and thus can anchor a dye to the substrate. The resulting precipitates are called lakes and are less soluble in water. In Gram's stain, iodine acts as a mordant because it forms an insoluble compound with the dye and the dye iodine complex is not soluble in water. Mordants combine with the dye. Mordants can be physical, e.g. heat, or chemical, e.g. iodine or phenol. They may be basic mordants, e.g. Alum, ferrous sulphate, antimonium tartrate, cetyl pyridinium chloride, etc. or acidic mordants, e.g. tannic acid or picric acid.

Examples of Gram-positive organisms: We shall study in great detail about Gram-positive and Gram-negative organisms in the later sections.

- Gram-positive cocci—Genus—*Staphylococcus and Streptococcus.*
- Gram-positive bacilli—Genus—*Clostridium and Bacillus.*
- Gram-negative cocci—Genus—*Neisseria.*
- Gram-negative bacilli—Genus—*Escherichia and Klebsiella* (Fig. 3.1).
- Not stained by Gram's stain—*Spores, Cell wall, Capsule.*

1. Gram reaction changes with age. In older cultures Gram-positive changes to Gram-negative.
2. If cell wall synthesis is defective the organism appears Gram-negative. Gram-positive and Gram-negative organisms not only differ in their Gram reaction but also in various other factors like susceptibility to antibiotics, pathogenicity etc. Given in the Table 3.2 are some differences between Gram-positive and Gram-negative organisms.

Precautions

1. Do not under/over decolorize.
2. Do not apply too much heat while fixation.

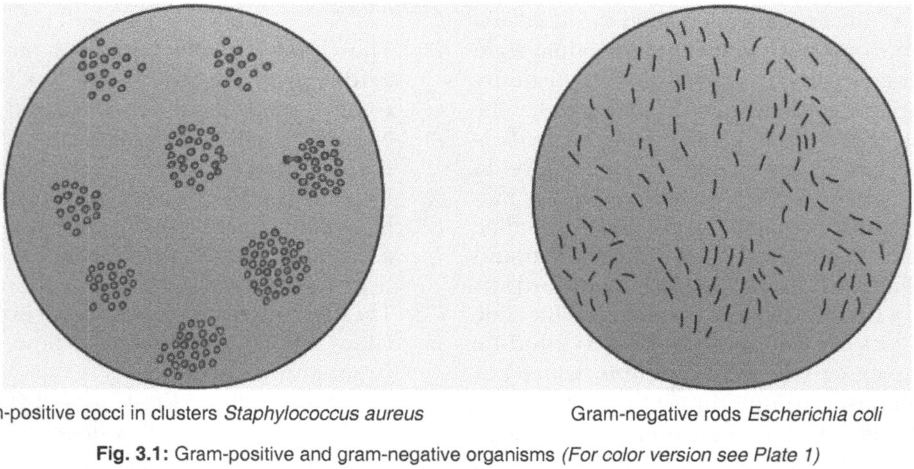

Gram-positive cocci in clusters *Staphylococcus aureus* Gram-negative rods *Escherichia coli*

Fig. 3.1: Gram-positive and gram-negative organisms *(For color version see Plate 1)*

Table 3.2: Differences between gram-positive and gram-negative organisms

	Gram-positive	*Gram-negative*
Cell wall thickness	Greater	Less
Cell wall ruptured by heat	No	Yes
Amino acids in cell wall	Few	Numerous
Separation of plasma membrane from cell wall	Difficult	Easy
Hexosamine content of cell wall	More	Less
Lipids in cell wall	None or low	Present
Phosphatidylcholine	Absent	May be present
Glycosyl diglyceride	Present	Absent
Mesosomes	Present	Absent
Magnesium content	Greater	Less
Lysozyme lysis	Very susceptible	Less so
Nature of toxins produced	Exotoxins	Endotoxins
Nutritional requirements	Generally complex	Relatively simpler
Susceptibility to penicillin	Greater	Less
Rupture by sudden changes in pressure and supersonic energy	More resistant	Less resistant

3. Do not wash with water after addition of crystal violet to prevent washing out of the dye.

Acid Fast Stain or the Ziehl-Neelsen Stain

Introduction

Certain bacteria called *acid fast bacteria* resist decolorization with strong acids, e.g. 20 percent H_2SO_4 after staining with a strong dye. For example, *Mycobacterium tuberculosis* which is also known as acid fast bacteria. This organism was first discovered by Robert Koch. In 1882 Ehrlich first noted that the application of strong acids did not result in decolorization when tubercle bacilli were stained with a chemical solution. Modifications were suggested by Ziehl and Neelsen and this stain came to be known as Ziehl-Neelsen stain.

Principle

Acid fast bacteria are relatively impermeable and resistant to simple stains but when stained with a strong reagent (hot basic fuchsin in aqueous 5 percent phenol), the dye penetrates the bacillus and once stained, the tubercle bacillus withstands the action of powerful decolorizing agents and retains the original stain. Here we are applying two kinds of mordants—physical mordant which is heat and chemical mordant which is phenol. With the combined action of the above, the fatty acids dissolve in the cell wall, and let the dye travel inside. Other bacteria which are not acid fast are decolorized and the original dye is removed. These are counterstained with methylene blue or malachite green.

What is the acid fastness due to:

a. There is a high content of lipids (fatty acids and higher alcohols) in tubercle bacilli. One of the lipids special to AFB is Mycolic acid. It is a hydroxy acid wax of high molecular weight containing carboxyl groups. It does not exist in the free state but exists in a bound state with carbohydrate. Because of the presence of mycolic acid, the solubility of the dye is not high in the decolorizer and very less quantity of color is lost to the decolorizer. The special anatomical distribution of the lipids also contributes to this.

b. The cell wall of the acid fast organism has the property of resisting the rapid movement of the dye out of the cell. This depends on cell wall integrity. If cell wall is lysed the cell loses its acid fastness. Both factors together contribute to the acid fast character.

Method

1. Cover the slide with carbol fuchsin, (which is basic fuchsin in absolute alcohol and 5 percent phenol) and heat until steam arises. Discontinue heating and then recontinue when steam stops arising. Continue this process for a period of 5 minutes. Stain must not be allowed to evaporate and dry. If necessary pour more carbol fuchsin to keep the whole slide covered with liquid.
2. Wash with water
3. Cover the slide with 20 percent H_2SO_4 (200 mL acid to be added to 800 mL of water from the side of the flask, 50 mL at a time, mix gently. Do not add water to acid). Keep for a minute. Wash the slide with water and pour on more acid. The dye is basic and its combination with acid produces a compound which is yellowish brown. The aim of washing is to remove the compound of acid and stain and allow fresh acid to react with the preparation. Decolorization takes a total time of 10 minutes and it is said to be over when after washing, the film is faintly pink.
4. Wash slide well with water.
5. Treat slide with 95 percent alcohol for two minutes (optional step). Then wash with water.
6. Counterstain with Loeffler's methylene blue for 15 to 20 seconds.
7. Wash dry. See in 100X.

Acid Fast Structures

Acid fast bacilli stain bright red while the other structures are stained blue. If tissue cells appear red, the preparation has not been adequately decolorized with H_2SO_4 (Fig. 3.2).

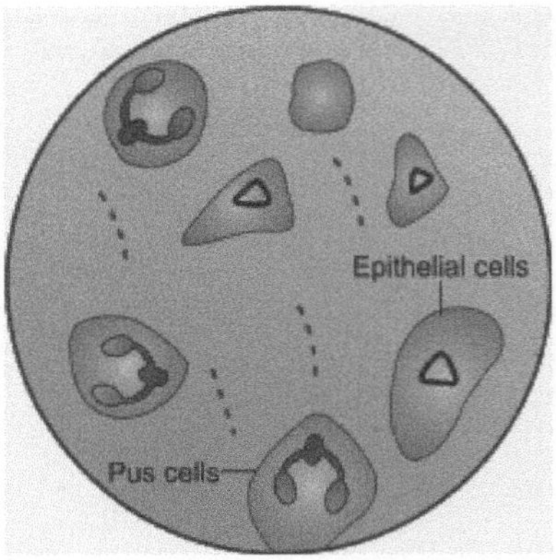

Fig. 3.2: Acid fast bacteria (*Mycobacterium tuberculosis*) *(For color version see Plate 1)*

Advantage of Using Alcohol as a Decolorizer

After primary decolourization with sulphuric acid, the film may be treated with 95 percent alcohol for two minutes (95 mL ethanol + water to make 100 mL) as a secondary decolorizer. The advantage of using alcohol is that:

1. Decolourization is completed more quickly and margins and the underside of the slide are more completely cleared and freed from deposits of stain.
2. Mycobacterium tuberculosis is acid and alcohol fast. Certain other acid fast bacilli which resist decolorization with acids may be seen in pathological specimens. They may be decolorized with alcohol. They are sometimes present in clinical samples and cause confusion.

Another decolorizer is 3 percent solution of HCl or HNO_3 [3 mL in 95 percent ethyl alcohol (97 mL)].

Precautions

1. Do not touch the smear
2. Do not blot as the bacilli may stick to the paper
3. Discard properly
4. Do not let the carbol fuchsin dry.

Concentration of acid used for decolorization:
- *Mycobacterium tuberculosis*—20%
- *Mycobacterium leprae*—5%
- *Nocardia*—1% or 0.5%
- *Actinomycetes*—1%
- *Spores*—0.25%

Other acid fast structures:
1. Some species of *Corynebacterium*
2. Posterior portion of the heads of human spermatozoa
3. Bacterial endospores
4. Ascospores of yeast
5. Exoskeleton of insects.

Fluorescent Stains

Auramine O can be substituted for carbol fuchsin in the Ziehl-Neelsen method.
The staining solution comprises of:
- Auramine O
- Phenol
- Distilled water
- Decolorizing solution is composed of industrial alcohol
  - 75 percent in water containing
  - 0.5% NaCl and 0.5% HCl.

We have dealt with this in Chapter 2 on Microscopy.

Albert Staining

Introduction

This stain is used to stain *Corynebacterium diphtheriae*. The body of the bacteria stains green and the volutin granules stain bluish black

Principle

What is metachromasia?
Metachromasia is the property of certain dyes which have coloured ions. When these dyes are used to stain certain bacteria, some parts of the bacteria appear a different colour from the background. This may be because certain sections of the bacteria affect the spread of the dye or have more affinity to the dye and so appear a different colour. An example of this is that ribonucleic acids have more affinity for metachromatic dyes like toluidine blue. Nucleic acid induces aggregation of the dye and hinders its diffusion so the bands of nucleic acid retain the dye strongly.

This property is especially made use of in *Corynebacterium diphtheriae* which has volutin granules also known as metachromatic granules. These take up blue black color whereas the rest of the body takes up a greenish color (Fig. 3.3).

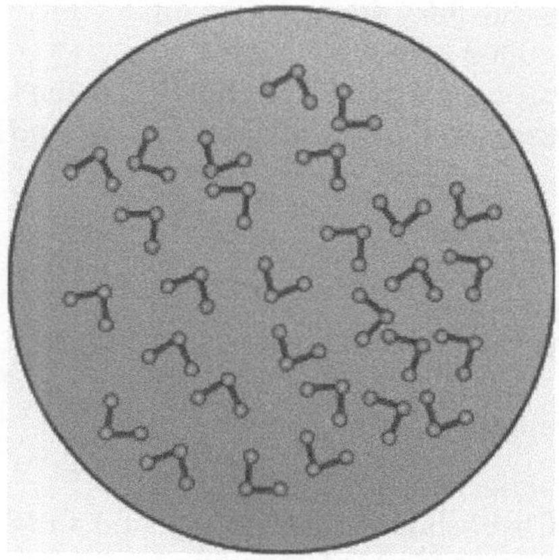

Fig. 3.3: *Corynebacterium diphtheriae* (Albert staining) *(For color version see Plate 1)*

What are volutin granules?
Volutin granules are well-developed granules of polymetaphosphate. In unstained preparations, they are seen as round refractile bodies within the bacterial cytoplasm. With basic dyes such as Gram's stain, they stain more strongly than the rest of the bacterium and with metachromatic dyes, they stain a reddish purple color while the rest of the bacterium is a greenish color. We shall also study about volutin granules on the chapter on *C. diphtheriae*.

Reagents

Albert I stain: This is Laybourn's modification in which malachite green is substituted for methyl green.

Staining solution I
- Toluidine blue 1.5 g
- Malachite green 2 g
- Glacial acetic acid 10 mL

- Alcohol (95% ethanol) 20 mL
- Distilled water 1 L

Dissolve the dyes in alcohol, add to the water and acetic acid. Allow to stand for a day and then filter.

Staining solution II

- Iodine 6 g
- KI 9 g
- DW 900 mL

Procedure

1. Make film, air dry, heat fix.
2. Cover slide with Albert's Stain I and allow it to act for 3 to 5 minutes.
3. Blot dry.
4. Cover slide with Albert's iodine II and allow to act for one minute.
5. Wash and Blot dry.

The granules appear bluish black; the protoplasm appears green.

Two other methods are used to stain metachromatic granules:

- Neisser's method.
- Ponder's method.

Neisser's Methylene Blue Stain

- Methylene blue—1 g
- Ethyl alcohol (95%)—50 mL
- Glacial acetic acid—50 mL
- Distilled water—1 L

Procedure

1. Stain with Neisser's methylene blue for three minutes.
2. Wash off with dilute iodine solution (Gram's iodine diluted 1 in 10) and leave some of this solution on the slide for 1 minute.
3. Wash with water.
4. Counterstain with neutral red solution for 3 minutes.
5. Wash in water and dry.
6. By this method, bacilli exhibit deep blue granules and remainder of this organism is pink.

Negative Staining—Capsular Staining

Introduction

Capsules of bacteria present in animal tissues, blood, serous fluids and pus are often clearly stained, when these samples are treated with one of the common stains such as basic fuchsin, methylene blue, Leishman's stain and Gram's stain (which colors them with red counterstain).

But when artificial cultures are examined, the capsules are not colored by ordinary staining methods and special methods must be employed for their demonstration, e.g. negative staining.

Dyes—India-ink, Nigrosin/Eosin.

India Ink Method

- Normal blue ink is used for this purpose. We can use a:
  - Wet India ink method
  - Dry India ink method

Wet India ink method

- Materials—India ink—dense, very finely granular and free from contamination.
- Culture plate.

Procedure

1. Carefully wipe a slide free from particles of dust.
2. Place a large loopful of undiluted India ink on the slide.
3. Emulsify a very small portion of solid bacterial culture or a small loopful of liquid culture in the ink. Rub the speck of solid material on the slide surface before mixing it into the ink (The fresh liquid cultures show the best capsule).
4. Place a clean cover slip on the ink drop and press it down through a sheet of blotting paper so that the film becomes very thin and pale in color. Neither too thick, nor too thin a film is to be made. If the film is too thick ink will cover the bacteria. If too thin the capsule will get crushed.

Appearance

On microscopic examination with oil-immersion, the highly retractile outline of the bacteria is seen. Between this retractile outline and the dark background of the ink particles, there is a clear space which is the capsule. Noncapsulated bacteria do not have this clear zone (Fig. 3.4).

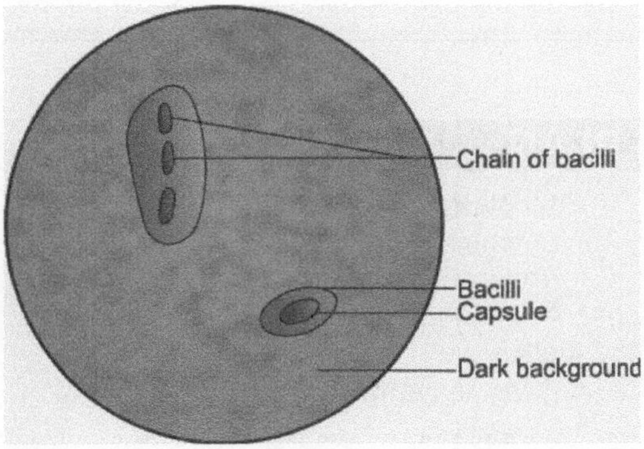

Fig. 3.4: Capsular staining chain of bacilli with capsule in wet film with India ink *(Bacillus species)*

Dry India ink method: Mix a bit of the growth of the culture plate with a drop of ink solution spread and dry the smear. Then observe under 100X.

Disadvantage of dry India ink method: In this method, shrinkage spaces give the appearance of capsules around bacteria that are non-capsulated and in thick films; capsules may be shrunken or obscured to the point that they are rendered invisible.

Nigrosin Staining

Ten percent solution of nigrosin and formalin is used. A small drop of dye is placed on a slide. Bacteria are mixed with it and a smear is made, dried and examined. Nigrosin gives a homogenous background and it is the simplest method of making a preliminary examination of a culture to show shape, size and arrangement of bacteria as also the capsule.

CHAPTER

4

Morphology of Bacteria

LESSON PLAN

- Introduction
- Some Definitions
  - Bacteria
  - Viruses
  - Fungi
  - Parasites
- Appearance of Bacteria
  - Size
  - Shape
  - Arrangement
- Structure of Bacterial Cell
  - Cell Wall
  - Cell Membrane
- Protoplasm
  - Cytoplasm
  - Vacuoles
  - Nucleus
- Additional
  - Capsule and Slimlayer
  - Flagella
  - Fimbriae
  - Spore
- Abnormal Forms of Bacteria
  - L Forms or Phase Organisms
  - Pleomorphism and Involution
  - Spheroplasts and Protoplasts

INTRODUCTION

Microorganisms which include bacteria, viruses, fungi and protozoa come under a kingdom called PROTISTA. The kingdom Protista has been divided into two groups—Prokaryotes and Eukaryotes. The differences between the two are given in Table 4.1. Bacteria come under the group prokaryotes while the other microorganisms of medical importance come under eukaryotes. Viruses form the boundary between living and nonliving.

SOME DEFINITIONS

Bacteria

Bacteria are unicellular, prokaryotic microorganisms that do not have chlorophyll. They have both DNA (single molecule) and RNA.

Viruses

Viruses are obligate intracellular parasitic microorganisms that do not have a cellular organization. They have one type of nucleic acid, never both. Viruses form the boundary between the living and nonliving. They are called living chemicals. They do not have the enzymes necessary for protein and nucleic acid synthesis and are totally dependent on the host cell machinery for survival.

Fungi

Fungi are eukaryotic unicellular/multicellular microorganisms that have rigid cell walls containing chitin.

Table 4.1: Differences between prokaryotic and eukaryotic cells

Property	*Prokaryotes*	*Eukaryotes*
Nucleus		
• Nuclear membrane	Absent	Present
• Nucleolus	Absent	Present
• Chromosome	One, circular	More than one, linear
• Mitotic division	Absent	Present
Cytoplasm		
• Cytoplasmic movement	Absent	Present
• Pinocytosis	Absent	Present
• Mitochondria	Absent	Present
• Lysosomes	Absent	Present
• Golgi apparatus	Absent	Present
• Endoplasmic reticulum	Absent	Present
• Ribosome	70 S	80 S
Chemical composition		
• Sterols	Absent	Present
• Muramic acid	Present	Absent
• Diaminopimelic acid	May be present	Absent
Approximate diameter of cell	1 μm	10 μm
Cilia	Absent	Present
Pili	Present	Absent

Parasites

Parasites are eukaryotic microorganisms that are unicellular or multicellular with a cellular organization and dependent on the host cell for its nutrition but not for reproduction. They can live outside the host too.

APPEARANCE OF BACTERIA

- Size
- Shape
- Arrangement.

Size

The unit of measurement in bacteriology is the micron (micrometer)

1 micron (μ) or micrometer $= \frac{1}{1000}$ of a mm or 10^{-3} mm or 10^{-6} m

- 1 millimicron mμ is also called nanometer

1 mμ or nm $= \frac{1}{1000}$ of a micron or 10^{-3} μ or 10^{-6} mm or 10^{-9}m

- 1 Angstrom unit (Å) $= \frac{1}{10}$ of a nanometer

The smallest object we can see with the naked eye is 200 microns. This is called the limit of resolution of the naked eye. Bacteria are much smaller than this and can be seen under a microscope. Bacteria of medical importance generally measure. 0.2 to 1.5 μ in diameter and 3 to 5 μ in length.

Shape

Depending on shape bacteria are divided into several varieties:

1. *Cocci*: Cocci are spherical or oval cells. They are derived from the word *kokkos* which means berry.

1 coccus   Many cocci

2. *Bacilli*: Bacilli are rod shaped cells. The word is derived from the word baculus meaning rod.

1 bacillus   Many bacilli

3. *Vibrios*: Vibrios are comma shaped, curved rods and derive their name from their vibratory motility.

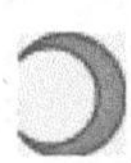

Vibrio

4. *Spirilla*: Spirilla are rigid spiral forms.

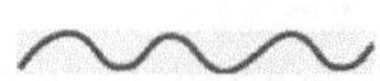

Spirillum

5. *Spirochetes*: Spirochetes are flexible spiral forms. They derive their name from *speira* meaning coil and chaite meaning hair.

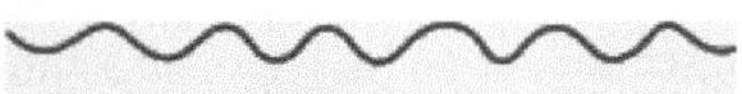

Spirochete

6. *Actinomyces*: *Actinomyces* are branching filamentous bacteria which look like radiating sun rays when seen in tissue lesions. The name is derived from actis meaning ray and mykes meaning fungus. The shape is due to a rigid cell wall.

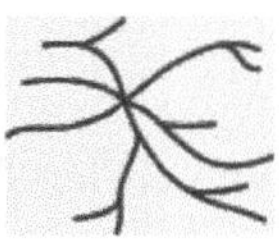

7. *Mycoplasmas*: Mycoplasmas are bacteria that are cell wall deficient and so do not have a stable morphology. They can occur as round oval bodies or filaments.

Arrangement

Bacteria sometimes show a special cellular arrangement or grouping. Usually the cocci show arrangements (Fig. 4.1). They can be arranged in:

Pairs	*Diplococci, e.g. Pneumococci, Gonococci or Meningococci*
Chains	*Streptococci*
In groups of 4 (Tetrads)	*Micrococci*
In groups of 8	*Sarcina*
Grape-like clusters	*Staphylococci*

- Some bacilli also show special arrangement.
- Certain bacilli are arranged at an angle to each other forming a chinese letter pattern (*Corynebacteria*) (Fig. 4.2).
- Some bacilli are arranged in chains (*Streptobacilli* or *Bacillus anthracis*).
- Some are arranged in pairs-diplobacilli (*K. pneumoniae*).

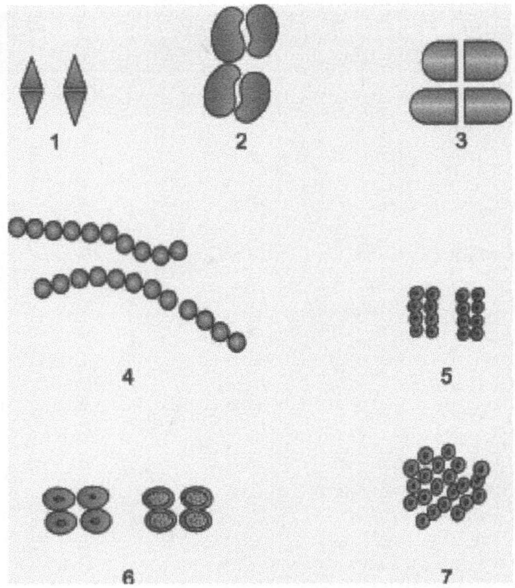

Fig. 4.1: Arrangement of cocci: (1) Pneumococci, (2) Gonococci, (3) Meningococci, (4) Streptococci, (5) Sarcina, (6) Micrococci, (7) Staphylococci

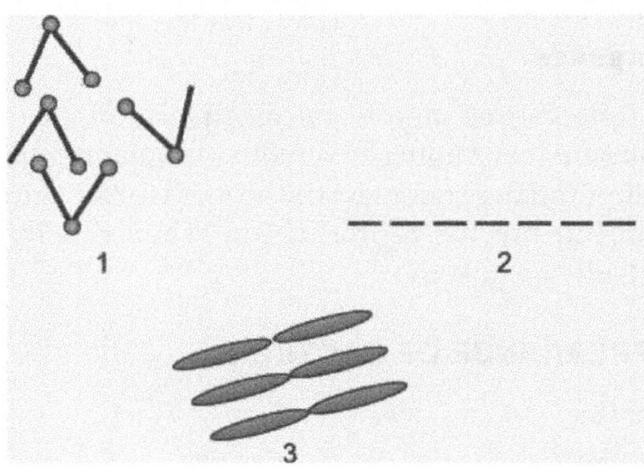

Fig. 4.2: Arrangement of bacilli: (1) Corynebacteria, (2) Bacilli in chains *B. anthracis*, (3) Diplobacilli (*K. pneumoniae*)

These arrangements of bacteria are characteristic of a bacterial group. This is due to the tendency of the daughter cells to remain attached to the parent cells even after repeated binary fission.

STRUCTURE OF BACTERIAL CELL

Figure 4.3 shows the structure of a typical bacterial cell. The principal structures of a bacterial cell can be divided into three main groups.

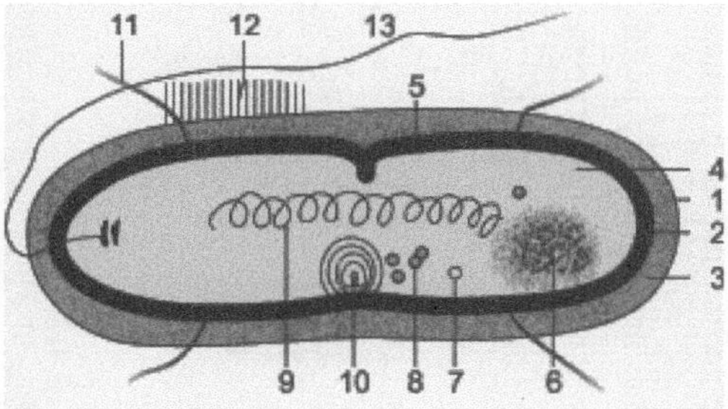

Fig. 4.3: Structure of bacterial cell dividing: (1) Capsule, (2) Plasma membrane, (3) Cell wall, (4) Cytoplasm, (5) Division septum, (6) Ribosome, (7) Fat globule, (8) Inclusion body, (9) DNA, (10) Mesosome, (11) Sex pili, (12) Common pili, (13) Flagella

CELL ENVELOPE

This consists of two components
- Cell wall
- Cytoplasmic membrane or plasma membrane.

PROTOPLASM

This consists of cytoplasm and nuclear body. The cytoplasm has within it:
- Ribosomes
- Mesosomes
- Inclusion granules
- Vacuoles.

ADDITIONAL COMPONENTS

- Capsule
- Fimbriae
- Flagella
- Spore

Cell Wall

Definition

Cell wall is the rigid outer covering of the bacterial cell.

Structure

- The bacterial cell wall is about 10 to 25 nm in thickness.
- Chemically it is composed of mucopeptide formed by N-acetyl glucosamine and N-acetylmuramic acid molecules linked alternately in a chain by peptides (Fig. 4.4).

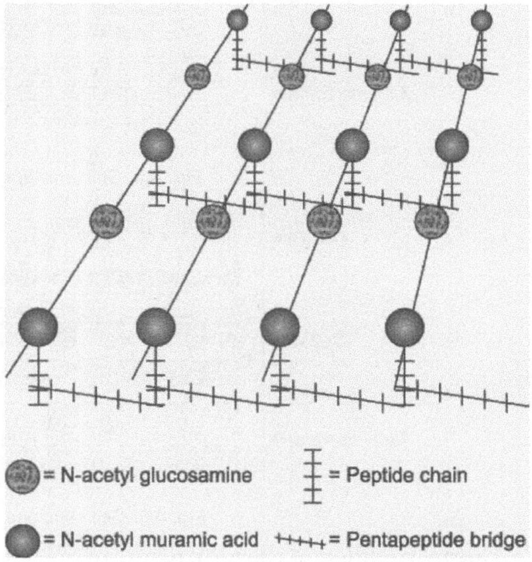

Fig. 4.4: The structure of cell wall mucopeptide

There are many differences between the cell wall of Gram-positive bacteria and Gram-negative bacteria (Table 4.2).

Table 4.2: Differences between cell wall of gram-positive and Gram-negative bacteria

	Gram-positive	*Gram-negative*
Thickness	Thicker	Thinner
Lipids	Absent or scanty	Present
LPS	Absent	Present
Teichoic acid	Present	Absent
Variety of Aa*	Few	Several

*Aa = Amino acids

The gram-positive cell wall is simpler than gram-negative cell wall.

Gram-negative bacteria have a special structure called lipopolysaccharide on the cell wall which is responsible for O antigen specificity and endotoxic activities like fever, tissue damage, etc. (Figs 4.5 and 4.6).

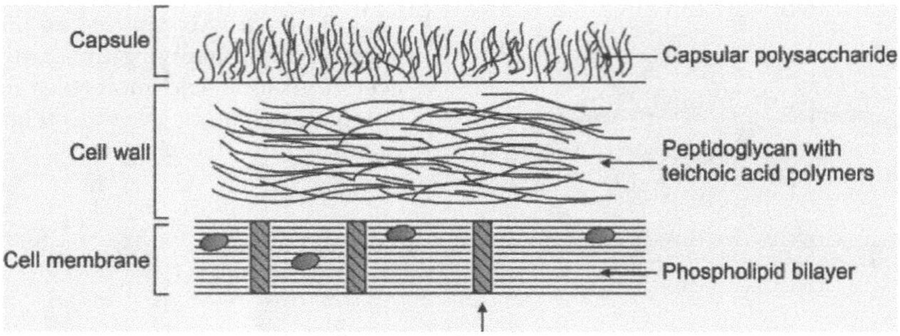

Fig. 4.5: Cell envelope of gram-positive bacteria

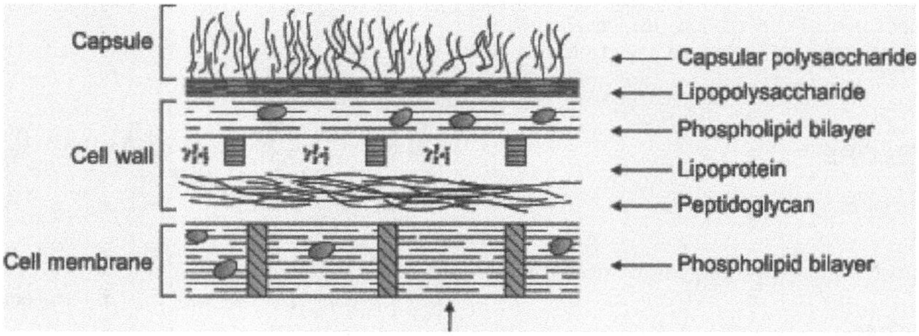

Fig. 4.6: Cell envelope of gram-negative bacteria

Due to the different chemical nature of the cell wall, the bacteria differ in their staining properties.

Certain acid fast bacteria contain mycolic acid in their cell wall.

Function

- It gives shape and rigidity to the bacterial cell.
- It also has antigens which are important in pathogenesis of diseases caused by bacteria.
- It supports the weak cytoplasmic membrane.
- It plays a major role in cell division.

Demonstration of Cell Wall

The cell wall cannot be seen by light microscope and does not stain with ordinary dyes. It lies invisible and unstained outside the shrunken bacterial protoplast. Direct and indirect methods to demonstrate its presence are:

a. Plasmolysis: When the bacterial cell is placed in a highly concentrated solution the cytoplasm loses water by osmosis and shrinks while the cell wall retains the original shape and size.
b. Reaction with specific antibody.
c. Mechanical rupture of the cell.
d. Special staining procedure.
e. Electron microscopy.

Cell Wall Deficient Forms

- Cell wall synthesis can be inhibited by antibiotics
- Cell wall can be lysed by an enzyme called lysozyme normally present in tissue fluids. When lysozyme acts on a gram-positive bacterium, a protoplast is formed consisting of a cytoplasmic membrane and its contents. When lysozyme acts on gram-negative bacteria, the result is a spheroplast which differs from the protoplast in that some cell wall material is retained. Both protoplasts and spheroplasts are spherical cell wall deficient forms and play a role in the persistence of chronic bacterial infections.

Cell Membrane

Definition

The cell membrane or cytoplasmic membrane or plasma membrane is a thin elastic layer (5 to 10 nm in thickness) lining the inner surface of the cell wall and separating it from the cytoplasm (Fig. 4.7).

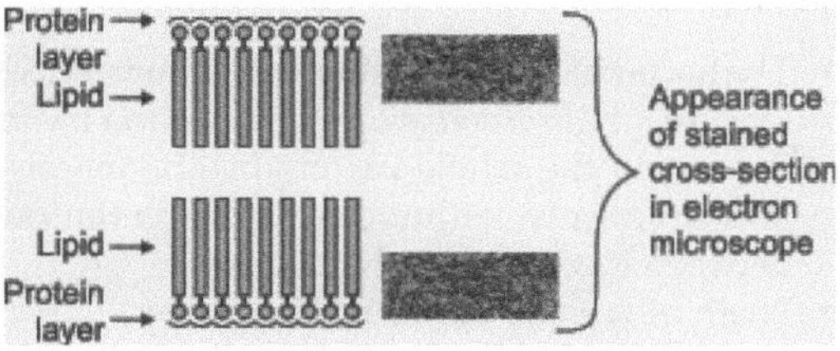

Fig. 4.7: A diagram of a unit membrane

Chemical Structure

Chemically, the membrane consists of lipoprotein with very small amounts of carbohydrate. In bacteria, the membrane does not have cholesterol which is found in animal cells.

Function

- It is a semipermeable membrane which controls the inflow and outflow of metabolites to and from the cytoplasm.
- It also has specific enzymes called permeases which control the passage of metabolites. The cytoplasmic membrane has other enzymes, e.g. respiratory enzymes, enzymes manufacturing substances of the cell wall, etc.
- The cell membrane gives rise to mesosomes and fimbria.

Demonstration

Through the electron microscope we can see the presence of three layers making up a unit membrane.

PROTOPLASM

Cytoplasm

Definition

It is a viscous watery solution which has many organic and inorganic solutes. It contains certain structures in it like ribosomes, mesosomes, inclusion granules and vacuoles.

Properties

- Bacterial cytoplasm does not have endoplasmic reticulum or mitochondria.
- Bacterial cytoplasm does not show motility called cytoplasmic streaming.
- The cytoplasm stains uniformly with basic dyes in young cultures but becomes granular with age.

Cytoplasmic Contents

Ribosomes

- They are the centers of protein synthesis.
- They are slightly smaller (10 to 20 nm) than the ribosomes of eukaryotic cells and are seen integrated in the linear strands of mRNA to form polysomes.
- Bacteria possess 70S ribosomes.

Mesosomes or Chondroids

- They are invaginations or ingrowths of the plasma membrane into the cytoplasm forming twisted multilayered vesicular structures.
- They have the respiratory enzymes of the bacteria and are similar to the mitochondria of eukaryotes.
- They are more common in gram-positive bacteria.
- Mesosomes are found near to the nuclear body and the site of synthesis of cross wall suggesting that they coordinate nuclear and cytoplasmic division during binary fission.

Intracytoplasmic Inclusions

These are certain bodies that are found inside the cytoplasm. They are different for different species and also depend on the age and condition of the culture. They are not permanent structures. They appear to be accumulations of excess metabolites within the cell and are present more, when the bacteria has access to abundant nutrition. They disappear under food starvation. They are useful for identification of bacteria.

These are:
- Volutin
- Polysaccharide—glycogen or starch
- Lipid
- Sulfur.

Volutin Granules

Also called metachromatic granules or Babès-Ernst granules.

- They are strongly basophilic bodies composed of polymetaphosphate.
- They appear blue black when stained with Albert's stain with the rest of the bacteria appearing green. This property of a part of the bacteria picking up a different colour from the rest of the bacteria is called metachromasia.
- Volutin granules are present in *Corynebacterium diphtheriae.*
- Their function is uncertain. They have been considered to represent a reserve of energy and phosphate for cell metabolism (Fig. 4.8).

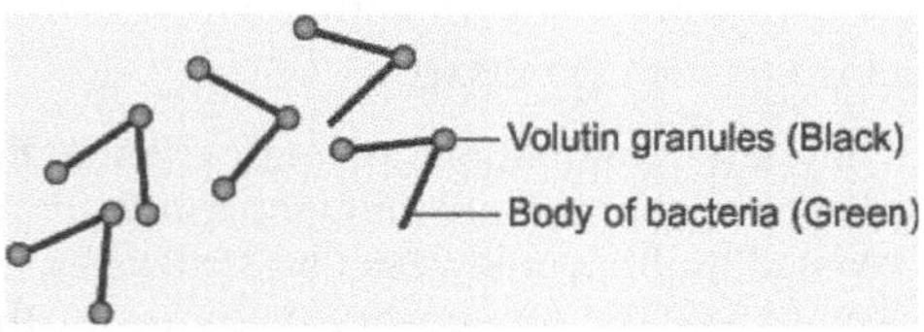

Fig. 4.8: *Corynebacterium diphtheriae* with volutin granules

Polysaccharide: Polysaccharide granules can be demonstrated by staining with iodine. These can be of either glycogen (red brown) or starch (blue) when stained with iodine.

Lipid inclusions: Lipid inclusions can be demonstrated by fat soluble dyes like, Sudan black.

Vacuoles

Vacuoles are fluid containing cavities separated from the cytoplasm by a membrane.

Nucleus

Structure

The bacterial nucleus has no nuclear membrane or nucleolus. The nuclear DNA does not appear to be associated with basic protein. The genome consists of a single molecule of double stranded DNA arranged in the form of a circle. Sometimes it opens in the form of a long chain about 1000 μ in length but usually it is tightly coiled and packed. The bacterial chromosome replicates by simple fission. It is always present in a bacterial cell.

Demonstration

- The bacterial nucleus cannot be demonstrated by direct light microscopy because the basic dyes stain the whole bacterial cell intensely and uniformly without any differentiation between cytoplasm and nucleus.
- It can be seen by electron microscopy.
- It can also be demonstrated by acid or ribonuclease hydrolysis and then staining for nuclear material.
- Bacteria may sometimes have extranuclear genetic elements consisting of DNA. These cytoplasmic carriers of genetic information are called plasmids. They can be transferred from one bacterium to another through conjugation. They are responsible for properties like toxigenicity and drug resistance which constitute a survival advantage.

ADDITIONAL

Capsule and Slime Layer

Definition

Capsule is a viscid gelatinous secretion of the bacteria which forms a defined organized coat around the cell wall, e.g. the capsule of *Pneumococcus*. When the same secretion is loose and undefined, it is called a slime layer, e.g. in leuconostoc. Some bacteria have both a capsule and slime layer, e.g. *Streptococcus salivarius*. When the layer can be seen with the light microscope ($\geq$0.2 μm) it is called capsule. If it is narrower and only detectable by serological techniques or electron microscopy they are called microcapsules.

Biochemical Structure

The capsular gel is made up of mostly water and has only 2 percent solids. The solids are:

- Polysaccharide as in *Pneumococcus*
- Polypeptide as in *Bacillus anthracis*
- Hyaluronic acid as in *Streptococcus pyogenes*.

Slime is generally:
- Polysaccharide, e.g. *Pneumococcus*
- Polypeptide, e.g. *Bacillus anthracis*

Bacteria which produce a lot of slime, produce mucoid growth on agar with a stringy consistency.

Demonstration

The capsule has less affinity for basic dyes and is not visible in Gram's stained smears. It can be demonstrated by:

a. *Negative staining* using India ink method where the capsules are seen as clear haloes around the bacteria against a black background.
b. *Quellung reaction*—Capsular material is antigenic and may be demonstrated by serological methods. When a suspension of a capsulated bacterium is mixed with its specific anticapsular serum and examined under the microscope, the capsule becomes very prominent and appears swollen. This is called Quellung reaction and is seen in *Pneumococcus*.
c. *Special capsule staining techniques* using copper salts as mordants.
d. The capsule cannot be visible easily by electron microscope, because they shrink a lot on drying.

Function of Capsules

Capsules protect bacteria from destruction by lytic enzymes. They also contribute to the virulence of pathogenic bacteria by inhibiting phagocytosis. Loss of capsule may render the bacterium avirulent. Capsules also have antigens.

- Repeated subcultures lead to a loss of capsule and also of virulence.
- Bacteria which are capsulated are:
  - *Pneumococcus*
  - *Bacillus anthracis*
  - *Streptococcus pyogenes*
  - *Klebsiella pneumoniae*
  - *Plague bacillus (Yersinia pestis)*

Flagella

Definition

Flagella are unbranched, long, wavy, filamentous structures which are the organs of movement in bacteria.

Structure

They are 3 to 20 μm long and 0.01 to 0.013 μm on diameter. They have a square tip. Each flagellum consists of three different parts:

- Filament
- Hook
- Basal body

The hook-basal body portion is embedded in the cell wall. The filament is external to the cell and joined to the hook at the cell surface. Different genera of bacteria have flagella of similar chemical composition but different thickness, different antigenic structure, different wave length and variation in number and arrangement of flagella. Figure 4.9 shows the different types of flagellar arrangement.

- If the flagella are arranged all around the cell they are called *peritrichous* as in typhoid bacilli.
- They may also be situated at one or both ends of the cell called polar. Polar flagella may be single (*monotrichous*) as in cholera vibrios, in a bunch (*lophotrichous*) as in *Spirilla* or with a flagella at both poles (*amphitrichous*).

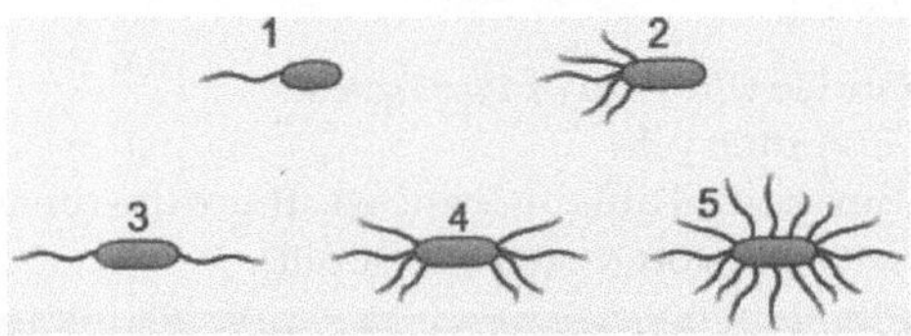

Fig. 4.9: Types of flagellar arrangement: (1) Single polar flagellum (Monotrichate), (2) Bunch of flagella at one pole (Lophotrichate), (3) Single flagellum at each pole, (4) Bunch of flagella at both poles, (5) Peritrichate

Demonstration of Flagella

- Flagella cannot be seen by light microscope
- They can sometimes be seen by dark ground microscopy or electron microscopy by metal shadowing or negative staining.

- Special staining techniques in which the thickness is increased by deposition of a substance onto the flagella called mordanting can be used to demonstrate flagella.
- Flagella can also be demonstrated indirectly by demonstration of motility under the microscope by a hanging drop preparation or by spread on semisolid agar.

Chemical Structure

Flagella are made up of a protein called flagellin.

Function

- They are responsible for bacterial movement which is helpful for bacteria to obtain nutrition in the environment.
- It also helps pathogenic bacteria in penetrating through barriers in the body.

Fimbriae

Definition

Some gram-negative bacilli carry very fine short hair like surface appendages called fimbriae or pili. They are shorter and thinner than flagella (0.1 to 1.5 μ long and 10 nm thick) and project from the cell surface as straight filaments. They originate in the cell membrane. They are best seen in liquid cultures and freshly isolated strains.

Types

Fimbriae (Pili) are of two types:
- Common pili.
- Sex pili (Table 4.3 shows the differences between common and sex pili).

Table 4.3: Differences between common and sex pili

Common pili	*Sex pili*
Help in attachment to the surface of the host so that bacteria can stick to the nutritionally favorable environments	Help in attachment of male bacteria to female bacteria by forming hollow conjugation tubes through which genetic material is transferred from the donor to the recipient cell
Shorter and more in number	Longer and fewer in number

Demonstration

- Fimbriae can be seen only under the electron microscopy by metal shadowing or negative staining.
- Many fimbriated cells agglutinate red blood cells of guinea pigs, fowls, horses and pigs strongly, human and sheep cells weakly and ox cells not at all. This gives us a simple method for detecting such fimbriae. Depending on the property of hemagglutination, we can have different types of fimbriae (6 types).
- They form a pellicle in liquid media.

Chemical Structure

Fimbriae are made up of a protein called **pilin**, and are best found in freshly isolated strains and in liquid cultures. They disappear following subcultures on solid media.

Fimbriae are antigenic. Different genera may have the same fimbrial antigen. So it is necessary to see that bacterial antigens used for serological tests should not have fimbriae. Table 4.4 shows the differences between flagella and fimbriae.

Table 4.4: Differences between flagella and fimbriae

Flagella	*Fimbriae*
• Flagella arises from cell protoplasm	Fimbriae arise from cell membrane
• They are longer and thicker than fimbriae 3-20 μm long and 0.01 to 0.013 μm thick	Fimbriae are shorter and thinner than flagella 0.1 to 1.5 μ long and 4–8 nm thick
• Responsible for movement	Responsible for adhesion to favorable environment and transfer of genetic material during conjugation
• Made up of a protein-flagellin	Made up of a protein-pilin
• Usually not straight (curved)	Always straight
• Less in number (1 to 20)	Numerous (100 to 500)
• Various positions of flagella	Peritrichous in common pili
• Found in both Gram-positive and negative bacteria	Found only in Gram-negative bacteria

Function

- They are organs of adhesion
- They help in conjugation
- They are antigenic
- They cause hemagglutination.

Spore

Definition

Spores are highly resistant resting stages of certain bacteria like members of genera *Bacillus* and *Clostridium*. Each bacterium forms one spore which on germination forms a single vegetative cell. As bacterial spores are formed inside the bacterial cell, they are called endospores.

Formation of Spores

Spore formation usually occurs after a period of vegetative growth and is related to the depletion of nutrients. There is production of many new structures, enzymes and metabolites along with disappearance of many vegetative cell structures. During sporulation some bacteria release antibiotics.

Structures of the Spore

At the center of the spore is the nuclear body and cytoplasm (spore core) surrounded by a spore wall, a delicate membrane called inner membrane from which the cell wall of future bacteria will develop. Outside this is the thick spore cortex which in turn is enclosed by a multilayered tough spore coat. Sometimes a loose outer covering called exosporium is found (Fig. 4.10).

New antigens appear on sporulation.

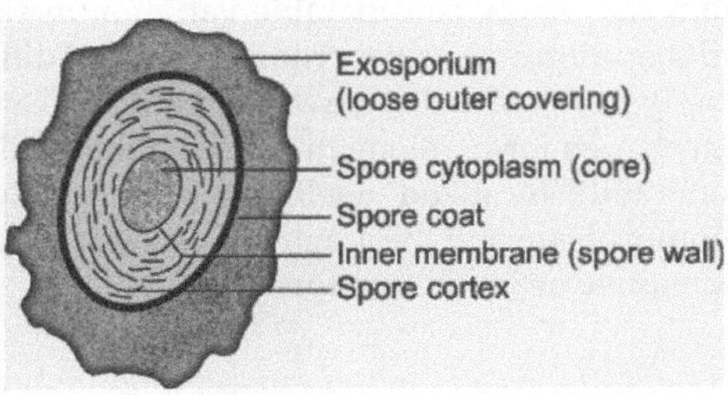

Fig. 4.10: Cross-section of a bacterial spore

The shape, position and size of the spore are different in different species. They may be central terminal or subterminal. They may be oval or spherical in shape and may or may not distend the bacillary body (Fig. 4.11).

Demonstration

- Spores are seen in unstained preparations as refractile bodies.
- In Gram's stained preparations, they appear as unstained areas.
- Spores can be stained by a modification of Ziehl-Neelsen technique.

Function of the Spore

- Bacterial spores are one of the most resistant forms of life.
- They may remain viable for centuries.
- Sporulation helps bacteria to survive for long periods under unfavorable environment.

When a spore is transferred to conditions helpful for vegetative growth, the spores germinate, the spore swells, the spore wall is shed and the germ cell appears by rupturing the spore coat. The germ cell elongates to form the vegetative bacterium. Spores of all medically important bacteria are destroyed by autoclaving at 121°C × 15 minutes.

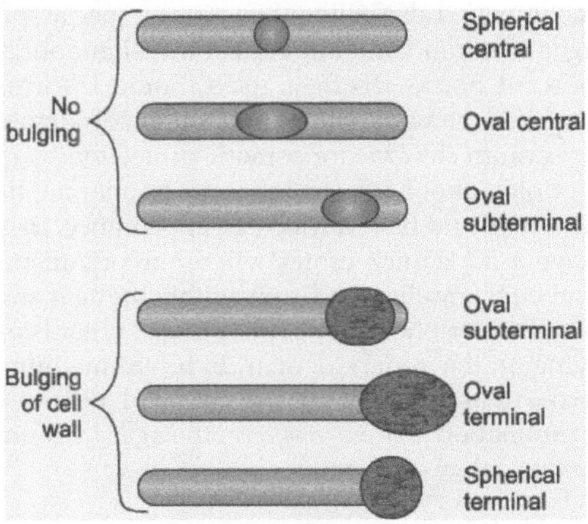

Fig. 4.11: The shape and situation of the spore in the bacterial cell

ABNORMAL FORMS OF BACTERIA

L Forms or L Phase Organisms

Definition

L forms are abnormal growth forms of bacteria, derived by variation, usually in the laboratory from bacteria of normal morphology. They are named after Lister Institute, London where they were first observed by Kleineberger Nobel who was studying cultures of *Streptobacillus moniliformis*.

Structure

They differ from the parent bacteria in lacking a rigid cell wall and hence have no regular size and shape. Some L forms may completely lack a cell wall and some may have a weakened cell wall like spheroplasts.

L forms are usually soft protoplasmic bodies spherical or disk like but sometimes extremely variable in shape. They range in size from minute bodies about 0.1 μm in diameter to large once of 10–20 mm. They can pass through bacteria stopping filters. L forms are viable and are capable of growing and multiplying on a suitable artificial nutrient medium.

Maintenance

Though L forms can grow on ordinary culture medium and also in liquid medium, a special soft agar medium containing meat infusion and 20 percent horse serum is used. Some L forms require a medium with a large content of sucrose or sodium chloride for osmotic protection.

Colonies of L phase organisms on agar media are small and have a fried egg appearance, they have a dark thick center where the organisms embed themselves and grow within the agar and a higher peripheral zone consisting of organisms lying on the surface of agar. In liquid medium, growth is usually in the form of clumps. Examination is done *in situ* on the agar medium because they are fragile.

Origin

Some bacteria, e.g. *Streptobacillus moniliformis* and *Bacteroides* give rise spontaneously to L forms even when grown in an optimal culture medium. L form growth may be induced by culture in the presence of an inhibitor of cell wall synthesis like penicillin, or by deprivation of a nutrient essential for cell wall synthesis, e.g. diaminopimelic acid or by destruction of the cell wall with antibody and complement.

Reversion to Bacterial Forms

L forms can be stable when they continue to reproduce as L forms even when the cell wall inhibitor is removed. Unstable L forms generally revert to the normal bacterial form within a few hours of culture in the absence of the inducing agent.

Role

L forms resemble mycoplasmas. It is possible that mycoplasmas represent stable L forms of as yet unidentified parent bacteria. But usually L forms are laboratory artifacts that do not survive to any important extent in natural habitats. They have been isolated from patients suffering from chronic urinary tract and pus forming infections. L forms could account for bacterial persistence during therapy with antibiotics L forms are non-pathogenic to laboratory animals.

Pleomorphism and Involution

In the course of their growth, bacteria of a single strain may show considerable variation in size and shape forming a proportion of cells that differ grossly from normal, e.g. swollen, spherical and pear shaped forms, elongated filaments and filaments with localized swellings. This is called pleomorphism and the abnormal cells are called degenerate or involution forms.

How are they Formed?

It can occur naturally in certain species, e.g. *Streptobacillus moniliformis or Yersinia pestis* in ageing cultures, or in the presence of antagonistic substances such as penicillin, glycine, lithium chloride, sodium chloride in high concentrations and organic acids at high pH.

The abnormal shape is due to defective cell wall synthesis or autolytic enzymes. The growing protoplasm expands the weakened wall to produce a swollen cell similar to spheroplast that later bursts and lyses. Others revert to normal form when transferred to a suitable environment.

Spheroplasts and Protoplasts

- When bacteria with their cell walls removed or weakened are held in a concentrated solution do not lyse and get converted into viable spherical bodies.
- If all the cell wall material has been removed from them, the spheres are free protoplasts. These are normally formed when gram-positive bacilli are treated with lysozyme.
- If they remain enclosed by an intact but weakened residual cell wall they are called spheroplasts. These are formed when gram-negative bacilli are grown in the presence of penicillin, bacitracin, oxymycin (cycloserine) or glycine that inhibit synthesis of mucopeptide component of cell wall. The same result may be obtained by culturing certain bacteria on medium lacking a nutrient, e.g. diaminopimelic acid, lysine or hexosamine derivative that they require specifically for cell wall synthesis.
- Protoplasts and spheroplasts are osmotically sensitive; if the medium is much diluted they swell up burst and perish by lysis. Spheroplasts are not as osmotically sensitive as protoplasts because they have a residual wall structure.
- If maintained in an osmotically protected agar medium both remain viable and continue to grow and metabolize. Protoplasts enlarge but do not multiply. Spheroplasts when kept on an osmotically protective agar medium containing a cell wall inhibitor like penicillin may multiply by fission or budding and reproduce through many serial subcultures. Spheroplasts revert back when transferred to culture medium lacking the cell wall inhibitor. Spheroplasts have sometimes been called unstable L forms. Protoplasts have not been found capable of reverting to normal bacterial morphology.

CHAPTER

5

Growth and Nutrition of Bacteria

LESSON PLAN

- Growth
- Bacterial Cell Division
- Growth Curve
  - Total Count
  - Viable Count
  - What is Continuous Culture?
- Growth Requirements of Bacteria
  - Nutrition
  - Physical Conditions Required for Growth

GROWTH

By growth we mean, an increase in size of all the parts of the bacterial cell under favorable conditions which are a suitable temperature and pH and a good culture medium. This is normally followed by multiplication. When a bacterial cell reaches a certain size it divides to form two daughter cells. Bacteria divide by binary fission.

BACTERIAL CELL DIVISION

Nuclear division occurs before cell division (Fig. 5.1). Then the cell divides by in growth of a transverse septum from both sides of the cell which meet in the center and result in two daughter cells. In some species, the daughter cells remain partially attached after cell division giving rise to special arrangement of bacteria.

The time required for a bacterium to give rise to two daughter cells under optimum conditions is known as *generation time or population doubling time*. In *Escherichia coli*, the generation time is about 20 minutes, in Tubercle bacilli it is 20 hours and in Lepra bacilli about 20 days. Generation time affects the time taken for visible growth to appear. Thus *Escherichia coli* grows after overnight incubation whereas tubercle bacilli take 4 to 6 weeks.

When bacteria grow on solid media, they form ***colonies***. Each colony represents a clone of cells derived from a single parent cell. In liquid media, the growth is diffuse.

As bacteria reproduce so rapidly, a single bacterial cell can give rise to 10^{21} bacterial cells in 24 hours weighing 4000 tons. But this does not happen because multiplication stops after few cell divisions due to depletion of nutrients or accumulation of toxic products. A similar situation occurs in the human body, the nutrients are in plenty but the body's defense mechanisms

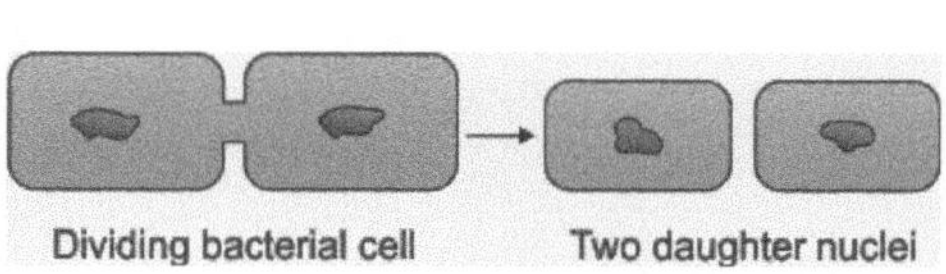

Fig. 5.1: Bacterial cell dividing by binary fission

fight against the bacteria. For industrial or research purposes we sometimes need a continuous culture of bacteria. This is done by continuously adding nutrients and removing bacterial cells.

GROWTH CURVE

When a bacterium is grown in a suitable liquid medium and incubated, the growth follows a definite pattern. If bacterial counts are made at intervals after inoculation and plotted in relation to time, a growth curve is obtained (Fig. 5.2).

Two types of growth curve can be drawn according to the measurement of cell numbers that are used.

Total Count

This is based on the number of cells present, whether living or dead. Living cells are those that divide. Dead cells are those that do not divide.

Viable Count

This measures only those cells capable of growing and hence producing a colony, four main phases are recognized in the growth curve:

1. Lag
2. Log
3. Stationary
4. Death/Decline.

Lag Phase

- There is no multiplication of cells.
- There is increase in size of the cell.
- There is more metabolic activity.
- The duration of this phase is dependent on the time taken for the organism to adapt itself to the new growth environment. In this period the bacteria builds up necessary enzymes and metabolic intermediates in adequate quantities for multiplication to proceed. Maximum cell size is achieved towards the end of the lag phase. The lag phase is different in different species of bacteria and depends on the species and the environment.
- A horizontal line is obtained on the graph.

Log Phase

- The cells divide at a constant rate.
- The cell numbers increase exponentially and a straight line is obtained in the graph.

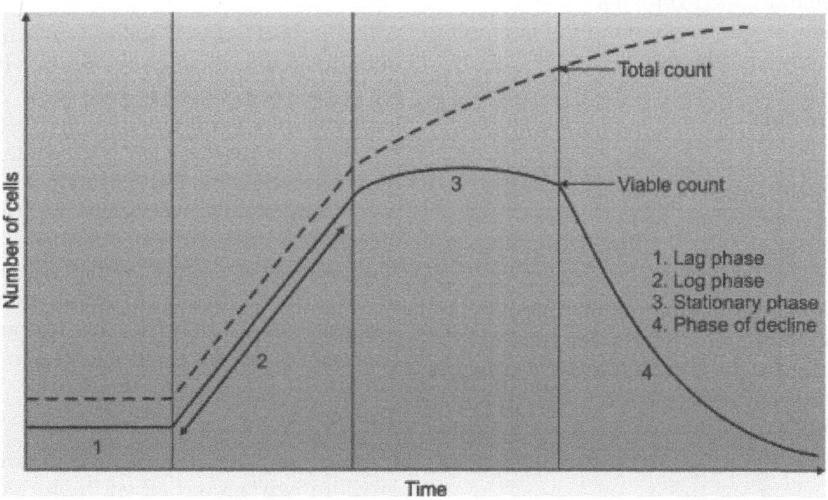

Fig. 5.2: Bacterial growth curve. The viable count shows lag, log, stationary and decline phases. In the total count, the phase of decline is not evident

At this time the bacteria overcome the body's defenses and the infection gets out of control. Total number of cells produced, depend on the generation time and also environmental conditions.

Stationary Phase

After some time, exponential growth is no longer possible and the rate of multiplication decreases and then stops when the cells pass into the stationary phase. This is because of exhaustion of nutrients or accumulation of toxic waste end products. In this situation, an equilibrium exists between the dying cell and the newly formed cell. Viable count remains stationary.

There are four changes in cells in this phase:
- The metabolism of the cell slows down, and they have a high level of intracellular storage products like, volutin granules or polysaccharide (Inclusion Granules).
- There is a variation in morphology and physiology of cells. The gram-positive cells may turn gram-negative.
- Many species of bacteria produce secondary metabolites which are natural products formed by cells that have stopped dividing like antibiotics and exotoxins.
- Formation of spores occurs at the beginning of the stationary phase.

Phase of Decline

- This is the phase when the population decreases due to death of cells.
- Death of cells can be due to:
  a. Nutritional exhaustion (finishing of nutrients).
  b. Accumulation of toxic metabolites.
  c. Autolytic enzymes: These enzymes lead to cell rupture (lysis) and release of contents into the environment.
- In the death or decline phase, the total count remains the same but the viable count decreases.
- In the decline phase highly abnormal morphological forms appear which are called involution forms.

As we have seen in the various stages, the morphology of the cell alters. The various changes are given in the Table 5.1 below:

Table 5.1: Morphological variation in bacterial cells during various stages of the growth curve

Stage of the growth curve	*Morphological variation*
• Lag phase	Cells have the maximum size towards the end of lag phase
• Log phase	The cells are smaller and stain more uniformly
• Stationary phase	Cells are gram variable and show irregular staining due to presence of intracellular storage granules, sporulation, etc.
• Phase of decline	Involution forms

What is Continuous Culture?

A continuous culture is a system in which there is a continuous production of bacteria for industrial or research purposes.

There is a continuous supply of fresh nutrients into the culture vessel and continuous removal of the grown bacteria. So, the phases are not observed as in the growth curve.

There are two methods to obtain a continuous culture:

Chemostat

As shown in Figure 5.3 there is constant addition of fresh medium through a pump into the fermenter vessel. Also the dead cells are continuously removed into a collector vessel. We control the system in such a way, such that the rate of production of new cells by multiplication is equal to the rate of removal of grown cells into the collector vessel. This state can be continued indefinitely. The presence of the nutrient is the limiting factor in this set up because once the nutrient is finished; it requires the addition of more nutrient (media) to be able to sustain continued growth.

Turbidostat

Here the addition of measured volume of fresh medium is triggered when the turbidity in the growth vessel reaches a predetermined value that is monitored by a photoelectric cell. As a result of the addition, the cells are diluted and continue

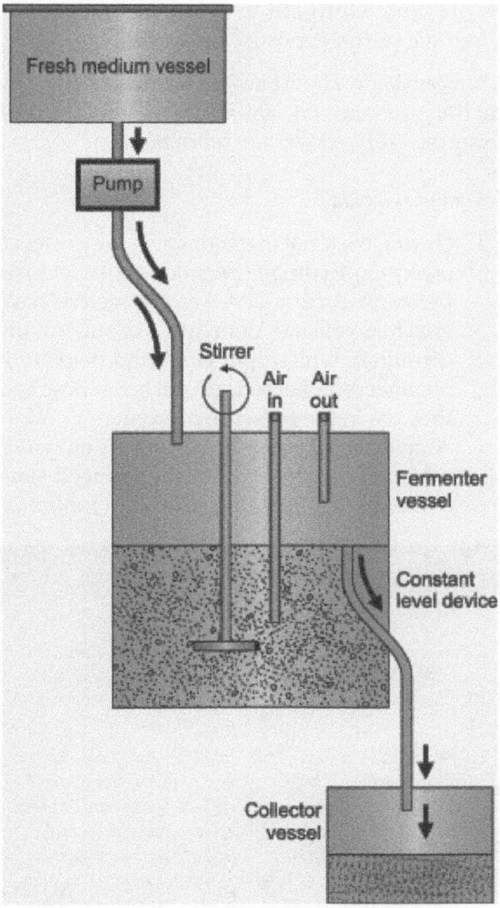

Fig. 5.3: Chemostat: An apparatus for the continuous culture of bacteria

to grow until they reach the critical turbidity and the process is repeated.

GROWTH REQUIREMENTS OF BACTERIA

For the study of a bacterial species it is necessary to grow the bacteria and for that we must know its growth requirements. Two important conditions must be fulfilled.

a. Suitable nutrition should be supplied.
b. Physical environmental conditions should be optimum.

Nutrition

The bacterial cell has the same approximate chemical composition as the cells of the higher organisms. The principal constituent of bacterial cells is water which forms 80 percent of the total weight of the cells. Proteins, polysaccharides, lipids, nucleic acids, mucopeptides and low molecular weight compounds make up the rest. Bacterial metabolism is also similar to the metabolism of higher organisms showing that there is unity of biochemistry. However, there are certain differences between the two and advantage is taken of these differences in selective killing of bacteria.

For growth and multiplication of bacteria, the minimum nutritional requirements are:

- Water
- Source of carbon
- Source of nitrogen
- Inorganic salts: Sulfur, phosphorus, sodium, potassium, magnesium, iron, manganese, calcium and cobalt.

Water is the vehicle for the entry of all nutrients into the cells and for the elimination of all waste products. It participates in the metabolic reactions and forms an integral part of the protoplasm.

On the basis of nutritional requirements bacteria can be divided into two major groups—Autotrophs and Heterotrophs.

Autotrophs: The bacteria which are able to utilize CO_2 as their main source of carbon. Energy is obtained in these organisms by either sunlight or by oxidation of inorganic compounds. They make all essential metabolites. Plants are examples of autotrophs but among bacteria the pigmented sulfur bacteria and iron bacteria are included in this category.

Heterotrophs: The bacteria which obtain their energy by breakdown of suitable organic nutrients. The majority of bacteria are heterotrophs. These are again divided into two groups.

a. *Nonexacting bacteria or Nonfastidious*: These are bacteria whose nutrition requirements are minimum or basic and are able to synthesize all their structural units from carbon, nitrogen and inorganic salts. Examples are *Pseudomonas and Staphylococcus aureus.*
b. *Exacting bacteria or Fastidious*: Some bacteria need different compounds besides a carbon and nitrogen source such as amino acids, nucleotides, lipids, carbohydrates and coenzymes. Other bacteria require certain organic compounds in minute quantities called growth factors or bacterial vitamins without which growth does not normally occur. They are vitamins of B group—thiamine, riboflavine, nicotinic acid, pyridoxine, folic acid and vitamin B_{12}. Such bacteria which require more than the basic nutrition are called exacting bacteria or fastidious bacteria. For examples, are genus *Streptococcus* and *Neisseria.*

Physical Conditions Required for Growth

Provided the nutrition is optimum, the rapid growth of bacteria is possible only under suitable environmental conditions.

Oxygen: Depending upon the influence of oxygen on growth viability, bacteria are divided into aerobes, anaerobes and microaerophilic bacteria.

Aerobic: These bacteria require oxygen for their growth. They may be divided into:

1. *Obligate aerobes*: Obligate aeorbes like, *Vibrio cholerae* grow only in the presence of oxygen. They will not grow if oxygen is not provided.
2. *Facultative anaerobes*: They are ordinarily aerobic but can grow in the absence of oxygen though less abundantly. Most bacteria of medical importance belong to this group.

Anaerobic bacteria: These bacteria grow only in the absence of oxygen. They cannot grow if oxygen is present. Obligate anaerobes like, genus *Clostridia* die on exposure to oxygen.

Microaerophilic: These bacteria are those that grow in the presence of low oxygen tension. For example—*Mycobacterium tuberculosis.*

Why is O_2 Toxic?

1. During bacterial metabolism in the presence of oxygen, hydrogen peroxide and other toxic peroxides accumulate. Aerobic bacteria have enzymes catalase, peroxidase or superoxide dismutase which split H_2O_2 and detoxify it but anaerobic bacteria do not have these and they die in the presence of oxygen.
2. Anaerobic bacteria have certain enzymes which are active only in the reduced state and oxygen makes them inactive (Table 5.2).

Table 5.2: Differences between aerobic and anaerobic bacteria

Aerobic	*Anaerobic*
1. Aerobic bacteria use oxygen as the ultimate hydrogen acceptor	In anaerobic bacteria, the hydrogen acceptors are other than oxygen (nitrates or sulfates)
2. The carbon and energy source may be completely oxidised to CO_2 and water and energy rich phosphate bonds (ATP) are fomed. This process is called oxidative phosphorylation	In anaerobic bacteria a process called fermentation takes place in which there is formation of several organic end products such as acids, alcohols and gas. Energy rich phosphate bonds are formed. This is called substrate phosphorylation

Carbon dioxide: All bacteria require the presence of a small amount of carbon dioxide for growth, an amount normally provided by the atmosphere or by reactions within the cell itself. Some bacteria like *Brucella abortus* and *Neisseria gonorrhoeae* require a higher concentration of CO_2 (5–10%) and this must be provided in the environment.

Temperature

For each species of bacteria there is a different and definite temperature range within which growth takes place. The limits are the maximum and the minimum temperature for each bacterium. The optimum temperature is that at which the growth is most rapid, 37°C is the optimum temperature at which most pathogenic bacteria grow. This is the temperature at which we incubate bacteria in an incubator.

Based on the temperature requirements bacteria are divided into three groups.

a. Mesophilic
b. Psychrophilic
c. Thermophilic

Mesophilic: These bacteria grow best at temperatures of 20 to 45°C. Most pathogenic bacteria belong to this group.

Psychrophilic: These bacteria grow best at temperatures less than 20°C. Some can even grow at temperatures less than 7°C. Their importance lies in their ability to cause spoilage of refrigerated and frozen food. They are not pathogenic. They are soil and water bacteria.

Thermophilic: These bacteria grow best at high temperatures between 55 to 80°C. They cause spoilage of underprocessed canned foods. For example, *Bacillus stearothermophilus*. Some can grow at temperatures as high as 250°C.

Heat also Kills Bacteria

- Heat kills microorganisms. As we shall see in later chapters this is widely used in sterilization and disinfection.
- At low temperatures, some species die rapidly but the majority survive well between 3 to 5°C in a domestic type refrigerator or in a deep freeze (-30-70°C) or in liquid nitrogen. Rapid freezing as with solid carbon dioxide or the use of a stabiliser such as glycerol minimises the death of cells on freezing.

H^+ Ion Concentration or pH

- A suitable environmental pH is very important for the growth of bacteria. The majority of commensal and pathogenic bacteria grow best at a neutral or slightly alkaline reaction pH (7.2–7.6).
- Some bacteria flourish in the presence of high degree of acidity. They are called Acidophilic bacteria like *Lactobacillus*. Others are sensitive to acid but tolerant to alkali. *Vibrio cholerae* tolerate great degrees of strong alkali solutions.

Light and Other Radiations

- Darkness is good for bacterial growth
- Bacteria are killed by ionizing radiations and ultraviolet radiations (Direct sunlight or radiation from a mercury vapor lamp).

Moisture and Drying

Water is a very important constituent of the bacterial cell. Therefore drying of the bacterial cell is lethal to bacteria. Some delicate bacteria like *Gonococcus*, *Treponema pallidum* or common cold virus die very rapidly. Others like, *Staphylococcus aureus* and *Mycobacterium tuberculosis* survive for weeks or months. Spores of *B. anthracis* survive for many years.

Freeze Drying or Lyophilization

This is the process in which the bacteria are dried rapidly and completely preferably while frozen and maintained in high vacuum (0.01 mm Hg or less) in a sealed glass ampoule stored at room temperature in the dark. It is in powder form. This is used for preservation of bacterial cultures.

Osmotic Pressure

Bacteria are very tolerant of changes in the osmotic pressure of their environment because of the strength of their cell wall. A concentration of 5 to 12 percent NaCl is tolerated by most bacteria. If a bacterium is suddenly exposed to solutions of higher salt concentration there is shrinkage of the protoplasm and water travels outwards. This happens more readily in gram-negative than in gram-positive bacteria. This is called Plasmolysis.

Sudden transfer of a bacteria from a concentrated to a weak solution or to distilled water may cause Plasmoptysis. This means swelling and bursting of the cell as a result of excessive osmotic taking in of water.

Mechanical and Sonic Stress

- Though the cell walls of bacteria have considerable strength and elasticity it is possible to rupture and kill bacteria by exposure to mechanical stress.
- A bacterial suspension may be disintegrated by vigorous shaking with pure glass beads or by supersonic vibration. (9000–200,000 cycles per second) or (ultrasonic vibration over 200,000 cycles per second). These methods are used to separate the large molecular components of the cell.

CHAPTER

6

Sterilization and Disinfection

LESSON PLAN

SOME DEFINITIONS

Sterilization

It is the process by which an article, surface or medium is made free from all microorganisms either in the vegetative or spore state.

Disinfection

It is the process by which an article, surface or medium is made free from all pathogenic micro-organisms (that is organisms that are capable of giving rise to infections).

Antisepsis

It is the process by which the growth of bacteria is inhibited but they are not killed.

Bactericidal

These are agents or processes by which the bacteria are killed.

Bacteriostatic

These are agents or processes which prevent the multiplication of bacteria.

Some chemicals may be bactericidal or bacteriostatic at different concentration.

USES OF STERILIZATION

Microorganisms are present everywhere. They can cause contamination, infection and decay. It becomes important therefore to destroy them in certain situations.

1. Operation theaters complete asepsis (absence of bacteria) is required to control infection.
2. Wound dressings and nursing. If aseptic conditions are not provided it would lead to wound infection.
3. Collection of samples for culture. Unwanted bacteria are not required as we want to grow the disease causing bacteria. Collection of samples should be under aseptic conditions.
4. Preparation of culture media. If the medium for the growth of bacteria is contaminated with unwanted bacteria we will not be able to grow the desired bacterium.
5. Food and drug manufacture.
6. Vaccine preparation.

In the last two situations contamination with bacteria would prove dangerous.

WHAT NEEDS TO BE STERILIZED?

1. Culture media
2. Fluids to be instulled in the patient
3. Reagents
4. Laboratory containers
5. Surgical instruments
6. Syringes
7. Surgical drapes
8. Catheters and tubings which are single use. These are industrially sterilized.
9. Industrial equipment.

METHODS OF STERILIZATION

The methods of sterilization chosen depend on:
1. Object to be sterilized
2. Number and kind of microorganisms that could be present (Table 6.1).

Table 6.1: Methods of sterilization

Physical	*Chemical*
• *Sunlight*	• Alcohols
• *Drying*	• Aldehydes
• *Dry Heat*	• Dyes
– Hot air oven	• Halogens
– Flaming	• Phenols
– Incineration	• Surfaces active agents
	• Metallic salts
	• Gases
• *Moist Heat*	
– Pasteurization	
– Boiling	
– Steam under normal pressure	
– Steam under high pressure	
• *Filtration*	
– Candles	
– Asbestos pads	
– Membranes	
• *Radiation*	
• *Ultrasonic and sonic vibration*	

PHYSICAL

Sunlight

- Sunlight has a bactericidal effect due to a combination of the effect of ultraviolet rays and heat rays.
- It is the natural method of sterilization in tanks, rivers and lakes.

For example, Typhoid bacteria exposed to the sun were killed in two hours where as controls kept in the dark were still alive after six days.

Drying

Drying can harm the bacteria in principle but it is not a practically used method for sterilization. However, drying can be used for storage of foods where the moisture is reduced to avoid multiplication of bacteria.

Heat

Most of the sterilization in the laboratory is by heat. It is most reliable. We either use dry heat or moist heat.

Dry heat is different from moist heat. The killing effect of dry heat is because of protein denaturation and destructive oxidation of essential cell constituents. The killing effect of moist heat is due to denaturation and coagulation of protein and enzymes.

Why is moist heat more effective?
1. Penetration of moist heat is better.
2. Bacteria are more susceptible to moist heat because coagulation of proteins occurs more readily and requires lower temperatures.

3. Moist heat releases latent heat which is the heat that is taken up by water when it changes into steam.
4. Moist heat increases the water content of a spore and helps in the breakdown.

The time required for sterilization depends on many factors:

1. *Temperature*—Higher the temperature lower the time required
2. *Spores*—Whether spores are present and the type of spores
3. *Organism*—The characteristics of the organisms.

Dry Heat

Flaming

Inoculating loops or wires, points of forceps, spatulas and scalpels are held in a Bunsen flame till they become red hot. Mouths of culture tubes, glass slides and cover slips are passed a few times through the Bunsen flame to sterilize them.

Incineration

Incineration means burning the material to ashes. It is a very good method for rapidly destroying material such as contaminated dressings, bedding and pathological material by burning them. It is widely used for the disposal of biomedical waste which needs destruction.

Hot Air Oven

Introduction: It is the most widely used method of dry heat sterilization.

Temperature and Time—160° × 1 hr

Principle: The principle of hot air oven is based on dry heat sterilization. It is accomplished by conduction where the heat is absorbed by the exterior surface of an item and then passed inward to the next layer. The bacteria are killed by oxidation of cell constituents. The oven is electrically heated and thermostatically controlled.

Structure

- The hot air oven is a metallic box usually white in colour (Fig. 6.1).

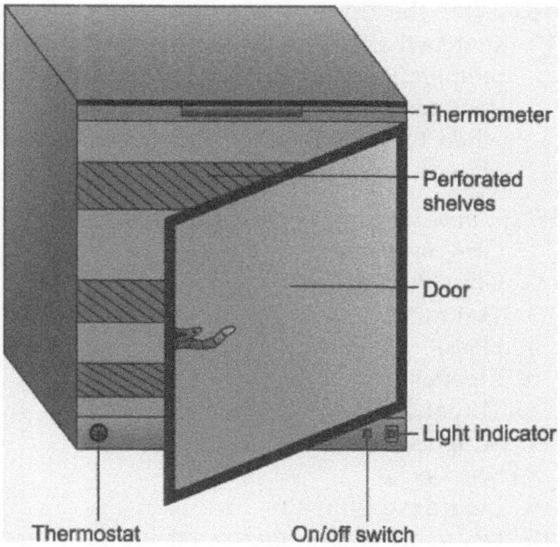

Fig. 6.1: Hot air oven

- The heating element is in the wall of the oven. There is a tight fitting door to allow no air leak.
- At the top front surface of the hot air oven is a thermometer which indicates the temperature inside the oven.
- At the bottom front surface is a thermostat to set the temperature, an indicator light and a switch.
- Inside the oven are two or three perforated shelves. The holes allow free circulation of air.
- There is a fan fitted inside to allow even distribution of hot air.

Working of the Hot Air Oven

1. The glassware is properly packed and arranged on the shelves. The Petri dishes and pipettes are packed in kraft paper. The test tubes and flasks are plugged with cotton wool. The glassware should be completely dry before putting it in the oven.
2. The door is closed and the oven is switched on.
3. The thermostat is set to the required temperature (160°C). The light bulb glows red.
4. When the required temperature is reached, the light bulb switches off and the holding time of one hour starts.

5. After the time of one hour the oven is switched off and allowed to cool. When the temperature reaches room temperature, the door can be opened. If the door is opened when the inside is hot there is danger of glassware cracking.

What can be sterilized in the hot air oven?

1. Glass syringes
2. Glass Petri dishes
3. Test tubes
4. Flasks
5. Pipettes
6. Throat swabs
7. Scalpels
8. Scissors
9. Liquid paraffin
10. Dry materials in sealed containers (powders, fats, oils and greases).

Precautions to be taken while working with the hot air oven:

1. The hot air oven should not be over loaded to allow for good circulation of air.
2. The holding time must be started from the time a temperature of 160°C is reached.
3. Oven must be allowed to cool before the door is opened to avoid cracking of glassware.

Sterilization control of the hot air oven

- The spores of a nontoxigenic strain of *Clostridium tetani* are used. Paper strips impregnated with 10^6 spores are placed in envelopes and inserted into the hot air oven. After sterilization is over, the strips are removed and inoculated into cooked meat media and incubated under anaerobic conditions for 5 days at 37°C. No growth should occur if sterilization is adequate.
- Brownie's tube is available for dry heat sterilization control. After proper sterilization, a green colour is produced after 60 minutes at 160°C.
- Thermocouples may be used.

Moist Heat

As we know, moist heat is quicker than dry heat and has greater penetrative power. Killing by moist heat requires the microorganisms to be in contact with steam. If the articles are sealed in a container, they cannot get moist heat. Moist heat coagulates the proteins in any organism and this is aided by the water vapor that has a very high penetrating property, leading to their death. It also causes oxidative free radical damage.

Moist heat is of three kinds:

a. Temperature below 100°C
b. Temperature at 100°C
c. Temperature greater than 100°C.

Temperature below 100°C

1. Pasteurization of milk: Temperature used is 63°C × 30 minutes (Holder method) or 72°C × (15 to 20 seconds) Flash method. This is followed by cooling quickly to 13°C or lower. There is an ultra high method which uses a temperature of 137.8° for two seconds. This method is used for tetra packs.
2. Vaccines of nonsporing bacteria are heat inactivated in special vaccine baths at 60°C × 1 hour.
3. Clothing, bed clothes, eating utensils and some equipment may be disinfected by washing in water at 70 to 80°C for several minutes.
4. Cystoscopes, specula and apparatus that may be damaged by boiling can be disinfected in a bath at 75°C × 10 minutes.
5. Inspissation is done at 80 to 85°C × 30 minutes to one hour. This is a method of solidifying culture media that are heat sensitive and cannot withstand autoclaving. We inspissate Löwenstein-Jensen medium (*culture medium for Mycobacterium tuberculosis*) to solidify it. A hot air oven fitted with a fan may be used for inspissation.

Temperature at 100°C

1. *Boiling*
   - Vegetative bacteria are killed almost immediately at 90 to 100°C but sporing bacteria require considerable period of boiling.

- Boiling should not be used as a method of sterilization, only as disinfection. Boiling should be done for a period of 10 to 30 minutes.

2. *Steam at atmospheric pressure (100°C)*: An atmosphere of free steam is used to sterilize culture media which may decompose if subjected to higher temperatures. A simple steamer is used for this purpose. Sugars used for biochemical tests are sterilized in this way.

   The steamer is a tinned copper cabinet. There is a perforated tray fitted above the water level. The material placed on the tray gets surrounded by steam. It is also used to melt pre sterilized agar containing media which has solidified.

3. *Tyndallization*: Usually an exposure of 90 minutes is enough for complete sterilization but an exposure of 100°C × 20 minutes on three successive days with incubation in between is used so that the vegetative bacteria are killed and the spores get enough time in between to germinate and then get killed by the next exposure next day. This is known as tyndallisation or intermittent sterilization. It is used for heat sensitive substances.

Temperature Greater than 100°C

Steam under pressure:

- The equipment which uses the principle is called autoclave and the procedure autoclaving.
- Autoclaving is the most reliable method of sterilizing culture media. It can be used for all materials that are water containing, permeable or wettable.

Principle of an Autoclave

Autoclave is a laboratory equipment which provides moist heat at temperatures greater than 100°C. Water boils when its vapor pressure is equal to that of the surrounding atmosphere. Hence when pressure inside a closed vessel increases the temperature at which water boils also increases. A temperature of 121°C at 15 pounds per square inch pressure for 15 minutes is used in the autoclave. Saturated steam has great penetrative power. When the steam comes in contact with a cooler surface it condenses into water and gives up its latent heat to that surface. Latent heat means hidden heat and 1600 mL of steam at 100°C and at atmospheric pressure condenses into 1 mL of water at 100°C and liberates 518 calories of heat.

Structure of an Autoclave

There are many kinds of autoclaves. In its simplest form, the autoclave consists of a vertical or horizontal cylinder of gunmetal or stainless steel. The lid or door is fastened by screw clamps and made airtight by an asbestos washer. On the lid of the autoclave are:

1. A manual discharge tap for the discharge of air and steam.
2. An automatic discharge tap for the steam to escape.
3. A pressure gauge which measures the pressure.
4. A safety valve which opens only under emergency if the pressure rises too much (Fig. 6.2).

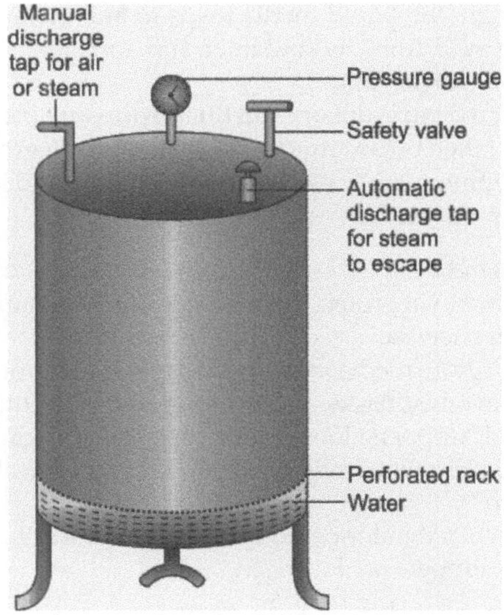

Fig. 6.2: Vertical autoclave

Working of an Autoclave

- Sufficient water is put at the bottom of the autoclave over which is placed a perforated tray. Heating is done by gas or electricity.
- The material to be sterilized is placed on the tray and heating is started. The lid is screwed tight with the discharge tap open.
- The safety valve is set to the required pressure.
- The steam and the air mixture is allowed to escape freely till all the air has been displaced.
- When no more air bubbles come out the discharge tap is closed.
- The steam pressure rises inside and when it reaches the desired set level the automatic steam release opens and steam escapes.

The pressure gauge should read 15 atmospheric pressure. From this time the holding time is calculated. When the holding period is over, the heater is turned off and the autoclave is allowed to cool, till the pressure gauge indicates that the inside is at atmospheric pressure. The dischange tap is opened slowly and air is allowed to enter the autoclave.

When the autoclave is sufficiently cool, the lid is opened and the contents are cooled. The loosely stoppered bottles are tightened.

If the tap is opened when the pressure inside is high, the liquid media tends to boil violently and spill from its container and sometimes an explosion occurs.

If the tap is not opened till the pressure inside has fallen below atmospheric pressure an excessive amount of water will be evaporated and lost from the media.

Preparation of the load: The aim is to allow steam to enter, yet protect the load from contamination with bacteria.

Culture media and liquid reagents are protected in tubes, flasks, and bottles closed with cotton wool, stoppers, loose metal caps or screw caps.

Instruments may be wrapped in permeable cloth.

When the stoppered bottles are to be sterilized the stoppers are loosened.

Sterilization control of autoclave: This is done for determining the efficacy of moist heat sterilization. The spores of *Bacillus stearothermophilus* are used as the test organism. This is a thermophilic organism with an optimum growth temperature of 55 to 60°C and its spores require an exposure of 12 minutes at 121°C to be killed. Paper strips impregnated with 10^6 spores are dried at room temperature and placed in paper envelopes. These envelopes are inserted in different parts of the autoclave and after sterilizing, the strips are inoculated into a suitable culture medium and incubated. Correct autoclaving should kill the spores following which there should be no growth on culture media. Apart from this, there are:

- Chemical indicators
- Autoclave tapes
- Thermocouples.

See Table 6.2 for the time and temperature required for sterilization of autoclave and hot air oven.

Table 6.2: Times and temperatures for heat sterilization (Recommendations of the medical research council)

Method	*Temperature*	*Holding time in minutes*
Autoclave	121	15
	126	10
	134	03
Hot air oven	160	60
	170	18
	180	7.5
	190	1.5

Filtration

- This is the method used for sterilization of heat sensitive liquids such as pharmaceutical ophthalmic solutions, oils, antibiotics, etc.
- Very useful to sterilize antibiotic solutions, sera and carbohydrate solutions which are used in the preparation of culture media.
- Also used to filter microorganisms which are present in very few numbers and can be obtained from the filter disc in a solution.
- We can obtain bacteria free filtrates of toxins and bacteriophages.

- Filters with varying pore size are used such as 0.2 micrometers and 20 nanometers to eliminate bacteria and viruses respectively.
- Four main types of filters are used for bacteriological proposes. The details given below are for optional reading:

Earthenware Filters

Earthenware filters are made in the form of a hollow candle and the fluid is forced from the inside to the outside by suction or pressure.

1. *Berkefeld filters*: These are made from Kieselguhr, a fossilised diatomaceous earth found in Germany. They are available in 3 grades of porosity:
   V (viel) — coarsest
   W (wenig) — finest
   N (normal) — intermediate
   V is the usual one used to clarify liquids but they are not fine enough to sterilize liquids by holding back bacteria. It does not let 0.75 μm diameter (*Serratia marcescens*) pass.
2. *Porcelain filters*: The most common type of porcelain filter is the Chamberland, a French filter made up of kaolin and sand and the English Doulton. The Chamberland filters are made of various porosities and are graded L_1, L_{1a}, L_2, L_3, L_5, L_7, L_9 and L_{11}. Excluding L_1 all are sterilizing. The Doulton filter candle range is P_2 P_5 and P_{11}, the latter two are sterilizing.
   For use the candle is mounted on a silicone rubber bung and filtration is effected from within outward.
3. *Mandler*: American Mandler filters are made from kieselguhr, asbestos and plaster of Paris. These are similar to Berkefeld filters.

Asbestos Filters (Seitz)

This is made from the chrysotile type of asbestos. Chemically it is composed of magnesium silicate. The asbestos discs are available in different grades. The important ones are:

1. HP/PYR — for removal of pyrogens.
2. HP/EKS — for absolute sterility using controlled standard conditions.
3. HP/EK — for clarifying.

After use the disc is discarded.

Sintered Glass Filters

These are made from finely ground glass fused sufficiently to make the particles stick. These may be supplied in the form of a disk fused into a glass funnel. These are available in different pore sizes as per British standards specification. After use they are washed with running water in the reverse direction and cleaned with warm strong sulphuric acid.

Membrane Filters (Millipore)

- These membranes are manufactured from a variety of polymeric materials such as cellulose nitrate, cellulose diacetate, polycarbonate and polyester. Being less absorptive than others, they have a faster rate of filtration for any given porosity. They are manufactured as disks of 13 to 293 mm in diameter and porosities from 0.015 to 12 μm.
- *Two types are available*: The older type, gradocol membranes (graded collodion membrane) are composed of cellulose nitrate whereas the modern membrane filters consist of cellulose acetate.
- These filters are sterilized by autoclaving.

HEPA Filters

HEPA filters are High-efficiency particulate air filters. HEPA is a screen that filters out particles in the air by forcing them through microscopic pores.

They remove at least 99.97% of airborne particles of 0.3 μm or less in diameter. HEPA filters are composed of a mat of randomly arranged fibers. The fibers are typically composed of fiberglass and possess diameters between 0.5 and 2.0 μm. Key functional components are fiber diameter, filter thickness and face velocity. They are designed to target much smaller pollutants and particles. These particles are trapped through a combination of the following three mechanisms:

1. Interception, where particles following a line of flow in the air stream come within one radius of a fiber and adhere to it.

2. Impaction, where larger particles are unable to avoid fibers due to curving contours of air stream and are forced to get trapped there.
3. Diffusion, an enhancing mechanism is a result of the collision with gas molecules by the smallest particles, especially those below 0.1 µm in diameter, which are stopped by the barriers of fibers and thereby do not follow a continuous path.

Uses of HEPA Filters

1. Used in prevention of the spread of airborne bacterial and viral organisms and therefore infections. They are extensively used in the operation theaters.
2. Used in vacuum cleaners and air purifiers.
3. They can help limit the amount of dust, mites, pollen, spores, and other allergens in the environment, making them useful in achieving greater asthma control.

Radiation

Two types of radiation are used for sterilization purposes:

a. Nonionizing
b. Ionizing

Nonionizing — Infra-red
Ultraviolet

Ionizing — Gamma rays, X-rays, cosmic rays
High energy electrons.

Nonionizing Radiation

Infrared radiation is used for mass sterilization of syringes. Ultraviolet radiation is used for disinfecting enclosed areas such as entryways, hospital wards, operation rooms, virus inoculation rooms and virus laboratories. This is called hot sterilization.

Ionizing Radiation

X-rays, cosmic rays and high energy electrons are highly lethal to DNA and other vital constituents. They have high penetrative power. This is called cold sterilization.

Large commercial plants use Gamma radiation for sterilizing most plastics, syringes, swabs, culture plates, catheters, various types of rubber, oils, greases and cardboards.

Ultrasonic and Sonic Vibration

This method is not in use.

CHEMICAL AGENTS

These are antiseptics and disinfectants.

Alcohols

- Three kinds of alcohol are used
  — *Ethyl alcohol* (ethanol)
  — *Isopropyl alcohol*
  — *Methyl alcohol*
- They are *skin antiseptics.*
- They *denature bacterial proteins.*
- There have *no action on spores or viruses.*
- *Cone of 60 to 70 percent in water is used.*
- Isopropyl alcohol is better than ethyl alcohol and is used for disinfection of clinical thermometers.
- They are widely used as hand hygiene agents (hand gels and hand rubs)
- Methyl alcohol is used against fungal spores and for cleaning cabinets. But it is toxic and inflammable.
- They should not be applied to wounds because they can cause tissue damage.

Aldehydes

Formaldehyde

It is:

- Bactericidal, sporicidal, virucidal
- It is used for preservation of anatomical specimens
- 10 percent formalin containing 0.5 percent sodium tetraborate is used to sterilize clean metal instruments.
- Formaldehyde gas is used for sterilising instruments and heat sensitive catheters used for fumigation.
- Toxic and irritant to eyes and skin and when inhaled.

Glutaraldehyde: It is especially active against tubercle bacilli, fungi and viruses:

- It is less toxic and irritant to the eyes and skin than formaldehyde.
- Used to treat cytoscopes and bronchoscopes, rubber anaesthetic tubes, face masks, plastic endotracheal tubes, metal instruments and polythene tubing.

Dyes

- Aniline dyes
- Acridine dyes
- Used as skin and wound antiseptics
- Bacteriostatic but low bactericidal activity.

Aniline dyes
Example

- Brilliant green, Malachite green
- Crystal violet
- The aniline dyes are more active against gram-positive than gram-negative organisms.
- They have no activity against tubercle bacilli and hence the use of Malachite green in Löwenstein-Jensen medium.
- They are used as selective agents in culture medium.
- They are inhibited by pus and hence not much role in skin infections.

Acridine dyes

- Proflavine, Acriflavine, Euflavine, Aminacrine
- They are not that inhibited by pus.
- They can be used in clinical medicine.

Halogens

Iodine

- Skin disinfectant
- Active bactericidal agent
- Moderate activity against spores
- Active against tubercle bacillus and a number of viruses.
- For example, betadine, isodine, tincture of iodine, etc.

Chlorine

- Bactericidal
- Virucidal
- Organic chloramines are used as antiseptics for dressing wounds
- Chlorine and its products are widely used for disinfection purposes.

Phenols

- Lister, the father of antiseptic surgery introduced their use in surgery.
- Lysol and cresol are powerful microbicidal agents
- Not inactivated by organic substances and are good general disinfectants.
- Chlorophenols and chloroxyphenols are less toxic and irritant than phenols but also less active and more readily inactivated by organic matter.
- All phenols are relatively inactive against *Pseudomonas*.
- Phenols are toxic to man.
- Hexachlorophene, a widely used phenolic preparation is effective against gram-positive organisms but less so against gram-negative organisms.
- Chlorhexidine (Hibitane) is a relatively non-toxic skin antiseptic, most active against Gram-positive organisms and fairly effective against gram-negative ones. It is used to treat wounds.

Gases

Ethylene oxide

- It is a sweet smelling penetrating gas.
- It has a boiling point of 10.7°C.
- It is highly inflammable and explosive. It is therefore mixed with less inert gases like CO_2 and N_2 in such a way that final concentration is 10 percent.
- It is virucidal and sporicidal.
- It penetrates plastics.
- It is specially used for sterilising heart lung machines, respirators, sutures, dental equipment, books, clothing, glass and metal surfaces, etc. in the ETO machines.
- It is unsuitable for fumigation because of its explosive property.
- It is carcinogenic.

Beta propiolactone

- It is more efficient for fumigation purposes than formaldehyde because it is less toxic.
- It is carcinogenic.

Surface Active Agents

- These agents reduce surface tension.
- They are used as wetting agents, detergents and emulsifiers.
- There are four groups of surface active agents.
  Anionic Cationic
  Nonionic Amphoteric

Cationic

- These are the most important.
- They are quartenary ammonium compounds.
- They are bactericidal.
- They are more active against gram-positive bacteria.
- There is no action on spores, tubercle bacilli and most viruses.
- Examples are—Cetavlon or cetrimide (cetyl trimethyl ammonium bromide).
- Benzalkonium chloride.

They are active at alkaline pH. Acid and inorganic matter inactivates them.

Anionic

These are the common soaps:

- Soaps prepared from saturated fatty acids (e.g. coconut oil) are more effective against gram-negative bacilli.
- Those that are prepared from unsaturated fatty acids work against gram-positive bacteria.

Metallic Salts

- Salts of copper, mercury, silver, etc. are used as disinfectants.
- They are weak bactericidal and weak fungicidal agents.
- Copper salts act as fungicides.

Testing of Disinfectants

Rideal-Walker test: Similar quantities of organisms are submitted to the action of varying concentrations of phenol and of the germicide to be tested.

The dilution of disinfectant X which sterilizes the suspension in a given time divided by the dilution of phenol which would do the same thing gives us the phenol coefficient.

Chick-Martin test: Here the disinfectant does not act in pure solution. The disinfectant is tested in water containing a suspension of 3 percent dried human feces.

Table 6.3 shows the important properties of chemical disinfectants.

Disinfection of Skin

- Soap and water removes the transient surface contaminants.
- Chlorhexidine and an iodine detergent scrub is used to remove pathogens.
- Phisohex (0.5% chlorhexidine and 1% glycerol in 70% isopropyl alcohol) is an important skin disinfectant.

Table 6.3: Showing important properties of chemical disinfectants

Carcinogenic	Ethylene oxide, Betapropiolactone (BPL)
Skin Antiseptics	Ethyl alcohol Aniline and acridine dyes Iodine in aqueous and alcoholic solution Organic chloramines Chlorophenols and chloroxyphenols
Bactericidal	Isopropyl alcohol Formaldehyde Iodine Chlorine Phenol Ethylene oxide BPL
Impairing DNA Complexes	Acridine dyes Ethylene oxide
Virucidal	Formaldehyde Glutaraldehyde Iodine Chlorine Ethylene oxide BPL Cationic quartenary ammonium compounds
Sporicidal	Formaldehyde, ethylene oxide
Fungicidal	Methyl alcohol, glutaraldehyde, mercury salts, copper

Table 6.4: Best method of sterilization

LJ medium *Loeffler's* medium	Solidified by Inspissation
Other culture media	Autoclave
Glassware	Hot air oven
Antibiotics, sera	Filtration
Throat swabs	Hot air oven
Rubber catheters	Irradiation, UV-rays
Endoscopes	Chemicals
Linen	Autoclaves
Not subjected to heat	Urea, protein, sugar

- If skin is broken, chlorhexidine + cetrimide is used for disinfection.
- If skin is contaminated phenolic or hypochlorite disinfectant, e.g. 2 percent Hycolin is used.

See Table 6.4 for the best method of sterilization, employed for different objects.

Blood is not sterilized

CHAPTER

7

Cultivation of Microorganisms-I: Culture Medium

LESSON PLAN

- Definition of Culture Medium
- Use of Culture Medium
- What are the Characteristics of an Ideal Culture Medium?
- Basic Requirements of Culture Media
- Some Common Constituents of Culture Media
  - Agar-agar
  - Peptone
- Dehydrated Culture Medium
- Classification of Culture Media
  - Based on Microorganism Involved
  - Based on Physical State of the Culture Medium
  - Based on Composition
  - Based on the Characteristics of the Medium
- Other Media
  - Media for Biochemical Tests
  - Media for Anaerobic Organisms
  - Media for Blood Culture
  - Media for Antibiotic Sensitivity Tests

DEFINITION OF CULTURE MEDIUM

The food material or substances required for growing microorganisms in vitro (outside the body) is called culture medium.

USE OF CULTURE MEDIUM

It is important to grow microorganisms outside the body for the following purposes:

1. To identify the cause of infection from the clinical sample, so that proper treatment can be given.
2. To study the characteristics or properties of microorganisms.
3. To prepare biological products like vaccines, toxoids, antigens, etc.
4. For antibiotic assays.
5. For research in the field of molecular biology and biotechnology.
6. For bacteriophage (viruses that infect bacteria) typing of bacteria.

WHAT ARE THE CHARACTERISTICS OF AN IDEAL CULTURE MEDIUM?

To get a good growth of the bacteria, outside the body, the culture medium should be similar in composition to the tissues and body fluids in which bacteria grow. It should have the following features:

1. Growth should be satisfactory even with a small inoculum (the material that is introduced on the culture plate for growth).
2. It should be easy to prepare.
3. There should be rapid growth.

4. It should be cheap and nontoxic.
5. It should be able to bring out the growth characteristics of the bacteria.

No single medium is perfect or can satisfy all requirements. There are many culture media and we have to choose between them.

BASIC REQUIREMENTS OF CULTURE MEDIA

- *Energy source*: Energy is obtained by the bacteria by oxidation and decomposition of proteins and carbohydrates.
- *Carbon source*: This is usually carbohydrate.
- *Nitrogen source*: The nitrogen source is usually peptone.
- *Special growth factors*: These are sometimes required for growth of some bacteria example, vitamin B_{12}, Riboflavin, etc.
- *Mineral salts*: Sulphates, phosphates, chlorides, carbonates, sodium, potassium, magnesium and calcium are added for the growth of some microorganisms.

SOME COMMON CONSTITUENTS OF CULTURE MEDIA

- Agar-agar
- Peptone.

Agar

Introduction

Agar-agar is a golden yellow granular powder that is used for solidification of culture media. It is prepared from sea weeds—*Gelidium, Eucheuma* and *Pterocladia*. It is extracted from the dried weeds by a hot water process. The product is clarified, dried and finally supplied as a powder.

Chemical Structure

The chief component of agar is a long-chain polysaccharide composed mainly of d-galactopyranose units. It also contains a variety of impurities including organic salts or long-chain fatty acids. The minerals present are Mg^{+2} and Ca^{+2}. Agar is thought to exist as magnesium or calcium sulphate esters of the polysaccharide.

Properties of Agar

- Agar melts at 95°C into a liquid form and sets at 42°C. For preparing culture media, the required amount of agar powder is added and dissolved by placing the mixture in a steamer at 100° × 1 hour. The usual concentration of agar is 2 percent. If it is used in the concentration of 0.25 to 0.5 percent, semisolid or sloppy agar is obtained.
- It is bacteriologically inert. It does not add to or subtract from the nutritive value of the medium, neither is it decomposed by bacterial growth.
- It is nontoxic
- It is cheap
- It is the most commonly used substance for solidifying culture media.

Peptone

Peptones are the breakdown products of proteins. Important constituents of peptone are peptones, proteoses, amino acids, inorganic salts like phosphates of potassium and magnesium and certain accessory growth factors like nicotinic acid and riboflavin.

- Peptone consists of water soluble products obtained from lean meat or other protein material such as heart muscle, casein, fibrin or soya flour by digestion with mainly proteolytic enzymes (pepsin, trypsin or papain).
- Peptone is supplied as a golden granular powder with a low moisture content.

DEHYDRATED CULTURE MEDIUM

Dehydrated culture medium is a composite medium in powder form containing each of the constituents in the correct proportion. The water has been extracted from it and it is, therefore, called dehydrated. Dehydrated culture medium is packed in boxed with an airtight lid to prevent it from getting bad during storage. The required amount of powder is weighed and mixed in distilled water by heating or boiling. It is then autoclaved and is ready to be used. It is very easy to make and convenient to use as opposed to the earlier days when the constituents had to be added separately and boiled.

CLASSIFICATION OF CULTURE MEDIA

There are many ways in which culture media can be classified:

Based on the Microorganism Involved

Based on the type of microorganism which is to be cultured, culture media can be classified as:

- Bacterial culture medium
- Fungal culture medium
- Protozoal culture medium
- Viral culture medium.

In this chapter we shall focus on bacterial culture mediums. In the laboratory, bacteria are the easiest to grow.

Based on Physical State of the Culture Medium

Based on the state of the medium, a medium can be solid, liquid or semisolid. Solid medium has an agar concentration of 2 percent. Semisolid medium results when the agar used is about 0.25 to 0.5 percent.

Examples of solid culture mediums are:

- Nutrient agar
- Blood agar
- MacConkey's agar

Examples of liquid culture mediums are:

- Peptone water
- Nutrient broth

Examples of sloppy agar is the medium used in Craige's tube. The comparative assessment of liquid and solid media is given in the Table 7.1.

Table 7.1: Comparison of solid and liquid culture mediums

Liquid culture media	*Solid culture media*
• The growth is very quick (6 to 8 hours)	The growth is slower (18 to 20 hours)
• Is used for antibiotic sensitivity tests for preparing bacterial inoculum	Is not commonly used
• Is used for studying biochemical reactions	Cannot be used for studying biochemical reactions
• Cannot identify the bacteria as there is uniform turbidity	Bacteria form solid colonies which helps in identification of bacteria
• Cannot isolate more than one bacteria	Can isolate more than one bacteria
• Used for studying motility of bacteria	Cannot be used for studying motility of bacteria

Based on Composition

Defined Synthetic Media

These are media in which the exact chemical composition of the constituents is known. These media are used for research purposes.

Semidefined

In these media the exact chemical composition of the constituents is not known because substances like meat and peptone are used. Most of the culture media used for routine diagnostic work is semidefined culture medium.

Based on the Characteristics of the Medium

Simple Media/Basal Media

Definition: Simple or basal media are culture media which contain the minimum adequate nutrition for nonfastidious organisms. Nonfastidious means bacteria which are not that fussy about their nutritional requirement. They require the basic nutrition provided to them by a simple or basal media.

Examples of simple or basal media are:

1. Peptone water Liquid
2. Nutrient broth Liquid
3. Nutrient agar Solid

Peptone water: Peptone water is a liquid medium. It is widely used to obtain a good growth of bacteria, for antibiotic sensitivity tests or biochemical reactions. Its constituents are sodium chloride and water. It is colorless or very light yellow in color. It is available in powder form which can be dissolved in water to form peptone water.

Nutrient broth: Nutrient broth is a simple or basal liquid medium which has meat, peptone, sodium chloride and water. It is very light yellow in color.

Nutrient agar: Agar is added to nutrient broth to make it solid, which is called nutrient agar. It is very light yellow in color.

Enriched Culture Medium

Definition: Enriched culture medium as the name suggests is a culture medium which is richer or has certain substances to increase the nutritive value of the medium for the growth of fastidious bacteria.

Examples: Blood Agar
Loeffler's serum slope
Chocolate agar
Löwenstein-Jensen medium

Blood agar: Blood agar is an enriched culture medium. Blood agar is formed when blood is added to nutrient agar. Sheep or horse blood is used. The concentration of blood used is 5 to 50 percent. Normally, a concentration of 5 to 10 percent is used, which means 10 mL or 5 mL of blood is added to nutrient agar (90 to 95 mL) to make it to a total of 100 mL. It is red in color.

It is widely used for the growth of fastidious bacteria.

Preparation of blood agar: Blood is collected from the sheep or horse veins with the help of a sterile needle attached to a sterile blood bag. This bag can hold about 500 mL to 1 liter of blood and can be stored in a refrigerator. Nutrient agar is prepared and autoclaved. To prepare blood agar (10%) 10 mL of blood is mixed with 90 mL of melted nutrient agar. The temperature of the nutrient agar should be about 50 to 60°C and the sterile blood should be at room temperature. The two are mixed and plates poured. If blood is added to very hot nutrient agar, the blood cells rupture and if the temperature of nutrient agar falls to very low, it solidifies before the blood can be mixed into it.

Loeffler's serum slope: This medium is used for the rapid growth of *C. diphtheriae*.

It has:
- Serum of ox, sheep or horse
- Nutrient broth
- Glucose
- 2.5 mL of it is poured into 6 mL screw capped bottles as slopes and inspissated
- It is creamish yellow in color.

Chocolate agar: If blood collected with sterile precautions is added to sterile nutrient agar at a higher temperature (> 50 to 60°C) then the blood cells rupture, the constituents are released and the color change into brown or chocolate. This agar is called chocolate agar.

Preparation of chocolate agar: There are two methods of preparation of chocolate agar:

1. Allow the melted, sterile nutrient agar to remain at 75°C and add blood. A water bath can be used to maintain temperature at 75°C. The blood and agar is mixed gently until the medium becomes chocolate brown in color.
2. Heating of already poured and set plates of ordinary blood agar in an incubator or hot air oven at 55°C for 1 to 2 hours.
   - Chocolate agar is more enriched than blood agar and it is used for the growth of *Neisseria meningitidis, Neisseria gonorrhoeae* and *Pneumococcus*.

LJ medium (Löwenstein-Jensen medium): LJ medium is an enriched medium used for the growth of *Mycobacterium tuberculosis*. A good pneumonic to remember the constituents of this culture medium is GAMES:
- Constituents of LJ medium
- G stands for glycerol
- Asparagine
- Malachite green
- Egg
- Salt solution

We will study about this medium in detail later. Each constituent of the medium is sterilized separately. The eggs are washed with soap and water, dried and cracked with a sterile knife into a sterile bowl and beat using a sterile beater. The medium is poured in 5 mL amounts into 28 mL

McCartney bottles (screw capped universal containers) and inspissated at 80°C for 1 hour to coagulate and solidify the medium. As the medium has been prepared with sterile precautions, this final heating is to solidify, not to sterilize it. It is bluish green in color.

Selective Medium

Definition: Selective medium is a medium in which certain substances are present which inhibit or poison all other bacteria except the desired bacteria. In other words it is selective for the growth of the desired bacterium. It encourages the growth of a particular species from a mixed inoculum. Selective medium are solid media and are used especially to find out the pathogenic bacteria from a clinical sample of mixed bacterial flora like stool.

Examples of selective media are:

Hoyle's Potassium-tellurite blood agar: This medium is a selective medium for *Corynebacterium diphtheriae*.

Complete medium is as follows:
- Agar base = 200 mL
- Blood = 10 mL
- Tellurite solution = 2 mL

When we add 0.03 to 0.04 percent potassium tellurite, it makes the medium selective for *Corynebacterium* by inhibiting most other pathogenic and commensal bacteria. It also gives a black color to the colonies of *C. diphtheriae*.

The color of the medium is red.

DCA (deoxycholate citrate agar): This is the selective medium for the isolation of *Shigella dysenteriae*, food poisoning salmonellae, *S. paratyphi B*, and *S. typhi*.

It is composed of:
1. Neutral red lactose agar—100 mL
2. Solution A—5 mL
3. Solution B—5 mL

Neutral red lactose agar:
- Meat extract
- Peptone
- Agar
- Neutral red (2% in 50% ethanol)
- Lactose
- Water.

Solution A:
- Sodium citrate
- Sodium thiosulphate
- Ferric ammonium citrate
- Sterile water.

Solution B:
- Sodium deoxycholate
- Sterile water

Basically this medium is the same as MacConkey's agar but it has deoxycholate in it. The color of the medium is pink. It is selective for intestinal pathogens from feces and inhibits the lactose fermenting coliform bacilli *Escherichia coli* and *Klebsiella species*. The colonies of salmonellae and shigellae appear as pale or colorless and can be differentiated from the pink colonies of *Escherichia coli* and *Klebsiella* which are smaller and lesser as they are inhibited.

Wilson and Blair BBSA: Brilliant green bismuth sulphite agar. This is a selective medium for the growth of *Salmonella typhi* and *Salmonella paratyphi B*. These two bacteria reduce sulphite to sulphide and form black colonies. Brilliant green inhibits *Escherichia coli*.

Enrichment Media

Definition: Enrichment media is the same as selective media but it is liquid. This favors the multiplication of a particular species either by selectively favoring it by providing enrichments or has inhibitory substances that suppress competitors. It improves the growth of the wanted bacteria sending it into log phase and suppresses that of unwanted bacteria by keeping them in the lag phase. Therefore, it results in an absolute increase in the number of wanted bacteria relative to other bacteria.

Examples:

Selenite F broth: The selenite in this medium inhibits the coliform bacteria while permitting salmonellae and many shigellae to grow.

Constituents of the medium:

- Sodium hydrogen selenite
- Peptone
- Lactose
- Disodium hydrogen phosphate
- Sodium dihydrogen phosphate
- Sterile water

Dissolve the ingredients in right proportion with sterile precautions and distribute the yellowish solution in 10 ml amounts into large test tubes or universal containers and steam for 20 minutes at 100°C.

Tetrathionate broth: It is selective for salmonella including *S. typhi* and sometimes shigella. It inhibits coliform bacteria.

Constituents:

- Calcium carbonate
- Nutrient broth
- Thiosulphate solution
- Iodine solution
- Phenol red.

This solution is reddish in color. After autoclaving, 10 mL amount is distributed in test tubes and stored for a maximum period of 1 week.

Indicator Medium

Definition: Indicator medium is a medium which has some substances that are changed visibly as a result of metabolic activities of particular organisms. Mostly they have indicator dyes which change their color by the change in pH caused by the growth and metabolic activity of the bacteria.

Examples:
- MacConkey's medium
- Wilson and blair bismuth sulphite medium

MacConkey's medium: This is a very useful medium as we shall study later to grow Enterobacteria. Constituents of MacConkey's medium can be remembered as *PLANT*.

- Peptone
- Lactose
- Agar
- Neutral red
- Taurocholate (Sodium taurocholate). This medium is pale pink in color.

Neutral red is an indicator dye which is pink in acidic pH and colorless in neutral pH. Certain bacteria breakdown lactose and produce acid. These bacteria are called lactose fermenting bacteria (LF). In acidic pH, the color of the colonies changes to pink. Those bacteria which do not breakdown lactose are called nonlactose fermenting bacteria (NLF), they appear colorless. Since, this medium indicates the growth of LF and NLF, MacConkey is called an indicator medium.

It also has taurocholate in it which inhibits the growth of other gram-positive bacteria. So it is mildly selective also.

Lactose fermenting bacteria are:

1. *Escherichia coli*
2. *Klebsiella* species

Nonlactose fermenting bacteria are:

1. *Salmonella* species
2. *Shigella* species

Wilson and Blair medium: As explained previously this medium indicates the growth of *Salmonella typhi* by the presence of black colonies.

Transport Medium

Definition: This medium is used to transport samples from one place to another especially in case of bacteria which die on prolonged exposure to the outside.

Characteristics of the transport medium:

1. It should be nontoxic.
2. It should not promote or inhibit the bacterial growth.
3. It should be easy to carry and transport.

Examples:

Stuart's transport medium: This is non-nutrient soft agar gel which contains a reducing substance to prevent oxidation and charcoal to neutralize bacterial inhibitors for gonococci. We use charcoal impregnated swabs for collection of sample.

Constituents:

- Sodium thioglycollate
- Sodium glycerophosphate

- Calcium chloride ($CaCl_2$)
- Agar
- Methylene blue
- Distilled water.

Amies transport medium: As patients dislike the use of swabs impregnated with charcoal in Stuart's transport medium, Amies transport medium incorporates the charcoal into the medium. Also used for gonococcus.

Constituents are:
- Sodium thioglycollate
- Sodium chloride
- Potassium chloride
- Calcium chloride
- Magnesium chloride
- Sodium hydrogen phosphate
- Potassium dihydrogen phosphate
- Charcoal (finely powdered)
- Agar
- Distilled water.

Pike's transport medium: This medium is used to preserve *Streptococcus pyogenes, Pneumococci and Haemophilus influenzae* in nose and throat swabs. It is blood agar containing crystal violet 1 in 1000000 and sodium azide 1 in 16000 distributed as stab cultures in tubes and bottles.

Buffered slycerol saline: If there is a delay of some hours, before the specimen of faces reaches the laboratory, this transport medium prevents other intestinal organisms from overgrowing the typhoid bacilli.

Constituents:
- Glycerol
- Sodium chloride
- Disodium hydrogen phosphate
- Phenol red
- Water.

PS—There is no need to memorize the names of the constituents of the mediums and their quantities. They have been given for better understanding.

Differential Culture Media

Definition: This is a medium which has substances incorporated in it which bring out different characteristics of the bacteria and differentiate between them.

Examples—MacConkey's medium:
MacConkey's medium differentiates between lactose fermenting and nonlactose fermenting bacteria.

Blood agar differentiates between hemolytic and nonhemolytic bacteria.

OTHER MEDIA

Media for Biochemical Tests

Special media are prepared for carrying out biochemical tests. For sugar reactions 1 percent sugar (glucose, lactose, sucrose or mannitol) is added to peptone water. Andrade's indicator is used in which acidic pH turns pink. Normally the biochemical tests carried out are:

Glucose	TSI
Lactose	Indole
Sucrose	
Mannitol	
Urease	
Citrate	

We shall study biochemical reactions in detail in the Chapter 10.

Media for Anaerobic Organisms

Anaerobic organisms as we shall later study do not tolerate oxygen at all. They require an atmosphere of no oxygen. Special media are required for their growth.

Cooked Meat Broth

This is the modified version of the original Robertson cooked meat medium. It has meat particles at the bottom to a depth of 2.5 cm and is covered with 15 mL of nutrient broth. The inoculum is introduced deep into the meat particles and they provide the anaerobic environment.

Thioglycollate Broth

In addition to a reducing agent and semisolid agar this medium contains methylene blue or resazurin.

Brain Heart Infusion Broth with Cooked Meat Particles

This medium allows the growth of nutritionally exacting aerobic and/or anaerobic bacteria. It is distributed into bottles containing meat particles prepared from fresh meat. The bottle contains a 2.5 cm layer of cooked meat particles overlaid with 70 mL BHI (brain heart infusion broth).

Media for Blood Culture

Special media are used for blood culture. The most commonly used culture media are:

1. Glucose broth—20 percent solution of glucose is added to nutrient broth.
2. Taurocholate broth

Others are:

1. Brain heart infusion broth
2. Cooked meat broth
3. Thioglycollate broth
4. Diphasic broth (Castaneda system)

Special media are used for examination of milk, water, etc. and for diagnosis of specific microorganisms.

Media for Antibiotic Sensitivity Tests

We use nutrient agar as well as Mueller Hinton agar for performing antibiotic sensitivity tests.

Mueller Hinton Agar

This medium was originally formulated for the isolation of pathogenic *Neisseria* species but now it is used for antibiotic sensitivity tests.

Constituents:

- Casein hydrolysate
- Agar
- Beef infusion
- Starch
- Distilled water

The medium is autoclaved and poured into plates. It is the same color as nutrient agar (very light yellow).

CHAPTER

8

Cultivation of Microorganisms-II: Inoculation Techniques

LESSON PLAN

- Introduction
- Culture Containers
  - Conical Flask
  - Round Bottomed Flasks
  - Test Tubes
  - Screw Capped Bottles
  - Petri Dishes
- pH Adjustment of Culture Media
- Distribution of Unsterilized Culture Media
- Sterilization of Prepared Media
- Distribution of Sterilized Media with Sterile Precautions
  - Liquid Media
  - Solid Media
  - Pouring Plates
  - Inspissation of the Serum and Egg Media
- Instruments Used for Culture
  - Inoculating Wires
  - Wire Loop
  - Scalpel
  - Sterile Pipettes
- Culture Procedures
  - Solid Media
  - Liquid Media
- Anaerobic Culture Methods
  - Cultivation in Vacuum
  - Displacement of Oxygen with Gases
  - Chemical or Biological Method
  - Reduction of O_2 in the Medium
- Methods of Isolating Pure Culture

INTRODUCTION

As we know it is important to grow the suspected bacteria in a sample on an artificial culture medium to diagnose it. In this process there are three main steps:

1. *Preparation*: The preparation of a suitable culture medium.
2. *Sterilization*: The removal of contaminating microorganisms from the culture medium and its containers so that the pathogenic bacteria can grow. This is known as sterilization.
3. *Inoculation*: The inoculation techniques by which we transfer the sample to the culture media for its growth.

In the last chapter we have learnt the types of culture medium and their preparation. We have also learnt sterilization procedures. This chapter deals with culture containers, dispensing and storage of culture media, inoculation techniques and special culture methods like anaerobic cultures.

CULTURE CONTAINERS

The following culture containers are used for preparation of culture media:

- Conical flasks
- Round bottomed flasks
- Beakers

The following culture containers are used for dispensing culture media:

1. Conical flasks
2. Test tubes
3. Screw capped bottles
4. Petri dishes

Conical Flask

Conical flasks of different capacities are used and stoppered with cotton wool. They are multipurpose because they can be used for preparation, sterilization and storage of culture media.

Round Bottomed Flasks

Large round bottomed flasks are used for preparation of culture medium.

Test Tubes

Test tubes of various sizes are used for dispensing media used in biochemical reactions. These can be liquid media such as peptone water and glucose broth stored in test tubes or solid agar slants such as urease, citrate, TSI or nutrient agar.

Screw Capped Bottles

The screw capped bottles normally used are:

- 6 mL capacity Bijou bottles used for dispensing Loeffler's serum slope
- 28 mL capacity universal containers (McCartney bottles) which are used to dispense LJ medium or blood culture
- 120 mL capacity flat bottles used for blood culture.

Screw capped bottles are made up of clear white flint glass. The caps are made of aluminum and each has a rubber washer 3 mm thick made of special rubber that is not inhibitory to bacterial growth. Screw capped bottles are air tight and do not allow their contents to dry out during storage. Media dispensed in screw capped bottles is used for inoculation.

Petri Dishes

Petri dishes are shallow flat bottomed circular glass or plastic containers with lids; they are normally 90 mm in diameter but smaller and larger dishes are available for special purposes. They provide a large surface area for the culture of bacteria or fungi. Approximately 20 to 22 mL of media is poured into plates for culture.

pH ADJUSTMENT OF CULTURE MEDIA

The pH of a culture medium should always be checked and adjusted. During autoclaving the pH falls by 1 unit. Also if the pH has been checked if the medium is hot, it will rise when temperature comes down. For these reasons we should check pH of the medium before autoclaving and keep it 1 unit higher. Checking the pH after autoclaving can also lead to contamination.

DISTRIBUTION OF UNSTERILIZED CULTURE MEDIA

Initially media are tubed, bottled or distributed in conical flasks without sterile precautions. Clean but unsterile glassware is used and the medium and the container are together sterilized by autoclaving. Liquid media may be distributed in test tubes or bottles. Generally, a test tube is only half full. Screw capped bottles can be filled upto 80 percent of their capacity. Solid media are generally initially prepared in liquid form by dissolving the agar powder. Distribution of the molten medium may be done at this stage as for liquid medium without careful sterile precautions, because after this the media is sterilized by autoclaving.

STERILIZATION OF PREPARED MEDIA

- If autoclaving will not damage the culture medium, it is the best method of sterilization
- The sterilization time required in the autoclave depends on the volume of the medium and also the type of container. For test tubes containing 10 mL of medium, a sterilization time of 15 minutes at 121°C is required and for McCartney bottles containing 10 mL of medium a time of 20 minutes at 121°C is required. The sterilization times are mentioned in Table 8.1:

Table 8.1: Sterilization time required in the autoclave at a temperature of 121°C

Volume of the medium	*Flask*	*Bottle*
10 mL	15 min	20 min
100 mL	20 min	25 min
500 mL	25 min	30 min
1 liter	30 min	40 min

Tubes and bottles must be kept in wire crates inside the autoclave so that steam has free access to them. Care must be taken that bottles of medium are not packed tightly otherwise they may break.

If any of the ingredients of the medium are liable to be spoiled by autoclaving, the complete medium should not be sterilized by heat. In such cases we autoclave the reagents which are stable to heat and add the heat sensitive ingredients with sterile precautions later. Some heat sensitive ingredients such as blood, serum or egg yolk can be obtained sterile. Others are filtered through a bacterial filter.

Sometimes lower temperatures such as 115°C for 10 to 20 minutes are recommended for sterilization of media containing ingredients that are not very stable to heat, e.g. sugar containing media.

DISTRIBUTION OF STERILIZED MEDIA WITH STERILE PRECAUTIONS

Liquid Media

As we have seen if the liquid media is heat stable, then it is distributed in unsterile but clean test tubes or bottles and sterilized along with the container. If the liquid medium is heat labile then it is presterilized by other methods and distributed into suitable sterile containers with sterile precautions.

Solid Media

Solid media may be distributed in test tubes bottles, or plates. This may be done for immediate use or storage. The most common shape of the media is the slope or slant which provides a large surface area for inoculation. For 150 mm × 16 mm test tubes 5 mL of medium is sufficient and it is allowed to set at such an angle that there is a thick butt at the bottom (Fig. 8.1).

After cooling, fresh agar slopes contain water of condensation at the foot of the tube, this should not be allowed to run over the surface of the medium or wet the plug/cap.

If the medium is to be used for a stab or shake culture, the test tube is half filled with the medium which is allowed to solidify in the upright position.

Screw capped bottles can be used. The amount of medium for slopes in Bijou bottles of 6 mL capacity is 2.5 mL. The medium must be allowed to set at an angle to form a butt as in test tubes.

Pouring Plates

- Solid media in Petri dishes are often called plates. For a dish of 90 mm diameter, 20 to 22 ml of medium is usually sufficient.
- Plates are always poured with sterile precautions. Bulk medium is prepared sterile and is poured into sterile Petri dishes. Care must be taken to avoid contamination from the air during pouring.
- We should pour plates on a bench in a small room free from air flow.
- To reduce condensation of water on the petri-dish lids, the medium should be cooled to 52°C before pouring. The melted medium is poured into dishes on a flat surface and the dishes are left undisturbed until the medium has set.

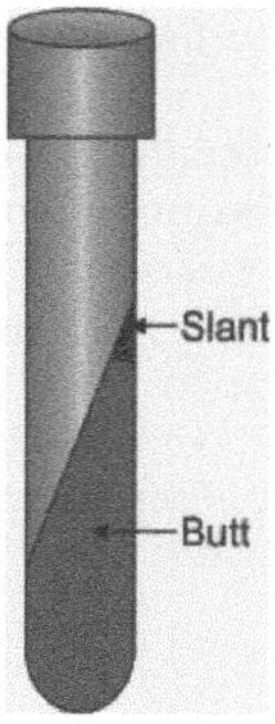

Fig. 8.1: Slope of a solid medium in test tube. A cotton wool plug or a slip on metal cap may be used

- To separate organisms from mixed cultures by plating it is essential that the surface of the medium should be dry.

When plates are poured the steam from the hot liquid condenses on the surface of the medium and this moisture is undesirable. It is removed by drying the poured and set plates in a warming or drying cabinet at 60°C for 15 to 30 minutes depending on the medium.

Inspissation of the Serum and Egg Media

The serum in Loeffler's media and egg in media such as Löwenstein-Jensen medium are usually solidified in an apparatus called the inspissator. It consists of a water jacketed copper box, the temperature of which is regulated automatically. The serum or egg media is put into tubes and placed in special racks so that the tubes are at the correct angle for forming slopes. The temperatures used is between 75°C to 85°C. At this temperature, the protein is completely solidified. Since we are using presterilized ingredients, inspissation is a method of solidification and not sterilization.

INSTRUMENTS USED FOR CULTURE

Inoculating Wires

These are very commonly used. The original type of inoculating wire was of platinum, No. 23 SWG, 2.5 inches (6.5 cm long) but others like Nichrome, Stainless steel or platinum iridium is a good choice. One end of the wire is inserted into a special aluminum holder.

The wire is sterilized by holding it vertically in a Bunsen flame so that the whole length becomes red hot at the same time.

Wire Loop

The free end is bent in the form of a flat circular and completely closed loop of 2 to 4 mm internal diameter. This is the most useful of the inoculating wires. Presterilized disposable loops are also available. The straight wire is used for stab cultures and also for picking up single colonies.

Scalpel

A sterile scalpel is used for making inoculations with scrapings from tissues and ulcers.

Sterile Pipettes

Graduated 1 mL or 10 mL glass pipettes can be used. These pipettes are stoppered with a cotton wool plug in their upper end to guard against contamination. They are wrapped in paper and sterilized in the hot air oven.

CULTURE PROCEDURES

1. The bench should be free from dust and wiped with disinfectant at least before the start of each day's work.
2. Air currents should be reduced to a minimum by closing windows and doors and restricting the movement of people in the room.
3. During inoculation, the culture medium should be uncovered only for a few seconds.
4. For right handed people, the following is the correct procedure which is followed. Place the burner and inoculating instruments to the right of the bench and cultures and media to the left. Culture plates and unseeded plates should be placed on the bench with the bottom containing the medium upper most. The caps of tubes and bottles should be loosened for easy removal.
5. Media should be labeled indicating the date and the bacterial sample with a glass marking pencil. Labeling should be done on the bottoms of Petri dishes, on tubes and on bottles rather than on lids or caps which can be mistakenly placed on other cultures.
6. During inoculation, the right hand holding the inoculating instrument charged with culture material from the specimen should be moved as little as possible and the left hand should bring the media to it.

Solid Media

Seeding the Plate

It is better to use a loop to seed the plate as a straight wire cuts the agar.

The methods of culture used in the lab are:
1. Streak
2. Lawn
3. Stroke
4. Stab
5. Pour plate
6. Sweep plate method

Streaking

Lift the bottom part of the Petri dish containing the medium with the left hand and hold it round the side with the thumb and middle finger. In most cases, the method of plating is shown in Figures 8.2A and B.

The inoculum is smeared over area A to give a well inoculum or well. The loop is resterilized and then drawn from the well in two or three parallel lines on to the fresh surface of the medium and then continued. At each step the inoculum is derived from the most distal part of the strokes which are preceding it.

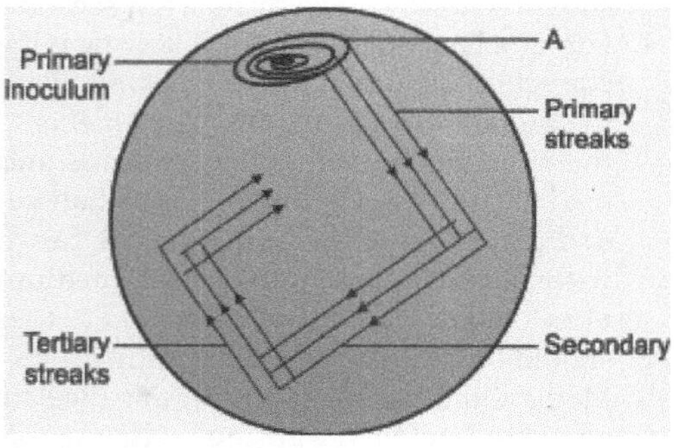

Fig. 8.2A: The method of streaking

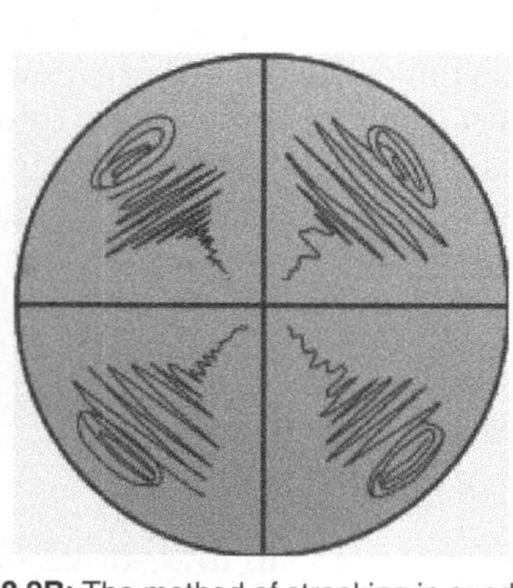

Fig. 8.2B: The method of streaking in quadrants

When the inoculum is small or the medium is selective it can be more heavily inoculated. Several loopfulls of the specimen are used to spread the well (A). The loop is then resterilized in a flame, recharged by rubbing it over area A and then used to seed the remainder of the plate by successive parallel strokes. Our main aim is to get discrete colonies. Sometimes when we have to put more than one cultures in a plate we use the following procedures, i.e. we divide the plate into quadrants and use one quadrant for one sample.

Plating machines are commercially available too.

After the plate has been seeded, the bottom of the Petri dish is returned to its lid and the loop is flamed. Plates are incubated in the inverted position with the lid underneath.

Lawn or Carpet Culture

Just like a lawn or carpet when we seed the entire plate it is called lawn or carpet culture. It provides a uniform surface growth of the bacterium and is useful for bacteriophage typing and antibiotic sensitivity testing (disc method). It is also used when a large amount of growth is required in solid media, e.g. in the preparation of bacterial antigens and vaccines. Lawn cultures are prepared in two ways.

i. *Flooding*: The surface of the plate is flooded with a liquid culture or suspension of the bacterium, pipetting off excess inoculum and incubating the plate.
ii. Application of swab soaked in the bacterial culture or suspension is applied in continuous lines all over the surface of the plate.

Stroke Culture

Stroke culture is made in tubes containing agar slope (slant) and is employed for providing a pure growth of the bacterium for slide agglutination and other diagnostic tests. It is also used to store the strain.

Stab Cultures

When we set the medium in the tube in an upright position providing a flat surface at the top of the medium, it can be used to pierce or puncture the medium for maintenance of stock culture, demonstration of gelatin liquefaction or to study oxygen requirement of bacteria.

The wire is plunged into the center of the medium and is withdrawn in the same line to avoid splitting of the medium.

Pour Plate Cultures

For preparing pour plate cultures, tubes containing 15 mL of the agar medium are melted and left to cool in a water bath at 45 to 50°C. Appropriate dilutions of the inoculum are added in 1 ml volume to the molten agar, mixed well and the contents of the tube are poured into a sterile Petri dish and allowed to set. After incubation, colonies will be seen distributed throughout the depth of the medium and can be enumerated using colony counters. The pour plate method gives an estimate of viable bacterial count in a suspension and is the method for quantitative urine cultures.

Sweep Plate Method

The edges of the Petri dishes containing the culture medium are rubbed over the fabric with the medium facing it. The dust particles from the cloth get settled on the culture medium and the colonies develop on incubation. They can be counted.

Liquid Media

How to Inoculate Liquid Cultures?

Liquid cultures in tubes, bottles or flasks may be inoculated by touching with a charged loop or by adding the inoculum with pipettes or syringes.

Advantages of liquid culture:

1. We use liquid cultures for blood culture and antibiotic sensitivity testing, where we require a large inoculum.
2. If the inoculum contains antibacterial substances or antibiotics, then liquid medium is preferable because it makes these substances ineffective by dilution.
3. Liquid cultures are also preferable when large yields of bacteria are required.

Inoculation from Liquid—Solid Media

Pick up the tube/bottle (Bottom part) with the left hand and remove the cap/plug with the crooked third/fourth fingers of the right hand. Then inoculate after flaming the mouth of the tube. Sterilize the loop by holding it in the right hand and pick up a drop from the liquid medium to plate on the surface of the solid media.

Inoculation from Solid—Liquid Media

Liquid cultures are usually inoculated from a solid medium by inclining the tube or bottle at an angle of 45° and depositing the inoculum on its wall above the surface of the medium at its lower end. When the container is returned to its vertical position, the inoculum is below the surface of the liquid. All aseptic precautions are observed.

ANAEROBIC CULTURE METHODS

Anaerobic bacteria differ in there requirement of and sensitivity to O_2. Some, such as *Clostridium histolyticum* are aerotolerant and may produce some growth on the surface of aerobic plates while others such as *Clostridium tetani* are strict anaerobes and form surface growth only if O_2 tension is less than 2 mm Hg.

Many methods have been described:

1. Cultivation in vacuum
2. Displacement of O_2
3. Chemical or biological methods
4. Reduction of O_2.

Cultivation in Vacuum

This was attempted by incubating cultures in a vacuum desiccator but this method is unsatisfactory as some oxygen gets left behind. Fluid cultures may boil over and media may get detached from the plates by the vacuum produced. This method is not in use now.

Displacement of O_2 with Gases

Displacement with gases such as H_2 N_2, Helium, or CO_2 is sometimes used but anaerobiosis is seldom complete by this method alone. This is a popular but ineffective method.

Candle jar: Here inoculated plates are placed inside a large air tight container and a lighted candle is kept in it before the lid is sealed. The burning candle is expected to use up all the O_2 inside before it goes off but some O_2 is always left behind. The candle jar provides a concentration of CO_2 while stimulates the growth of most bacteria.

Chemical or Biological Method

In the chemical/biological method alkaline pyrogallol absorbs O_2.

The method first introduced by Buckner has been employed with different modifications for providing anaerobiosis. Pyrogallic acid added to a solution of NaOH in a large test tube placed inside an air tight jar provides anaerobiosis but a small amount of carbon monoxide formed during the reaction may be inhibitory to some bacteria.

Instead of alkaline pyrogallol, anaerobiosis has been produced within jars with a mixture of chromium and sulphuric acid (Rosenthal method) or with yellow phosphorus.

Absorption of O_2 from a small closed system has been attempted by incubation along with aerobic bacteria, germinating seeds or chopped vegetables. Anaerobiosis produced by such biological methods is slow and ineffective.

McIntosh and Fildes Jar

The most reliable and widely used anaerobic method is McIntosh and Fildes anaerobic jar (Fig. 8.3).

The jar is a strong metallic or glass jar with a lid that can be screwed on tightly. The lid has terminals which can be connected to an electrical supply. It also has 2 tubes with taps, one acting as a gas inlet and the other as an outlet. On the underside of the lid is a small groove in which a small catalyst is placed (palladium + asbestos).

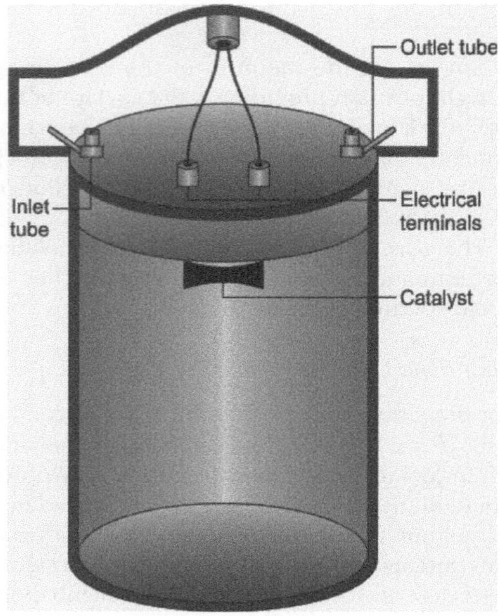

Fig. 8.3: McIntosh-Fildes jar

Inoculated culture plates are placed inside the jar with the medium in the bottom half of the plates and the lid clamped tight. The outlet tube is connected to a vacuum pump and the air inside is evacuated. The outlet tap is then closed and the inlet tube connected to a H_2 (hydrogen) supply. After the jar is filled with H_2, the electrical terminals are connected to a current supply so that palladinised asbestos is heated. This acts as a catalyst for the combination of H_2 with the remaining O_2 present in the jar. This method ensures complete anaerobiosis but carries the risk of explosion which may rarely occur. This risk can be eliminated by modification of the catalyst. Alumina pellets coated with palladium and contained in a gauze sachet placed on the underside of the lid of the jar acts as a catalyst at room temperature as long as it is day.

Gaspak

Gaspak is now the method of choice for preparing anaerobic jars. The gaspak is commercially available as a disposable envelope containing chemicals which generate H_2 and CO_2

on the addition of water. After the inoculated plates are kept in a jar, the gaspak envelope with water added is placed inside and the lid screwed tight. H_2 and CO_2 are liberated and the presence of a cold catalyst in the envelope permits the combination of H_2 and O_2 to produce an anaerobic environment. The gaspak is simple and effective, eliminating the need for drawing a vacuum and adding H_2.

An indicator should be employed for verifying anaerobic condition in the jars. Reduced methylene blue is generally used for this purpose. It remains colorless anaerobically but turns blue on exposure to O_2.

Reduction of O_2 in the Medium

Reduction of O_2 in the medium is achieved by the use of various reducing agents including 1 percent glucose, 1 percent thioglycollate, 0.1 percent ascorbic acid, and 0.05 percent cysteine.

An easily prepared anaerobic medium is broth into which are introduced pieces of red hot mettalic iron, the broth being then layered over with sterile vaseline. Broth containing fresh animal tissue such as rabbit kidney, spleen, testis/heart (Smith, Noguchi medium) supports the growth of many anaerobes.

Robertson cooked meat medium is probably the most widely used fluid medium for the culture of anaerobes. It consists of fat free minced cooked broth with a layer of sterile vaseline over it. It permits the growth of even strict anaerobes and indicates their saccharolytic or proteolytic activities by meat being turned red or black, respectively. For fastidious anaerobes particularly for quantitative cultures, pre-reduced media and anaerobic chamber (glove box) may be used. The anaerobic chamber is an air tight glass fronted cabinet, filled with inert gas with an entry lock for the introduction of materials.

METHODS OF ISOLATING PURE CULTURE

The following methods may be employed for isolating pure cultures of bacteria from mixtures:

1. Surface plating is the method routinely employed in clinical bacteriology from which colonies can be picked.
2. Enrichment, selective and indicator media are widely used for the isolation of pathogens from specimens such as feces.
3. Pretreatment of specimens with appropriate bacterial substances which destroy unwanted bacteria, is the standard practice for isolation of tubercle bacilli from sputum and other clinical specimens by treatment with alkali, acid or other substances to which most commensals are susceptible but tubercle bacilli are resistant.
4. Separation of bacteria with different optimum temperature can be done by incubation at different temperatures. Only thermophilic bacteria grow at 60°C. A mixture containing *N. meningitidis* and *B. catarrhalis* can be purified by incubation at 22°C when only the latter grows.
5. By heating at 80°C, a mixture containing vegetative and spore forming bacteria, the former can be eliminated. This method is useful for isolation of tetanus bacilli from dust.
6. Separation between motile and nonmotile bacteria can be effected using Craigie's tube. It consists of a tube of semisolid agar with a narrow tube open at both ends placed in the center of the medium in such a way it projects above the level of medium. The mixture is inoculated into the central tube. On incubation, the motile bacteria alone traverse the agar and appear on the top of the medium outside the central tube. A U-tube also serves the same purpose, inoculation being performed in one limb and the subculture taken from the other. This can also be used to obtain phase variants in *Salmonella* species.
8. Pathogenic bacteria may be isolated from mixtures by inoculation into appropriate animals.
9. Bacteria of different sizes may be separated by the use of selective filters. Filters are widely used for separating viruses from bacteria. Single cell methods using micromanipulators by which single bacterium can be separated or cultured are too complicated for routine use but may find application in research situations.

CHAPTER

9

Classification of Microorganisms

LESSON PLAN

- Introduction
- Basic Groups
  - Bacteria
  - Mycoplasms
  - *Rickettsia*
  - *Chlamydia*
  - Viruses
  - Protozoa
  - Fungi
- Morphological Classification of Bacteria
  - Filamentous Bacteria
  - True Bacteria
- Biological Classification
  - Pure Culture
  - Strain
  - Isolate
  - Species
  - Genus
- International Classification
- Numerical Classification
- Biochemical Classification
- DNA Composition as a Basis for Classification

INTRODUCTION

As we know, microorganisms are defined as living creatures that are microscopic in size and simple in structure. The diameter of the smallest body that can be seen clearly with the naked eye is about 200 μm. Most of the microorganisms are smaller than this and a microscope is required for their study. The light microscope can resolve bodies down to 0.2 μm in diameter. This includes all microbes with the exception of viruses most of which are smaller than 0.2 μm. The electron microscope has a limit of resolution smaller than 0.5 μm (0.0005 μm) and can resolve even the smallest virus (0.01 μm in diameter).

We must classify microorganisms in order to understand them.

BASIC GROUPS

Microorganisms are divided into prokaryotes and eukaryotes. The prokaryotes include blue green Algae, Bacteria, *Mycoplasma*, *Rickettsia*, *Chlamydia*, and Viruses. The Eukaryotes include Algae, Protozoa, Slime Moulds and Fungi.

Bacteria

Bacteria are prokaryotic microorganisms, which are unicellular and have both DNA and RNA.

Mycoplasms

They are prokaryotic cellular organisms that differ from bacteria in their smaller size, their lack of rigid cell wall, extreme variability in shape and size and extreme sensitivity to osmotic pressure of the environment. They are the smallest and simplest organisms capable of independent growth.

Rickettsia

They are simple, unicellular organisms that are rod shaped, spherical or pleomorphic. They are slightly smaller than bacteria but can be seen by light microscope. They are strict parasites that can grow only in living tissues of a suitable animal host.

Chlamydia

Chlamydia are smaller prokaryotes, that are obligate intracellular parasites. They exist in two forms—one is the infectious, extracellular transport form or elementary body and the other is the larger intracellular and the multiplying form of the organism. They cause trachoma and inclusion conjunctivitis in humans and a variety of other diseases in animals.

Viruses

They are the smallest and simplest of all microorganisms and different species range in size from 0.01 to 0.3 µm in diameter. Most are ultramicroscopic [they are smaller than can be resolved by light microscope (< 0.2 µm in diameter)]. All species are strictly parasitic and are capable of growth only within the living cells of plant, animal or bacterial host. The viruses depend completely on the synthetic machinery of the host. The viruses that infect and parasitize bacteria are called bacteriophages.

Protozoa

Non-photosynthetic unicellular organisms with protoplasm clearly differentiated into nucleus and cytoplasm. They are larger microorganisms with transverse diameter in the range of 2 to 100 µm. Some free living protozoa are saprophytic. Many protozoa are parasitic and live in and derive their nourishment from the body of an animal host.

Some reproduce by binary fission and some by a sexual mechanism. Some form resting stages called cysts.

Fungi

These are non-photosynthetic microorganisms possessing rigid cell walls. They may be saprophytic or parasitic. They can grow as unicellular cells or multicellular moulds.

MORPHOLOGICAL CLASSIFICATION OF BACTERIA

This classification is based on the morphology and the staining of the bacteria.

The bacteria are divided into 2 main classes-the filamentous bacteria and the true bacteria, (Flow chart 9.1).

Filamentous Bacteria

Filamentous bacteria are the:

1. *Actinomyces*
2. *Nocardia*
3. *Streptomyces*
4. *Micropolyspora*

Actinomyces

- Gram-positive
- Non acid fast
- Anaerobic
- Fragment into short coccal and bacillary forms
- Do not form conidia

Nocardia

- Similar to *Actinomyces*
- Aerobic
- Acid fast

Streptomyces

- Vegetative mycelium, not fragmenting into short forms.
- Conidia formed in chains from aerial hyphae.

Flow chart 9.1: Morphological classification of bacteria

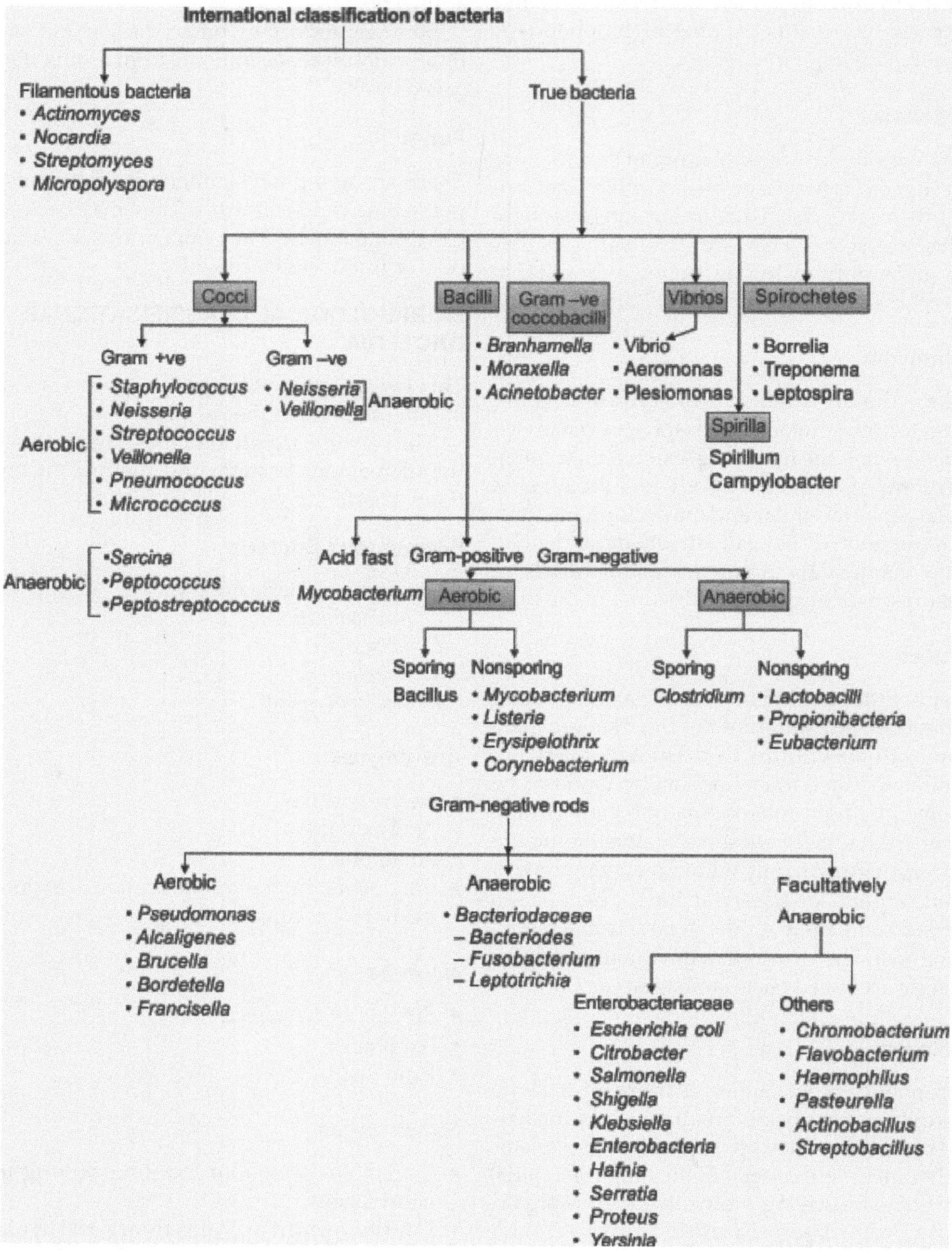

Micropolyspora

- Gram-positive
- Aerobic
- Nonacid fast
- Mycelium forming spores on substrate.

True Bacteria

These are simple, generally unicellular structures. They never occur in the form of a mycelium. They can be further divided into groups on the basis of their shapes.

- Cocci (spherical)
- Bacilli (rod shaped)
- *Vibrio* (comma shaped)
- Spirochetes
- *Spirilla* (spirally twisted rods).

Cocci

They are divided into two groups on the basis of their staining reaction with Gram's stain:

- Gram-positive
- Gram-negative.

Gram-positive cocci

- *Staphylococcus*—gram-positive cocci in clusters.
- *Streptococcus*—gram-positive cocci in chains
- *Micrococcus*—gram-positive cocci in tetrads
- *Sarcina*—gram-positive cocci in groups of eight.

Gram-negative cocci

- *Neisseria* — *Neisseria gonorrhoeae*
  — *Neisseria meningitidis*
- *Veillonella* — These are very small cocci arranged in clusters and pairs.

Bacilli

Just like cocci, bacilli are divided into:

- Acid fast
- Gram-negative
- Gram-positive.

Acid fast bacteria

These belong to the group mycobacteria. The two important groups are:

- *Mycobacterium tuberculosis*
- *Mycobacterium leprae*

Gram-positive rods

These can be further divided into aerobic and anaerobic rods.

Aerobic: Aerobic gram-positive rods can be further divided into:

- Spore forming—*Bacillus species*
- Nonspore forming
  - *Mycobacterium tuberculosis*
  - *Listeria*
  - *Erysipelothrix*
  - *Corynebacterium*
  - *Nocardia, Streptomyces.*

Anaerobic bacilli: These can again be divided into spore bearing and nonspore bearing:

Spore bearing → *Clostridium*
Nonspore bearing → *Lactobacilli*
Propionibacterium

Gram-negative rods

These can be divided into:

- Aerobic
- Anaerobic
- Facultatively anaerobic

Aerobic gram-negative rods

Alcaligenes *Pseudomonas*
Bordetella *Brucella*
Francisella.

Anaerobic gram-negative rods

Bacteroidaceae: Family which includes:

- Bacteroides
- *Fusobacterium*
- *Leptotrichia.*

Facultatively anaerobic gram-negative rods

- *Enterobacteriaceae*: This is a family which includes:
  - *Escherichia*
  - *Salmonella*
  - *Shigella*
  - *Klebsiella*
  - *Proteus*
  - *Yersinia*
  - *Citrobacter*
  - *Enterobacter*
  - *Hafnia*
  - *Serratia*

Other gram-negative rods are: *Chromobacterium, Flavobacterium, Hemophilus, Pasteurella, Actinobacillus, Streptobacillus.*

Vibrios

These are short nonflexous gram-negative rods. They show very active movement.

Spiral Bacteria

These are nonflexous, spiral filaments, gram-negative and mostly motile having polar flagella and show very active motility. For examples, are *Campylobacter*.

Spirochetes

These are slender, flexous, spiral filaments. They differ from the *Spirilla* in being capable of active flexion of the cell body and in being motile without possession of flagella.

Flow chart 9.2 shows a separate classification of anaerobic bacteria.

BIOLOGICAL CLASSIFICATION

The biological classification is based on characters which can be demonstrated like serological, physiological and ecological. At present no standard classification is universally accepted and applied.

Pure Culture

These are young colonies that are exclusively the progeny of a single cell and there are no mutant cells. These are described as clones.

Strain

A line or population of bacteria which descends from a single ancestral bacterium which is found in the natural habitat and in primary cultures from that habitat and subcultures from the primary cultures is called a strain.

Isolate

Each primary culture isolated from a natural source is called an isolate. Even in the same patient if the culture is isolated at different times it will be a different isolate.

Species

The species is defined as a group of individuals that are generally similar in major characters though they differ in minor characters.

Flow chart 9.2: Anaerobic bacteria

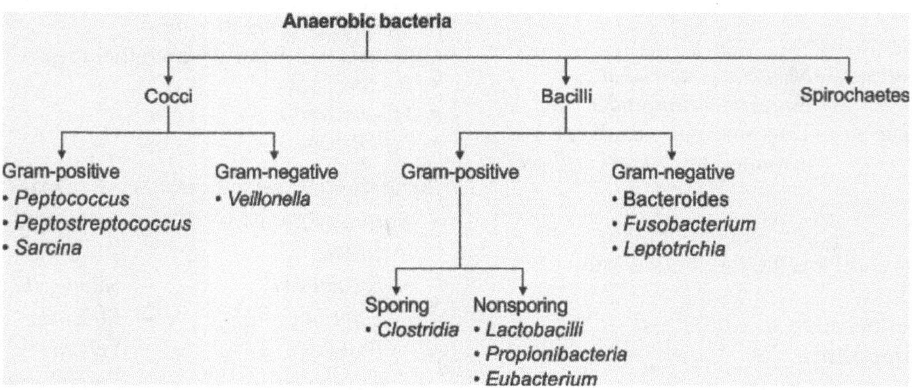

Genus

It includes many species sharing common characteristics.

INTERNATIONAL CLASSIFICATION

This classification was started by American microbiologists and is given in Bergey's Manual of Determinative Bacteriology. It is similar to the biological classification and it shows families and genera [Table 9.1 —*This is reproduced from Medical Microbiology (Mackie and McCartney vol I)*].

In the international system the major groups, e.g. orders and families are distinguished by characters, e.g. cell shape, Gram reaction, spore formation and flagellation, that are considered to be of major importance, and the minor groups, e.g. genera and species by characters considered to be of less importance e.g. fermentation reactions, nutritional requirement and pathogenicity.

NUMERICAL CLASSIFICATION

In this classification numbers are given to the characteristics of the organisms and the organisms are compared by their numbers. The classification thus depends upon total scores of as many similarities and differences as can be observed. A similarity index is then taken out to find out how similar one strain is to another.

BIOCHEMICAL CLASSIFICATION

The chemical constitution of the prokaryotic cell wall is different from that of eukaryotic cell walls. Also the chemical constitution of the gram-negative and gram-positive cell differs. Chemical analysis using chromatographic methods is used to differentiate between genera and species.

Table 9.1: International classification

Major group	*Family*	*Genus*	*Species examples*
1. Spirochetes	Spirochaetaceae. Slender, flexuous, helically coiled, unicellular bacteria that are motile but non-flagellate	*Borrelia* *Treponema* *Leptospira*	*Borr. recurrentis* *Tr. pallidum* *Lepto. interrogans*
2. Spiral and curved bacteria	Spirillaceae. Rigid, helically curved rods with polar flagella	*Spirillum* *Campylobacter*	*Sp. minor* *Camp. fetus*
3. Gram-negative aerobic rods	Pseudomonadaceae. Straight or curved, but not helical rods; motile by polar flagella; strict aerobes; usually oxidase positive	*Pseudomonas*	*Ps. aeruginosa* *Ps. cepacia* *Ps. mallei*
	Genera of uncertain affiliation. Motile by peritrichous flagella (Alcaligenes, Bord. bronchiseptica) or non-motile; strict aerobes	*Alcaligenes* *Brucella* *Bordetella* *Francisella*	*Alc. faecalis* *Br. melitensis* *Bord. pertussis* *Fr. tularensis*
4. Gram-negative facultatively anaerobic rods	Enterobacteriaceae. Motile by peritrichous flagella or non-motile; ferment carbohydrates; oxidase negative	*Escherichia* *Citrobacter* *Salmonella* *Shigella* *Klebsiella* *Enterobacter* *Hafnia* *Serratia* *Proteus* *Yersinia*	*Esch. coli* *Cit. freundii* *S. typhi* *Sh. dysenteriae* *Kl. pneumoniae* *Enter. cloacae* *Hafnia. alvei* *Serr. marcescens* *Pr. mirabilis* *Y. pestis*
	Vibrionaceae, rigid straight or curved rods, usually motile by polar flagella; farment carbohydrates; oxidase positive	*Vibrio* *Aeromonas* *Pleisiomonas*	*V. cholerae* *Aeromonas hydrophila* *Pleis. shigelloides*

Contd...

Contd...

Major group	Family	Genus	Species examples
	Genera of uncertain affiliation. Motile with polar or peritrichous flagella or non-motile ferment carbohydrates; oxidase positive or negative	*Chromobacterium* *Flavobacterium* *Haemorphilus* *Pasteurella* *Actinobacillus* *Streptobacillus*	*Chr. Violaceum* *Fl. meningosepticum* *H. influenzae* *Past. multocida* *Act. lignieresi* *Str. moniliformis*
5. Gram-negative anaerobic bacteria	Bacteroidaceae. Uniform or pleomorphic rods; motile by peritrichous flagella or non-motile; strict anaerobes	*Bacteroides* *Fusobacterium* *Leptotrichia*	*Bact. fragilis* *Fus. nucleatum* *Leptotrichia buccalis*
6. Gram-negative aerobic cocci and coccobacilli	Neisseriaceae. Cocci in pairs or masses, or plump rods in short chains; non-flagellate; most are oxidase positive	*Neisseria* *Branchamella* *Moraxella* *Acinetobacter*	*N. gonorrhoeae* *Bran. catarrhalis* *Mor. lacunata* *Acin. calcoaceticus*
7. Gram-negative anaerobic cocci	Veillonellaceae. Small to large cocci, often in pairs; strict anaerobes	*Veillonella*	*Veill. parvula*
8. Gram-positive cocci	Micrococcaceae. Cocci in regular or irregular clusters; aerobic or facultatively anaerobic	*Micrococcus* *Staphylococcus*	*Micro. luteus* *Staph. aureus*
	Streptococcaceae. Cocci in pairs, chains or tetrads; facultative anaerobes; nutritionally exacting	*Streptococcus* *Aerococcus* *Gemella*	*Strept. pyogenes* *Aerococcus. viridans* *Gem. haemolysans*
	Peptococcaceae. Cocci in pairs, masses or chains; strict anaerobes; nutritionally exacting	*Peptococcus* *Peptostreptococcus* *Sarcina*	*Peptococcus. aerogenes* *Peptostreptococcus anaerobius* *Sarc. ventriculi*
9. Endospore-forming rods	Bacillaceae. Most are Gram-positive, some variable or Gram-negative; Motile by peritrichous flagella or non-motile	*Bacillus* *Clostridium*	*B. anthracis* *Cl. tetani*
10. Gram-positive non-sporing rods	Lactobacillaceae. Rods single or in chains; usually non-motile; anaerobic or facultative; Nutritionally exacting	*Lactobacillus*	*Lacto. acidophilus* *Lacto. casei*
	Genera of uncertain affiliation. Aerobic Listeria motile; Erysipelothrix non-motile	*Listeria* *Erysipelothrix*	*List. monocytogenes* *Ery. rhusiopathiae*
11. Actinomyces and related organisms	Coryneform group of bacteria. Gram-positive rods; mostly non-motile; aerobic or facultative	*Corynebacterium* *Arthrobacter* *Kurthia*	*C. diphtheriae* *Arthrobacter. globiformis* *K. zopfi*
	Propionibacteriaceae. Gram-positive, anaerobic to aerotolerant rods	*Propionibacterium* *Eubacterium*	*Prop. acnes* *Eubacterium alactolyticum*
	Actinomycetaceae. Gram-positive non-acid-fast branched filaments which fragment into coccoid and diphtheroid forms; non-motile; no aerial spores; anaerobic or facultative	*Actinomyces* *Arachnia* *Bifidobacterium*	*Actinomyces. israelii* *Arach. propionica* *Bifido. bifidum*

Contd...

Contd...

Major group	Family	Genus	Species examples
	Mycobacteriaceae. Acid-fast rods, rarely filamentous or branching; aerobic	*Mycobacterium*	*Myco. tuberculosis*
	Nocardiaceae. Gram-positive branched filamentous, some acid-fast; aerobic	*Nocardia*	*Noc. asteroides*
	Streptomycetaceae. Gram-positive non-acid-fast mycelium forming aerial spores; aerobic	*Streptomyces*	*Streptomyces. griseus*
	Micromonosporaceae. Gram-positive non-acid-fast mycelium forming spores on substrate or aerial hyphae; most are aerobic	*Micropolyspora*	*Micropolyspora. faeni*
12. Rickettsias			
Gram-negative rod-shaped, coccoid or pleomorphic organisms that are smaller than most other bacteria, but have typical bacterial cell walls and reproduce by fission. The majority are obligatory intracellular parasites.			
	Rickettsiaceae. Rod-shaped or coccoid; non-motile; multiply only in living tissue cells other than erythrocytes; transmitted by arthropods	*Rickettsia* *Rochalimaea* *Coxiella*	*R. prowazekii* *Roch. quintana* *Cox. burnetii*
	Bartonellaceae. Coccoids, rings or filaments; some have flagella; parasitise erythrocytes; cultivable on inanimate media	*Bartonella*	*Bart. bacilliformis*
	Chlamydiaceae. Coccoid and non-motile; multiply only in living cells; small elementary bodies develop into larger initial bodies which multiply by fission and re-organise into elementary bodies	*Chlamydia*	*Chlam. trachomatis* *Chlam. psittaci*
13. Mycoplasmas			
Gram-negative pleomorphic, coccoid to filamentus organisms bounded by a single triple-layer membrane and lacking a rigid, peptidoglycan-containing cell wall; some forms ultramicroscopic. They are cultivable on inanimate cell-free media.			
	Mycoplasmataceae. Require sterol for growth	*Mycoplasma*	*Mycoplasma pneumoniae*
	Acholeplasmataceae. Do not require sterol for growth	*Acholeplasma*	*Achol. laidawii*

* This table is for optional reading.

DNA COMPOSITION AS A BASIS FOR CLASSIFICATION

The hydrogen bonding between guanine and cytosine (G-C) base pairs in DNA is stronger than that between adenine and thymine (A-T) pairs. Thus, the melting or denaturation temperature of DNA (at which the two strands separate) is basically determined by the G + C content. We can indirectly measure the G + C content by measuring the changes in light absorption characteristics brought about at melting temperature.

The G + C component of DNA in bacteria differs from about 25 to 80 moles percent. However, for one species the G + C content is fixed or falls within a narrow range and this provides a basis for classification.

CHAPTER

10

Bacterial Identification

LESSON PLAN

- ➢ Introduction
- ➢ Direct Staining of the Sample
- ➢ Culture
- ➢ Biochemical Tests
  - Oxidative Fermentative Test-O/F Test
  - Sugar Fermentation Reactions
  - Tests to Show Ability of the Bacteria to Utilize a Particular Substrate
  - Tests for Specific Breakdown Products
  - Enzymes of Bacteria
  - Complete Sugar Set
- ➢ Antigenic Characters
- ➢ Typing of Bacteria
- ➢ Animal Pathogenicity and Toxigenicity
- ➢ Molecular Biology Techniques
- ➢ Antibiotic Sensitivity Test

INTRODUCTION

Our main aim in diagnostic microbiology is to identify the disease causing (pathogenic) bacteria from the sample of the patient so that effective treatment can be given for cure. For this we follow a system of identification of the pathogenic bacteria in the sample.

DIRECT STAINING OF THE SAMPLE

We stain the sample depending on the type of bacteria one is suspecting.

- *Gram's stain*: For most bacterial infections, a Gram's stain is done. The Gram's stain divides the bacteria into gram-positive and gram-negative groups.
- *Ziehl-Neelsen stain*: This stain is used to differentiate between acid fast and non-acid fast bacteria. This is mostly used for the diagnosis of *Mycobacterium tuberculosis*.
- *Albert's stain*: This stain is used to stain *Corynebacterium diphtheriae*
- *Fluorescent stain*: Fluorescent stains are special stains which when exposed to ultraviolet light absorb energy and emit visible light. A dye that becomes luminous in this way is said to fluoresce. When tissue cells or organisms are stained with such a dye and examined with UV light in an adapted microscope they are seen as fluorescent objects. The fluorescent dyes have selective staining affinities for example, auramine can be used to stain *Mycobacterium tuberculosis*.
- *What can we see by staining reaction?* We can see the morphology of bacteria—the shape, size and arrangement. Use of special staining methods and special microscopes help us to observe other structural characteristics like flagella, spores, capsules, etc.

CULTURE

Since direct staining does not give a conclusive evidence of the identity of the bacteria we need to grow it in a culture medium to see the appearance of colonies and also carry out further tests for final identification. Without a culture we cannot prove that a particular bacterium is the causative agent of a disease.

We should always put up a culture first from the sample and then do the direct staining to minimize contamination.

When we study colonies (clones of single bacterial cells on solid media) we look for following:

Shape — circular, irregular, radiate, rhizoid

Size — in mm

Elevation — convex, concave

Margins — entire, bevelled

Surface — smooth, wavy, rough, granular.

Edges — entire, crenated, curled

Color— white, golden, pink, black, etc.

Structure — opaque, transparent or translucent

Consistency — membranous, friable, butyrous or viscid

Emulsifiability — whether it can be mixed in normal saline easily

Smell — of the colonies may sometimes help, e.g.,

Proteus group of bacteria have a typical fishy smell.

The following features are observed in a liquid medium.

- **Degree of growth** — Absent (clear liquid medium) / Scanty / Moderate / Abundant
- **Presence of turbidity**
- **Presence of deposit**
- **Nature of surface** growth such as pellicle

Based on the colony characteristics we are able to identify the major group to which the bacterium belongs.

For confirmation, we again do a staining and a hanging drop preparation. This is a slide and cover slip preparation of a liquid bacterial culture to observe motility in the bacteria. The next step in the identification are the biochemical tests.

BIOCHEMICAL TESTS

These are called biochemical tests because they are tests which identify the bacteria on the basis of the presence of certain enzymes and other biochemical properties. There are four types of biochemical reactions.

- To differentiate between aerobic/anaerobic breakdown of a carbohydrate.
- Tests to show how many carbohydrates can be attacked.
- Tests to show ability of the bacteria to utilize a particular substrate like citrate or urea.
- Tests for specific breakdown products like indole, H_2S.
- Tests to detect presence of enzymes in bacteria.

Species that cannot be differentiated by morphology and cultural characters may have differences in biochemical reactions.

Hugh Leifson Test O/F Test (Oxidative Fermentative Test)

- To differentiate between aerobic and anaerobic breakdown of a carbohydrate
- Bacteria breakdown glucose either fermentatively or oxidatively. The end products of fermentation are strong mixed acids that can be detected in a conventional fermentation test medium. However, the acids formed in oxidative degradation of glucose are extremely weak and a more sensitive medium is required for their detection. Hugh and Leifson first designed such a medium. The O/F medium of Hugh and Leifson differs from the carbohydrate fermentation media as follows:
- The concentration of peptone is decreased from 1 to 0.2 percent.
- The concentration of carbohydrate is increased from 0.5 to 1 percent.
- The concentration of agar is decreased to 0.2 percent from 0.3 percent making it semisolid.

The lower amount of peptone reduces the formation of alkaline amines which can neutralize small quantities of weak acids that may form from oxidative metabolism. The larger amount of carbohydrate serves to increase the amount of acid that can be formed. The semisolid consistency of the agar permits the acid that forms on the surface of the agar to permeate throughout the medium making interpretation of the pH shift easier to visualize.

Medium	*Conventional*	*OF*
Peptone	10 g	2 g
Sodium Chloride	5 g	5 g
D-glucose	5 g	10 g
Agar	15 g	2.50 g
Indicates	Andrade's	Bromothymol blue
Distilled water	1000 mL	1000 mL
pH	7.0	7.1

Procedure: When preparing the medium, the pH is adjusted to 7.1 before adding bromothymol blue and the medium is autoclaved in a flask at 121°C for 15 minutes. The carbohydrate to be added is sterilized separately and added to give a final concentration of 1 percent. The medium is then tubed to a depth of about 4 cm. Duplicate tubes of medium are inoculated by stabbing, 1 to 2 times. One tube is quickly covered with a layer of sterile petroleum jelly to a depth of 5 to 10 mm and both are incubated for up to 30 days.

Results

1. Fermenting organisms produce acid reaction throughout the medium in the covered as well as the open tube, e.g. *Enterobacteriaceae*.
2. Oxidising organisms produce an acid reaction only in the open tube, this begins at the surface and gradually extends downwards, e.g. *Pseudomonas*.
3. Organisms that cannot breakdown the carbohydrates aerobically/anaerobically produce no change, e.g. *Acinetobacter*.

Sugar Fermentation Reactions

General Sugar for Fermentation Reactions

The sugars which are used for fermentation reactions are:

1. Glucose
2. Lactose
3. Mannitol
4. Sucrose

The complete sugar medium is prepared by adding Andrade's indicator solution to the sugar solution.

A small inverted tube (Durham's tube) completely filled with liquid and containing no air bubbles is usually included in each culture bottle to detect gas.

Each liquid culture medium is inoculated with a speck of colonies and incubated for 24 to 48 hours. Next day we look for color change and gas production. If a bacterium ferments the sugar it produces a change in pH and the indicator turns pink, changing the color of solution.

Methyl Red Test

Introduction: Methyl red is a pH indicator dye with a range between 6.0 (yellow) and 4.4 (red). The pH at which methyl red detects acid is lower than the pH for other indicators used in other culture media. Thus, to produce a color change the organism must produce large quantities of acid from the carbohydrate substrate being used.

Principle: The methyl red test is a quantitative test for acid production. Those organisms which produce strong acids (lactic, acetic and formic) from glucose through the mixed acid fermentation pathway and then maintain the low pH give a positive MR reaction.

Medium: Glucose phosphate peptone water

- Polypeptone 5 g
- Glucose 5 g
- Dipotassium phosphate 5 g
- Distilled water 1 liter
- Final pH 6.9
- Methyl red indicator
  - Methyl red 0.1 g in 300 mL of 95% ethylalcohol
  - Distilled water = 200 mL

Procedure: Inoculate the MR-VP broth with a pure culture of the test organism. Inoculate the broth for 48 to 72 hours at 35°C. At the end of this time add 5 drops of methyl red reagent directly to the broth.

Interpretation: The development of a stable red color in the surface of the medium indicates sufficient acid production to lower the pH to 4.4 and constitutes a positive test.
Positive control → *Escherichia coli*
Negative control → *Enterobacter aerogenes*

Voges-Proskauer Test

Introduction: Voges-Proskauer is named after two microbiologists working at the beginning of the 20th century. They first observed the red color reaction when some bacteria were grown in the VP medium, for 48 to 72 hours and KOH was added to it. It was later discovered that the active product in the medium formed by bacterial metabolism is acetyl methyl carbinol.

Principle: Pyruvic acid, the compound formed in the fermentative degradation of glucose is further metabolized by certain bacteria into an end product called acetoin or acetyl methyl carbinol. It is a neutral end product.

In the presence of atmospheric O_2 and 40 percent KOH acetoin is converted to diacetyl and α napthol serves as a catalyst to bring out a red color complex.

Media and Reagents:

α Napthol (5%)	= 5 Grams
Absolute ethyl alcohol	= 100 mL
KOH (40%)	= 40 g
Distilled water	= 100 mL

Procedure: Inoculate a tube of MR and VP broth with a pure culture of the test organism. Incubate for 24 hours at 35°C. At the end of this time, take 1 mL of the broth in a clean test tube. Add. 0.6 mL of 5 percent a napthol followed by 0.2 mL of 40 percent KOH. It is essential that the reagents be added in this order. Shake the tube gently to expose the medium to atmospheric oxygen and allow the tube to remain undisturbed for 10 to 15 minutes.

Interpretation: A positive test is represented by the development of a red color 15 minutes or more after addition of the reagents indicating the presence of diacetyl, the oxidation product of acetoin. The test should be read after standing for more than one hour because negative Voges-Proskauer cultures may produce a copper like color giving it a false positive interpretation. There are two types of methods used to do it.
a. O' Meara's method
b. Barrit's method

These methods differ somewhat in the procedures, but the final result is the same.

Tests to Show the Ability of the Bacteria to Utilize a Specific Substrate

To show the ability of a bacterium to use a specific compound as their sole source of carbon and energy, we make a medium with only that compound in it. The organism is inoculated on that. After a suitable period of incubation, the plate is examined and the appearance of bacterial growth indicates that the bacteria has been able to utilize the test compound.

Citrate Test

Introduction: Sodium citrate is a salt of citric acid. Some bacteria instead of using carbohydrates as a source of energy use citrate as the sole source of carbon. This is an important identification test for bacteria. Any medium used to detect citrate utilization by test bacteria must be devoid of protein and carbohydrates as sources of carbon.

Principle: When a test bacteria utilizes citrate as the sole source of carbon it also utilizes ammonium as the sole source of nitrogen and leads to the production of alkaline end products. Bromo-thymol blue is the indicator which is yellow below the pH 6.0 and blue when pH > 7.6.

Medium:
Simmons citrate medium

• Ammonium dihydrogen phosphate	1 g
• Dipotassium phosphate	1 g
• Sodium chloride	5 g
• Sodium citrate	2 g
• Magnesium sulphate	0.20 g
• Agar	15 g
• Bromothymol blue	0.08 g
• Distilled water	1 liter

Procedure: A single colony is streaked on the slant surface of an agar medium. The tube is incubated at 35°C for 24 to 48 hours.

Interpretation: A positive test shows deep blue color in 24 to 48 hours indicating that the test organism has been able to utilize the citrate contained in the medium with the production of alkaline end products.

A positive test may also be read without blue color if there is a visible colonial growth along the inoculation streak line. If we incubate this tube for another 24 hours a blue color usually develops.

Controls:
- +ve control — *Klebsiella spp.*
- –ve control — *Escherichia coli*

Urease

Introduction: Urea is a diamide of carbon. All amides are easily hydrolyzed with the release of ammonia and carbon dioxide.

Principle: Many bacteria have an enzyme urease that hydrolyzes urea to release ammonia and carbon dioxide. Ammonia in solution reacts with carbon dioxide to form ammonium carbonate and it increases the pH of the medium. This change in pH is detected by an indicator dye.

Media:

Christensen's medium
- Peptone 1 g
- NaCl 5 g
- K_2HPO_4 2 g
- Phenol red (1 in 500 aqueous sol) 6 mL
- Agar 20 g
- Distilled water 1 liter
- Glucose 10% sterile sol (10 mL)
- Urea 20% sterile sol (100 mL)

We prepare the base solution without glucose or urea and adjust the pH to 6.8 to 6.9. Glucose and urea solutions are sterilized by filtration. The base solution is sterilized by autoclaving in a flask at 121°C for 30 minutes which is cooled to 50°C. Then glucose and urea solution is added and the medium is poured as deep slopes.

Procedure: The surface of the agar slant is streaked with the test organism and incubated for 18 to 24 hours.

Interpretation: Organisms that hydrolyze urea rapidly may produce a positive reaction within 1 to 2 hours. Less active species may require three or more days.
- Rapid urea splitters → Pink color throughout. (*Proteus*)
- Slow urea splitters (*Klebsiella*) → Pink color initially in slant, gradually covers entire tube
- No urea hydrolysis → Original yellow color.

Controls:
- *Positive* *Proteus spp*
- *Negative* *Escherichia coli*

Tests for Specific Breakdown Products

Indole Test

Introduction: Indole, a benzyl pyrrole is one of the metabolic degradation products of the amino acid tryptophan. Bacteria that have the enzyme tryptophanase breakdown tryptophan with the production of indole, pyruvic acid and ammonia. This test is very useful to differentiate *Escherichia coli* from *Klebsiella spp*.

Principle: The indole test is based on the formation of a red color complex when indole reacts with the aldehyde group of paradimethyl amino benzaldehyde. This is the active chemical in Kovács and Ehrlich's reagents.

Media: *Kovács* reagent has amyl or isoamyl alcohol, and paradimethyl aminobenzaldehyde.

Ehrlich's reagent has paradimethyl amino benzaldehyde, absolute ethyl alcohol and concentrated hydrochloric acid.

Procedure: Inoculate peptone water with the test organism and incubate at 35°C for 18 to 24 hours. At the end of this time add 15 drops of reagent down the inner wall of the tube. If Ehrlich's reagent is used this step is preceded by the addition of 1 mL of chloroform. This is not necessary with Kovács reagent.

Interpretation: Development of a bright red fuchsia color at the interface of the reagent and the broth within seconds after adding the reagent is indicative of the presence of indole and is a positive test.

Controls:
- +ve control — *Escherichia coli*
- –ve control — *Klebsiella pneumoniae*

Enzymes of Bacteria

Oxidase Test

Introduction: Some bacteria have an enzyme oxidase that catalyzes the transport of electrons between electron donors in the bacteria and a redox dye, which shows a deep purple color in the reduced state, i.e. after accepting electrons.

Principle: The oxidase test or cytochrome oxidase test (as it is called) utilizes certain reagent dyes such as tetramethyl paraphenylene diamine that substitute for oxygen as artificial electron acceptors. When it accepts electrons it is in the reduced state and develops a deep purple color.

Media and Reagents: There are two reagents
- *Kovács reagent*: This is tetramethyl paraphenylene diamine dihydrochloride 1 percent
- *Gordon and McLeod's reagent*: Dimethyl para phenylene diamine dihydrochloride 1 percent.

Procedure:

a. *Direct plate method*—Cultures are made on a suitable growth medium. A freshly prepared 1 percent solution of tetramethyl-p-phenylene-diamine hydrochloride is poured on to the plate so as to cover the surface and is then decanted. The colonies of oxidase positive organisms rapidly develop a purple color.
b. *Filter paper method*—Dry, wet.

Dry

The dry filter paper method is very convenient. Strips of Whatman's no.1 filter paper are soaked in a freshly prepared solution of tetramethyl-p-phenylene diamine dihydrochloride. After draining for about 30 seconds, the strips are freeze dried and stored in a dark bottle tightly sealed with a screw cap. The papers have a light purple tint and will keep for several months in an air tight container at room temperature. For use, a strip is removed, laid in a Petri dish and moistened with distilled water. The colony to be tested is picked up with a platinum loop and smeared over the moist area. A positive reaction is indicated by an intense purple hue appearing within 5 to 10 seconds, a delayed positive reaction by coloration in 10 to 60 seconds and a negative reaction by absence of coloration or by coloration later than 60 seconds.

Wet

A strip of filter paper is soaked with a little freshly made 1 percent solution of the reagent and then at once used by rubbing a speck of culture on it with a platinum loop. The result is read as for the dry filter paper method.

Precautions:
1. The reagent must be freshly prepared.
2. The bacterial growth must be transferred to the test paper with a clean platinum loop or a clean glass rod since traces of iron will catalyze the reaction and give false positive results.
3. Avoid testing from MacConkey's medium because a pink violet color is due to carry over from the medium and is not a true oxidase reaction. The true reaction gives an intense purple hue.
4. The tetramethyl derrivative of p-phenylene diamine is recommended because the reagent is more stable in storage and is more efficient for the detection of cytochrome oxidase and less toxic than the dimethyl derrivative.

Oxidase Positive Organisms

- *Neisseria spp*
- *Vibrio spp*
- *Pseudomonas*

- *Alcaligenes faecalis*
- *Aeromonas*
- *Campylobacter.*

PPA Test

Introduction: Phenylalanine is an amino acid that upon deamination forms a ketoacid-phenyl pyruvic acid. This requires the enzyme deaminase. Members of the *Proteus, Morganella* and *Providencia* genera possess the deaminase enzyme.

Principle: The phenylalanine test depends upon the detection of phenyl pyruvic acid in the test medium after growth of the test organism. Phenyl pyruvic acid reacts with ferric chloride to form a green colored complex.

Media and Reagents: The phenylalanine agar is poured as a slant into a tube.

Constituents:
- DL-Phenylalanine
- Yeast extract
- Sodium chloride
- Disodium hydrogen phosphate
- Agar
- Distilled water.

Procedure: The agar slant of the medium is inoculated with a single colony of the test organism isolated in pure culture. After incubation at 35°C for 18 to 24 hours 4 to 5 drops of the ferric chloride reagent are added directly to the surface of the agar. As reagent is added, the tube is rotated to dislodge the surface colonies.

Interpretation: Immediate appearance of an intense green color indicates the presence of phenyl pyruvic acid.

Controls:
- Positive—*Proteus*
- Negative—*E.coli*

Catalase Test

Principle: This demonstrates the presence of catalase, an enzyme that catalyzes the release of oxygen from hydrogen peroxide.

Method: There are two methods to demonstrate catalase.

a. 1 ml of H_2O_2 is poured over a 24 hours nutrient agar slope culture of the test organism and the tube is held in a slanting position. If bubbles are formed, it indicates the presence of catalase.
b. A drop of H_2O_2 is taken on a slide. With the help of a cover slip, a bit of the colony is scraped and placed on the drop. The development of bubbles under the edge of the cover slip demonstrates the presence of enzyme catalase.

Controls:
- Positive—*Staphylococcus*
- Negative—*Streptococcus*

A false positive reaction may be obtained if the culture medium contains catalase, e.g. blood agar or if an iron wire loop is used.

Combined Test—TSI (Triple Sugar Iron)

Introduction: Triple sugar iron medium has three sugars—glucose, lactose and sucrose. It is a combined test to indicate the ability of a bacteria to breakdown either glucose or all the sugars with or without gas. It also indicates the presence of H_2S. It can be used in addition to individual sugar tests or can be used instead of them when facilities are not available to include the sugar tests.

Principle: The concentration of glucose is one-tenth of that of lactose or sucrose. So, the amount of acid produced by the fermentation of only glucose is less as compared to the acid produced when all the three sugars are fermented.

Phenol red is the indicator. If the acid is produced it turns the color of the medium yellow. The test medium is poured as a slant. Depending on the color change in the slant or the butt the interpretation of the medium is done. The uninoculated medium is light orange in color. There are special chemicals to detect the presence of H_2S.

Media: The media has the following chemicals:
- Peptone
- NaCl
- Lactose

- Sucrose
- Glucose
- Ferric ammonium citrate
- Sodium thiosulphate
- Phenol red
- Agar.

Interpretation: There can be three situations.

If there is no fermentation of any sugar: If there is no fermentation of any sugar then peptones are broken down aerobically to amino acids shifting the pH to alkaline direction and in the presence of phenol red the color of the medium changes to red on the slant. There is no change in the butt, because, anaerobic environment exists here and peptones are broken down anaerobically to a lesser extent (Fig. 10.1).

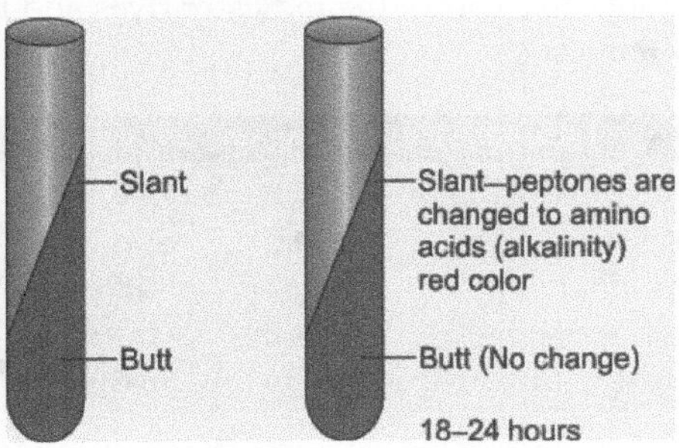

Fig. 10.1: Uninoculated medium

Examples
- *Pseudomonas*
- *Acinetobacter*
- *Alkaligenes faecalis.*

If only glucose is fermented: Glucose is present in lesser quantity. Hence, it is fermented but it gets finished. So in the first 6 to 12 hours, there is yellow color throughout but later on after 18 to 24 hours the peptones change to amino acids producing alkalinity and the acidity produced is counteracted at the slant. Therefore we get red color. Anaerobically peptone breakdown is less and is not enough to counteract the acid produced. So after 18 to 24 hours we get red color at the slant with yellow at the butt (Fig. 10.2).

If H_2S is produced we can suspect salmonella except *Salmonella paratyphi* A. If no H_2S is produced then shigella should be suspected.

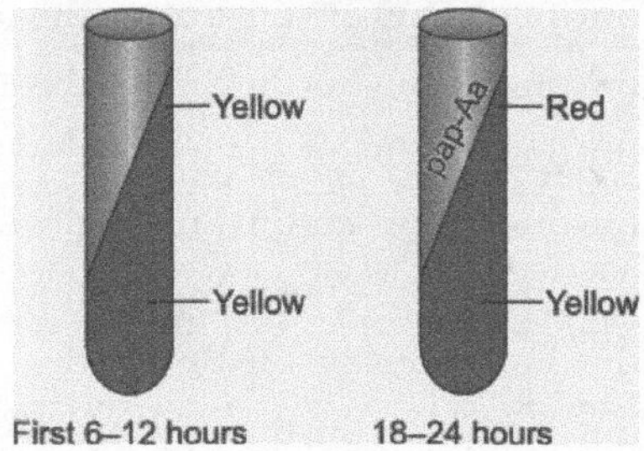

Fig. 10.2: If glucose is fermented

If all the three sugars are fermented: If all the three sugars are fermented, the total tube is yellow. This is in case of *Escherichia coli* and *Klebsiella spp* (Fig. 10.3).

If H_2S is positive too we should suspect *Proteus vulgaris* and *Proteus mirabilis.*

The results should be read at 18 to 24 hours. If more than 48 hours have passed the slant turns red due to utilization of peptone.

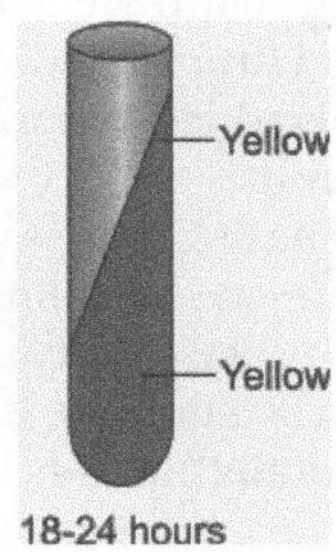

Fig. 10.3: If all the three sugars are fermented

Detection of H_2S: H_2S is a colorless gas and an indicator is necessary for its identification.

H_2S + Sodium thiosulphate + ferric ammonium citrate = Black precipitate of ferrous sulphide.

Coagulase Test

Principle: Coagulase is an enzyme found in *Staphylococcus aureus* which has the property of clotting human or rabbit plasma. It takes the help of a coagulase reacting factor (CRF) and converts the fibrinogen present in plasma to fibrin. Clotting does not occur with the plasma of certain species (e.g. guinea pig) because they lack CRF.

Types of coagulase: There are two types of coagulase enzyme-free and bound (Table 10.1).

Table 10.1: Types of coagulase	
Free coagulase	*Bound coagulase*
• It is a heat labile enzyme secreted free into the medium	• It is a heat stable constituent of the cell wall
• The tube coagulase detects the free coagulase	• The slide test detects the bound coagulase
• Requires CRF for its action	• Does not require CRF for its action
• Seven antigenic types are described	• Only one antigenic type is identified.

Method

Slide Method

- Detects bound coagulase.
- Pick up few colonies of the bacteria from an agar culture and emulsify in two drops of saline placed on a slide.
- After verifying that there is no spontaneous agglutination, a drop of undiluted human/or rabbit plasma is added to one of the emulsions and mixed gently.
- Prompt clumping in (5 to 10 sec) of the organism indicates the presence of bound coagulase.

False positive tests are caused by citrate utilizing bacteria such as *Enterococci* and *Pseudomonas*. In doubtful cases tube test should be done.

Tube Test: The tube test detects free coagulase.

Approximately 0.1 mL of an overnight broth culture or an agar culture suspension of the organism is added to 0.5 mL of citrated, oxalated or heparinized human/rabbit plasma (diluted 1 in 5 with saline) in a narrow test tube. Diluted plasma alone in a similar tube serves as a control. The tubes are incubated in a water bath at 37°C for 3 to 6 hours. If positive the plasma clots and does not flow when the tube is inverted. The grading is given as follows:

+ 4 → The clot remains in place when inverted
+ 3 → Large clots
+ 2 → Small clots
Negative → Free flowing

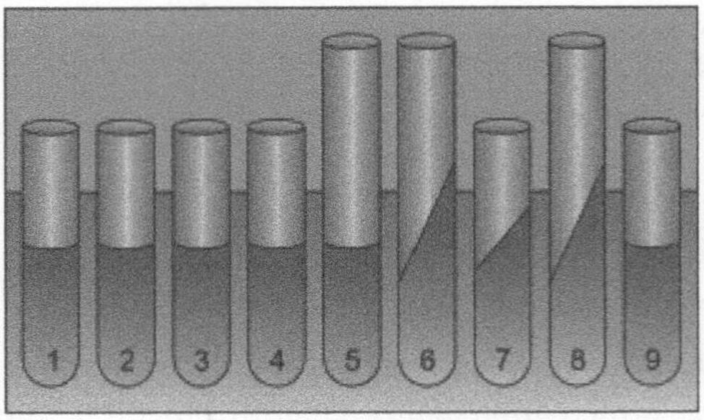

Fig. 10.4: (1) Glucose, (2) Lactose, (3) Sucrose, (4) Mannitol, (5) Peptone water for Indole test, (6) Citrate, (7) Urease, (8) TSI, (9) PPA test

Complete Sugar Set

The following is the usual sugar set used for biochemical testing (Fig. 10.4).

Table 10.2 shows the indicator dyes and the pH ranges.

Table 10.2: Indicator dyes and pH range	*pH range*	*Acid-alkaline*
Methyl red	4.4–6.2	Red-yellow
Phenol red	6.8–8.4	Yellow-pink
Bromocresol purple	5.2–6.8	Yellow-violet
Bromothymol blue	6.0–7.6	Yellow-blue

ANTIGENIC CHARACTERS

In bacteriology, species and types can often be identified by specific antibody reactions. These antibodies are raised in animals and used for diagnosis of an unknown bacterium.

TYPING OF BACTERIA

A single bacterial species with a particular set of pathogenic activities may include strains of different types that differ in minor characters. Recognition of the type of strain isolated from a patient may be of epidemiological value in tracing sources of infection and the various modes of spread of infection. There are various methods to type bacteria:

- When we distinguish them on the basis of biochemical reactions (metabolic characteristics) we call them biotypes.

- When we distinguish them on the basis of serological reactions (antigenic characteristics) we call them serotypes.
- Another important method of typing is by testing the susceptibility of a bacterial culture to lysis by of a set of type specific lytic bacteriophages. This is called phage typing. The phage type of the culture is identified according to its pattern of susceptibility to the different phages.
- Bacteriocins are naturally occurring antibacterial substances produced by many members of the family *Enterobacteriaceae* and some other bacteria. They are active mainly against strains of the same genus. Depending upon the ability of the strains of bacteria to produce one or other of a series of bacteriocins we type them into bacteriocin types. This is especially useful for strains which are serologically homogenous. They are used for subtyping *Shigella sonnei* and *Pseudomonas aeruginosa* isolates.

ANIMAL PATHOGENICITY AND TOXIGENICITY

Pathogenic bacteria produce characteristic lesions in lab animals. Based on this, we can identify the organism. In cases where a specific toxin is involved in the mechanism of pathogenesis, we can inoculate the culture material of the suspected bacterium into the animal to look for it's toxicity. It is specially used for *Corynebacterium diphtheriae*, *Clostridium tetani* and *Mycobacterium tuberculosis*.

MOLECULAR BIOLOGY TECHNIQUES

Special molecular biology techniques are used to diagnosis certain bacteria like *Mycobacterium tuberculosis* from clinical samples. These include the PCR (Polymerase chain reaction) which magnifies the DNA of the bacteria if present and makes it easier to diagnose.

ANTIBIOTIC SENSITIVITY TEST

The bacterium is grown on nutrient agar or Mueller Hinton agar and its growth is tested by adding the paper discs containing antibiotics. If the antibiotic kills the bacteria, they do not grow and this is called the zone of inhibition. These antibiotics are suitable for treatment. Antibiotic sensitivity test helps us in treatment and also serves as an epidemiological marker.

PS—There is no need for students to memorize the constituents of the media used for biochemical tests.

CHAPTER

11

Infection

LESSON PLAN

INTRODUCTION

Microorganisms are divided into saprophytes and parasites based on their relationship with the host.

Saprophytes

Saprophytes (Sapros-Decayed, Phyton-Plant) are free living microbes that live on dead or decaying organic matter. They are found in soil and water and play an important role in the degradation of organic materials in nature. They do not generally multiply in living tissues and are of not much importance in disease. When they infect humans who have low immunity they are called opportunistic.

Parasites

Parasites are microbes that can multiply and establish themselves in the host. Parasitic microbes may be **pathogens** or **commensals**. Pathogens produce diseases in the host but commensal microbes live in complete harmony with the host without causing damage to it. The normal bacterial flora is mostly of commensals. Many commensals behave as facultative pathogens or opportunistic pathogens and produce diseases only when host resistance is lowered.

WHAT IS INFECTION?

Infection means the lodgement and multiplication of a parasite in or on the tissues of a host. It does not always result in disease.

CLASSIFICATION OF INFECTIONS

- *Primary infection*: Initial infection with a parasite in a host is called primary infection.
- *Re-infection*: Subsequent infections by the same parasite in the host are called re-infections.
- *Secondary infection*: When in a host whose resistance is lowered by a preexisting infectious disease, a new parasite sets up infection, it is called secondary infection. This is also known as superinfection. Examples are the bacterial infection in a preexisting viral infection or tuberculosis in an AIDS patient.
- *Focal infection*: Focal infection indicates a condition where the infection is at a local site such as appendix or tonsils.
- *Cross infection*: When a patient is already suffering from disease, a new infection is set up from another host or an external source it is termed cross infection.
- *Nosocomial infection*: Cross infections occurring in hospitals are called nosocomial or hospital acquired infection.
- *Based on the source of infection*: Depending on whether the source of infection is from the host's own body or from external sources, infections are classified as *endogenous* or *exogenous*, respectively.
- Based on the clinical effect of infections they may be classified into:
  - Inapparent infection is one where clinical effects are not apparent or not seen. It is also called subclinical infection.
  - Atypical infection is one in which the typical clinical manifestations of a disease are not present.
  - Latent infection is one in which some parasites following infection remain in the tissues in a latent or hidden form. They multiply and produce clinical disease when host resistance is lowered. This is termed as latent infection.

SOURCES OF INFECTION

The various sources of infection for a man could be:

a. Man b. Animals
c. Insects d. Food
e. Water f. Soil

We shall discuss this one by one.

Man

The commonest source of infection for a man is another man. He can be a patient who is suffering from the disease or a carrier. A carrier is a person who harbors the pathogenic microorganism without suffering from any ill effect.

A healthy carrier is one who harbors the pathogens but has never suffered from the disease caused by the pathogen.

A convalescent carrier is one who has recovered from the disease but continues to have that pathogen in his body. Depending on how long a particular person has had the pathogen they can be classified as temporary or chronic carriers. The temporary carrier state lasts less than 6 months while chronic carrier state may last for several years or even for one's complete life (Flow chart 11.1).

Flow chart 11.1: Man as a source of infection

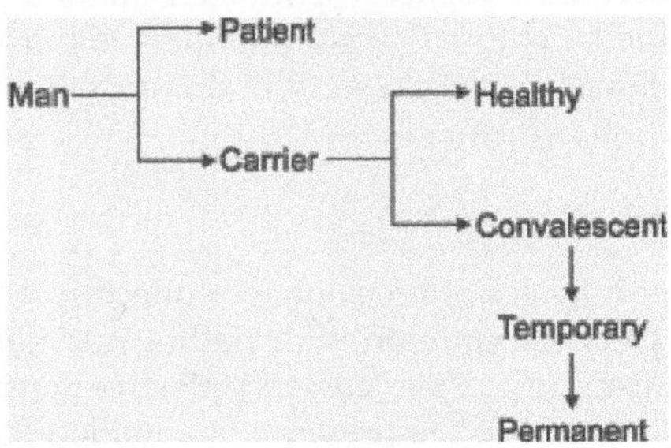

Animals

Many pathogens are able to infect both animals and man. Animals may therefore act as sources of infection. Infectious diseases transmitted from animals to man are called zoonosis. In some cases the infection in animals may be asymptomatic and they serve to maintain the parasite in nature and acts as a resevoir of human infection.

Zoonotic diseases may be:
- Bacterial (Plague from rats)
- Viral (Rabies from dogs)
- Protozoal (Leishmaniasis from dogs)
- Helminthic (Hydatid disease from dogs)
- Fungal (Dermatophytosis from cats/dogs)

Insects

Blood sucking insects may transmit pathogens to man. The diseases so caused are called arthropod borne diseases.

Insects such as mosquitoes, ticks, mites, fleas and lice that transmit specific infections are called vectors.

Vectors may be of two types:

Mechanical vectors: Transmission of dysentery or typhoid by domestic fly.

Biological vectors: These are vectors in which the pathogen multiplies and undergoes a part of the developmental cycle, e.g. *Aedes aegypti* mosquito in yellow fever and *Anopheles* in malaria. Some insects maintain the infection in nature, e.g. ticks in relapsing fever and spotted fevers.

Food

Contaminated food materials may act as sources of infection. Presence of pathogens in food may be due to external contamination, e.g. (food poisoning by *Staphylococcus*) or due to preexistent infection in meat.

Water

Water may act as the source of infection either due to contamination with pathogenic micro-organisms (e.g., *Vibrio cholerae*, infective hepatitis virus) or due to the presence of aquatic vectors (e.g. cyclops in guinea worm infection).

Soil

Some pathogens survive in soil for a long period. Examples are spores of tetanus bacillus, fungus and parasites such as roundworm and hookworm.

METHODS OF TRANSMISSION OF INFECTION

Contact

Diseases can be transmitted by direct contact as in syphilis and gonorrhoea or indirect contact by fomites which means non-living objects like clothing, toys, pencils or face towels which can transmit infection. An example of this would be Influenza illnesses where droplets fall on the surface of objects can be transmitted to persons coming in contact.

Inhalation

Respiratory infections such as influenza and tuberculosis are transmitted by inhalation of the pathogen. These microbes are shed into the environment by patients through secretions from the nose or throat. During sneezing, speaking or coughing large drops of secretions fall to the ground and dry there and some of the pathogens remain viable in the dust. Smaller droplets under 0.1 mm in diameter evaporate immediately and become droplet nuclei usually 1 to 10 μ in diameter which remain suspended in air for long periods acting as sources of infection.

Ingestion

Intestinal infections are generally acquired by the ingestion of food or drink contaminated with the pathogens.

Infection transmitted by ingestion may be water borne (cholera), food borne (food poisoning), or hand borne (dysentery).

Inoculation

Pathogens in some instances may be inoculated directly into the tissues of the host. Tetanus spores implanted in the depth of wounds, rabies virus deposited subcutaneously by dog bites and arboviruses injected by insect vectors are examples. Serum hepatitis and AIDS is transmitted by transfusion of contaminated blood.

Insects

May act as mechanical or biological vectors of infectious disease.

Congenital

Some pathogens are able to cross the placental barrier and infect the fetus in utero. This is known as vertical transmission. For examples, rubella virus, syphilis, toxoplasma, herpes virus, etc.

Iatrogenic and Laboratory Infections

Infection can sometimes be transmitted during procedures such as injections, lumbar puncture and catheterization. Other methods of treatment such as exchange transfusion, dialysis, heart and transplant surgery increase the possibilities of getting infections. Laboratory personnel handling infectious materials are at risk and special care should be taken to prevent lab infection.

OUTCOME OF AN INFECTION

The outcome of an infection will depend on the interaction between microbial factors which predispose to pathogenicity and host factors which contribute to resistance.

FACTORS WHICH CONTRIBUTE TO MICROBIAL PATHOGENICITY

The terms pathogenicity and virulence refer to the ability of a microbe to produce disease or tissue injury. The difference between them is that pathogenicity refers to the ability of a microbial species to produce disease while the term virulence is applied to the same property in a strain of microorganism. Virulence is not constant and may undergo changes. When it increases it is called exaltation and when it decreases it is called attenuation.

Virulence in turn is dependent on various factors.

Adhesion

The initial event in the pathogenesis of many infections is the attachment (adhesion) of the bacteria to body surfaces. The bacteria have special adhesive structures called adhesins. Adhesions may be fimbriae or colonization factors. They attach to special receptors present on the surface of the epithelial cells. Adhesins are virulence factors and loss of adhesins makes the strain avirulent. Adhesins are antigenic and specific immunization can be given against them.

Invasiveness

This indicates the ability of an organism to spread in the host tissue after establishing infection. Highly invasive pathogens produce generalized lesions while less invasive pathogens cause more localized lesions (staphylococcal abscess).

Toxigenicity

Bacteria produce two types of toxins—exotoxins and endotoxins.

Exotoxins are heat labile proteins which are secreted by certain species of bacteria and diffuse readily into the surrounding medium. They are mostly produced by gram-positive bacteria.

Endotoxins are heat stable polysaccharide-protein-lipid complexes which forms an integral part of the cell wall of gram-negative bacteria. Their toxicity depends on lipid component (lipid A).

The differences between the two are given in Table 11.1.

Communicability

The ability of a parasite to spread from one host to another is called communicability. Infections in which the pathogen is shed in secretions as in respiratory and intestinal diseases are highly communicable. When a microorganism is virulent as well as possesses communicability it can cause pandemics and epidemics.

Other Bacterial Products

Other bacterial products may contribute to virulence by inhibiting the mechanisms of host resistance. Examples of these are coagulase, fibrinolysin, hyaluronidases, hemolysins, etc.

Table 11.1: Differences between exotoxins and endotoxins

Exotoxins	*Endotoxins*
1. Proteins	Protein-polysaccharide-lipid complexes
2. Heat labile	Heat stable
3. Actively secreted by cells; diffuse into surrounding medium	Form part of cell wall, do not diffuse into surrounding medium
4. Readily separable from cultures by physical means such as filtration	Obtained only by cell lysis
5. Specific pharmacological effect for each toxin	Effect nonspecific, action common to all endotoxins
6. Specific tissue affinities	No specific tissue affinity
7. Action enzymic	No enzymatic action
8. Highly antigenic	Weakly antigenic
9. Active is very minute doses	Active only in very large doses
10. Action specifically neutralized by antibody	Neutralization by antibody ineffective
11. Can be toxoided	Cannot be toxoided
12. Produced mainly by gram-positive bacteria but also negative bacteria such as *Shigella, Cholera* and *enterotoxigenic Escherichia coli.*	Produced by Gram-negative bacteria

Bacterial Appendages

Capsulated bacteria such as *Pneumococci, Klebsiella pneumoniae* and *Haemophilus influenzae* are not readily phagocytosed. Some bacteria have surface antigens such as the Vi antigen of *S. typhi* and K antigens of *Escherichia coli*. They help the bacteria to withstand phagocytosis and lytic activity of the complement.

TYPES OF INFECTIOUS DISEASES

Infectious diseases may be localized or generalized. Localized infections may be superficial or deepseated. Generalized infection involves the spread of the infecting agent through lymphatics or blood stream.

Circulation of bacteria in the blood is known as bacteremia. Temporary bacteremia is a very common event, even in healthy individuals. The bacteria are immediately mopped up by phagocytic cells and are unable to initiate infection.

Bacteremia of greater severity and longer duration is seen during generalized infections as in typhoid fever.

Septicemia is the condition where bacteria circulate and multiply in the blood, form toxic products and cause high swinging type of fever. Pyemia is a condition where pyogenic bacteria produce septicemia with multiple abscesses in internal organs such as spleen, liver and kidneys.

Depending on the spread of infectious diseases in the community, they may be classified into different types:

- Endemic diseases are those which are constantly present in a particular area, e.g. typhoid fever.
- Epidemic disease is one that spreads rapidly involving many people in an area at the same time.
- Pandemic is an epidemic that spreads through many areas of the world involving very large numbers of persons within a short period. Influenza, cholera, plague and viral conjunctivitis are pandemic diseases.

CHAPTER

12

Antibiotic Sensitivity Test

LESSON PLAN

- Introduction
- Definition of Antibiotic Sensitivity Test (AST)
- Aim of AST
- Limitation of AST
- Other uses of AST
- Types of Sensitivity Tests
  - Diffusion Tests
  - Dilution Test

INTRODUCTION

The main aim of bacterial culture is to diagnose the pathogenic bacteria which cause the infection, but diagnosis is not enough because we have to cure the infection. For that, we have to give appropriate drugs. The drugs or medicines that act against bacteria are called antibiotics. But we cannot use any antibiotic against any bacteria because bacteria are sensitive to or get killed only by a particular group of antibiotics. To find out which antibiotics kill a particular pathogenic bacteria, we perform an antibiotic sensitivity test which determines the sensitivity or resistance pattern of a bacteria to the various antibiotics.

DEFINITION OF ANTIBIOTIC SENSITIVITY TEST

An antibiotic sensitivity is an *in vitro* test to determine the sensitivity or resistance of a particular bacterium to the group of antibiotics that we have tested. In other words it finds out which antibiotic can kill the test bacteria and cure the infection.

AIM OF ANTIBIOTIC SENSITIVITY TEST

The aim of antibiotic sensitivity test is to prescribe antibiotics which can kill the bacteria and cure the infection. The appropriate antibiotic should produce at the site of infection a concentration high enough to kill or inhibit the growth of the pathogenic bacteria without having a significant toxic effect.

The different strains of a few pathogenic species have constant sensitivity characters like *Streptococcus pyogenes* but strains of most pathogenic bacteria have to be tested each time.

LIMITATION OF ANTIBIOTIC SENSITIVITY TEST

We must remember that the *in vitro* antibiotic sensitivity test may not always reflect the same results as *in vivo*. Therefore, treatment given to a particular pathogen found sensitive to a drug *in vitro* may fail because the drug is not properly absorbed by the patient or it is unable to penetrate in an effective concentration. Therefore, the results of an antibiotic sensitivity test should be viewed along with the clinical response of the patient.

OTHER USES OF ANTIBIOTIC SENSITIVITY TEST

1. The accumulated results of sensitivity tests tell us the treatment we should start for a particular bacterial infection before the results of tests on the individual patients strains are available. Thus, we can save valuable time.
2. Sensitivity tests also are the main way in which we can assess the potential value of new antimicrobial drugs before they are put to clinical trial.
3. Antibiotic sensitivity test results enable us to adjust the dosage level of antibiotics.

If the antibiotic taken by the patient, has toxic effects on the body, its dosage schedule can be adjusted by doing repeated in vitro antibiotic sensitivity tests and keeping the concentration at a nontoxic but effective level.

TYPES OF SENSITIVITY TESTS

Antibiotic sensitivity tests are of two types:

- Diffusion
- Dilution.

Diffusion Tests

The diffusion method is the most widely used test for routine sensitivity testing of isolates from patients.

Principle

Here the drug is allowed to diffuse through a solid medium so that a gradient is established, the concentration being highest near the site of application of the drug and decreasing with distance. The test bacterium is seeded on the medium and its sensitivity to the drug is determined by inhibition of its growth. The drug is incorporated into discs and applied on the surface of the medium.

Two types of disc diffusion tests are used:

1. Stokes' method
2. Kirby-Bauer's method.

Stokes' Method

This is a comparative method in which we divide the culture plate into three parts. In the central portion is plated the control organism and on the other two sides, the test organism. The area where no bacterium grows after overnight incubation is called the zone of inhibition. The report of sensitive, resistant or intermediate resistant is given after comparing the zone of inhibitions of the test and the control organisms.

Preparation of Discs: Whatman no. 1 filter paper is used. 6 mm diameter filter paper discs are cut out. They are arranged in a big plate and sterilized by the hot air oven. Sterile antibiotic solutions are then prepared and 0.01 mL of antibiotic solutions is then put on the discs using a sterile syringe. Commercially prepared antibiotic discs can also be used. These should be stored in a refrigerator between 4 to 8°C and brought to room temperature before use.

Preparation of bacterial inoculum: The bacterial inoculum should ideally give an evenly spread growth. Too heavy an inoculum reduces the size of the inhibition zones produced by many antibiotics, too light an inoculum makes the zone diameters difficult to read. The inoculum should be prepared from material picked up with a loop from 5 to 10 colonies of the species to be tested. The density of the inoculum is prepared with Mcfarland standard 0.5. It should be inoculated into peptone water and incubated for 4 to 6 hours.

Method of inoculation: The inoculum can be distributed evenly over the test plate by flooding the plate with the bacterial suspension and drying its surface while it is in horizontal position before applying the antibiotic discs. This method is time consuming, hence it is not done. We normally take a sterile swab dipped into the suspension squeezed free from excess fluid against the side of the tube and rub it over the plate in the form of a lawn culture on the upper and lower thirds of the plate. The standard strain is inoculated over the middle thirds of the plate, uninoculated gaps 2 to 3 mm wide are left to separate the test from the control areas.

Medium used for antibiotic sensitivity test: Mueller Hinton agar—This medium was originally formulated for the isolation of pathogenic *Neisseria* species, but nowadays it is more commonly used for antibiotic sensitivity patterns. Nutrient agar can also be used alternatively in Stokes' method.

The composition of Mueller Hinton is as follows:

- Beef infusion 300 mL
- Casein hydrolysate 17.5 g
- Starch 1.5 g
- Agar 10 g
- Distilled water 1 liter

Emulsify the starch in a small amount of cold water, pour into the beef infusion and add the casein hydrolysate and the agar. Make up the volume to one liter with distilled water. Dissolve the constituents by heating gently at 100°C with agitation filter if required. Adjust the pH to 7.4. Dispense in screw capped bottles and sterilize by autoclaving at 121°C × 20 min. Pour plates.

Control strains: Four control strains are usually recommended for use with the comparative method.

- *Escherichia coli* NCTC (10418) for tests of coliform bacilli from the urinary tract.
- *Pseudomonas aeruginosa* NCTC (10662) for tests of this species.
- *Clostridium perfringens* NCTC (11229) for tests of clostridia against metronidazole and other anticlostridial antibiotics.
- *Staphylococcus aureus* NCTC (6571) for gram-positive cocci.

Interpretation of stokes' method: The basic principle of Stokes' method is based on the comparison between the zone of inhibition of the test and the control organism. The following rules are to be kept in mind (Fig. 12.1).

1. The control strain should show a zone of inhibition to all the antibiotics. If not then we should check whether the antibiotic itself is not working or that the control strain is contaminated.
2. If the zone of inhibition (ZI) of the test strain is less than 3 mm, then the test strain is resistant to that particular antibiotic and the antibiotic will have no effect on it.
3. If the zone of inhibition of the test strain is > 3 mm the test strain is sensitive to that antibiotic.

There are subgroups within this group:

Sensitive

The test organism is sensitive to the antibiotic if the following conditions are fulfilled.

1. If ZI of test organism = ZI of control organism (4).
2. If ZI of test organism is > that of control organism (3).
3. If ZI of test organism < ZI of control but the difference between the two is < 3 mm (5).

Intermediate Resistant

The ZI of test organism is < ZI of control and the difference is > 3 mm.

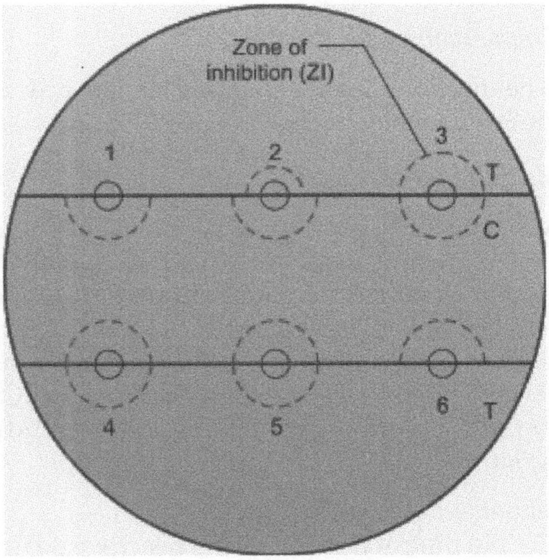

Fig. 12.1: Diagram showing interpretation of Stokes method *(For color version see Plate 1)*

C = Control; T = Test; ZI = Zone of inhibition; 1 = Resistant; 2 = Intermediate resistant; 3 = Sensitive; 4 = Sensitive; 5 = Sensitive; 6 = Resistant

How to Take the Reading?

The zone of inhibition is the distance in mm from the edge of the disc to the zone edge (if that is clear). If the zone of inhibition is not very clear it is measured to the point of 80 percent inhibition of growth. The measurement should be made with the help of a scale or a vernier calliper. The width of the zone outside the disc is measured.

Advantage of Stokes' Method

1. Since the control is taken into account, it produces dependable results.
2. We can always detect whether the antibiotic disc is working because if not, it will not give a zone of inhibition in the control.

Kirby-Bauer Method

The Kirby-Bauer method is the official method of the USA Food and Drugs Administration. Here the principle is the same but the method of interpretation is different. Discs of high content of antibiotic are placed on an inoculum of strictly standardized density on Mueller Hinton agar.

Preparation of the Inoculum

The inoculum is prepared in a similar way as for Stoke's method.

Method of Inoculation

A lawn culture is prepared on Mueller Hinton agar plate and discs are placed in a circular fashion leaving a minimum distance of 20 mm between two adjacent discs.

The zones of inhibition of the test organisms are compared to the standard charts of the ICS method (International Collaborative Study Group).

Advantages of Kirby-Bauer method:

1. No control is required and hence we do not have to maintain it.
2. It is easy to interpret from standard charts and does not require expertise as in Stokes' method.

Disadvantage of Kirby-Bauer method: The Kirby-Bauer method uses no control. A control strain is sensitive to all the antibiotics and hence confirms the potency of the disc.

Therefore, in this method we cannot find out if the antibiotic disc is not working and it will give the same picture as resistance.

Dilution Test

In this method serial dilutions of antibiotic solutions are made and inoculated with over night broth culture of the test strain. The minimum inhibitory concentration of the antibiotic, that is the minimum concentration of the antibiotic which can kill the microorganism is calculated. The tests can be carried out in agar or broth. Dilution tests are not used routinely for determination of antibiotic sensitivity or resistance but only for standardization of procedures, or for regulation of therapeutic dose accurately.

Some Commonly Used Antibiotics

Depending on the clinical isolate a selection of antibiotics is made. The common antibiotics in use are:

1. Penicillin
2. Cloxacillin
3. Ampicillin
4. Cephalexin
5. Amoxacillin
6. Agumentin
7. Cephaloridine
8. Cefotaxime
9. Cefuroxime
10. Sparfloxacin
11. Ciprofloxacin
12. Ofloxacin
13. Lomefloxacin
14. Gentamicin
15. Amikacin

There are many others.

CHAPTER 13

Bacterial Genetics

LESSON PLAN

- Introduction
- Basic Principles of Molecular Biology
  - DNA
  - RNA
  - Extrachromosomal Genetic Elements
- Genotypic and Phenotypic Variation
- Mutation
  - Definition
  - Types of Mutation
- Transmission of Genetic Material
  - Transformation
  - Transduction
  - Conjugation
- Genetic Mechanisms of Drug Resistance in Bacteria
- Transposable Genetic Elements
- Genetic Engineering

INTRODUCTION

Genetics is that branch of science which deals with the study of heredity and variation and the principles that govern them. It helps us to understand the basis of resemblance between parents and children and also the differences between them. Like other organisms, bacteria basically remain the same and retain their characteristics from generation to generation, yet at the same time, show differences in some properties in a small proportion of their progeny. So, bacteria also obey the laws of genetics. With the growth of knowledge in genetics, a new branch of science called molecular biology has emerged.

BASIC PRINCIPLES OF MOLECULAR BIOLOGY

The basic principle of molecular biology is that DNA (deoxyribonucleic acid) carries genetic information which is transcribed on to RNA (ribonucleic acid) and then converted into polypeptides which form the enzymes and proteins.

Hence, the DNA is the store house of all information for protein synthesis.

Let us learn a bit about RNA and DNA.

DNA

The DNA molecule is made up of two chains of nucleotides wound together to form a right handed double helix. Each chain has a backbone of deoxyribose and phosphate residues arranged alternately. Attached to each deoxyribose sugar is one of four nitrogenous bases, the purines—adenine (A) and guanine (G) and the pyramidines-thymine (T) and cytosine (C). Adenine is always linked to thymine and guanine to cytosine (Figs 13.1 and 13.2).

Thus, they form complementary base pairs. There is hydrogen bonding between the bases on opposite strands. The ratio of each pair of bases, i.e. A + T/G + C. is constant for each

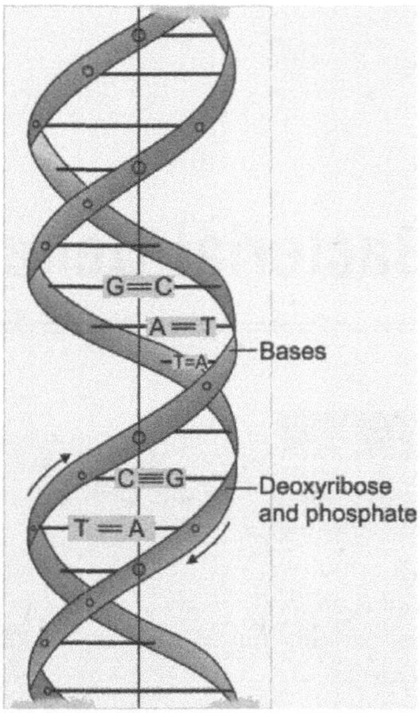

Fig. 13.1: DNA double helix

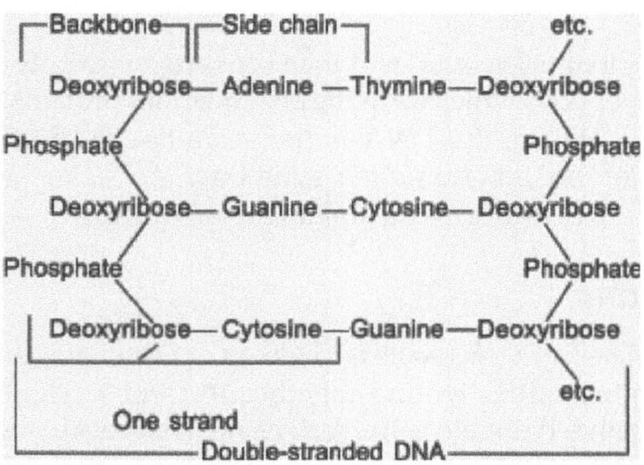

Fig. 13.2: A segment of double-stranded DNA illustrating its chemical structure

species but varies widely from one bacterial species to another. The DNA replicates by first unwinding at one end to form a fork, each strand of the fork acting as the template for the synthesis of a complementary strand with which it forms a double helix.

RNA

RNA is structurally similar to DNA except:

1. It contains the sugar ribose (instead of deoxyribose present in DNA).
2. It contains base uracil instead of thymine present in DNA.

Three types of RNA can be seen on the basis of structure and function:

- messenger RNA (m-RNA)
- ribosomal RNA (r-RNA)
- transfer RNA (t-RNA).

DNA acts as the template for the synthesis of m-RNA and so the bases are complementary to each other.

The genetic information in bacteria as in all cells is contained in the specific sequence of nucleotides in the cellular DNA. The sequence of nucleotides in the DNA determines the corresponding sequence of nucleotides in the RNA and this is translated into the appropriate sequence of amino acids by ribosomes. The sequence of amino acids in the resultant polypeptide chain in turn determines the specific configuration into which the chain folds itself while forming the completed molecule of protein. As we all know, the character of a cell is basically determined by the specific polypeptides that make up its enzymes and proteins and the genetic code is finally translated into proteins.

The unit of the code (codon) consists of a sequence of 3 bases, i.e. the code is triplet. Each codon specifies for a single amino acid, but more than one codon can exist for the same amino acid. Three codons (UAA, UAG, UGA) do not code for any amino acid and are called nonsense codons. They act as punctuation marks (stop codons) terminating the message for the synthesis of a polypeptide.

A segment of DNA carrying codons that specifies the production of a particular polypeptide chain is called a gene or cistron, which has hundreds to thousands of nucleotides.

The total complement of genes in a cell is called the cell's genome. Most bacteria contain enough DNA to code for the production of 1000 to 3000 genes.

In *Escherichia coli* which has been extensively studied, it has been found that the DNA is present as a single circular double stranded molecule about 1000 to 1300 μm long. The DNA is not associated with proteins and histones as in the eukaryotic cell.

Since, the DNA is 1000 times longer than the cell it is not arranged as a simple circle but in a coiled form. There are many differences in detail between the organization and control of DNA in prokaryotic and eukaryotic cells but basic functions are the same. The nuclear body is equivalent to the nucleus and the single circular molecule of naked DNA is the functional equivalent of a chromosome.

Eukaryotic cells have multiple chromosomes held together in a nuclear membrane and they have a complex mitotic apparatus for separating the two sets of chromosomes after replication. The advantage of the eukaryotic type of organization is that it can handle much more genetic information—this has permitted the evolution of complex multicellular organisms. Prokaryotic cells (haploid) have the advantages of simplicity, small size and rapid replication. In eukaryotes, several stretches of DNA that do not appear to function as codons occur between the coding sequences of genes. These useless noncoding intrusions are called introns while the structures of coding genes are called exons. During transcription, the genome is copied in its entirety, i.e. both introns and exons. The introns are then excised from the RNA copy before being translated by the ribosome into proteins.

Extrachromosomal Genetic Elements

- Besides the chromosomal DNA, bacteria may also have extrachromosomal genetic elements.
- They are called plasmids when they consist of DNA situated in the cytoplasm in the free state which reproduces independently.
- Genetic elements that exist in one of two alternate states either independently in the cytoplasm or integrated into the chromosome are called episomes.
- Plasmids and episomes are not essential for normal life and function of the host bacterium though they may give properties such as drug resistance and toxigenicity.
- Some plasmids can be transferred from one bacterium to another. They are called transmissible plasmids. They can be transmitted by either:
  1. Conjugation
  2. Transduction
- Some plasmids give the host cell the property of maleness or the ability to *conjugate* with other cells. Following conjugation, the recipient cell acquires the plasmid; becoming a male or donor cell in the process. The basis of becoming a male cell is the ability to forms special pili (sex pili) which are coded for by the plasmid. Sometimes plasmids are conveyed from cell to cell through the agency of bacteriophages. Transduction, for example, Penicillinase plasmid which induces penicillin resistance in *staphylococci* is an example of transducible plasmid.
- If we introduce genes from eukaryotic cells into plasmids they can replicate in *E. coli*. These are called recombinant DNA molecules which are powerful tools for genetic manipulation with application in medicine.

GENOTYPIC AND PHENOTYPIC VARIATION

The genotype: The sum total of genes that make up the genetic apparatus of a cell is called its genotype. The expression of the genotype is influenced by the environment.

The phenotype: It is the physical expression of the genotype in a given environment. A cell may exhibit different phenotypic expression in different environments.

The variations that occur in the phenotype are influenced by the environment, limited in range by the genotype, temporary and not heritable. On the other hand the genotypic variations are stable, heritable and not influenced by the environment. They may occur by:

1. Mutation
2. Genetic transfer or exchange—transformation, transduction, lysogenic conversion and conjugation.

How phenotypic variations influence genotype, is illustrated by regulation of enzyme induction. Studies by Jacob and Monod on the synthesis of betagalactosidase by *E. coli* led to the operon concept which explains the regulatory mechanism involving two types of genes—structural and regulatory. The genes determining the structure of a particular protein are called structural genes. The activity of structural genes is controlled by regulator genes which lie adjacent to them.

The lac operon is formed of three structural genes.

lac Z lac Y and lac A

These are arranged linearly and the regulator gene is lac I which codes for repressor gene which attaches to the operator (lac O) or the inducer (in this case)—lactose.

lac I	lac P	lac O	lac Z lac Y lac A
Regulator	Promoter	Operator	Structural genes (lac operon)

Regulator: Codes for repressor which can attach to lactose or to the operator

For transcription of RNA for enzyme synthesis, the RNA polymerase has to attach to the promoter region and travel along with the structural genes in sequence.

In the resting stage the repressor molecule is bound to the operator, preventing the passage of RNA polymerase from the promoter to the operon. The repressor molecule has an affinity for lactose, in the presence of which it leaves the operator region free enabling transcription to take place. When the lactose which is present is finished, the repressor again attaches to the operator switching off transcription.

The structural genes code for three enzymes:
- Betagalactosidase
- Galactoside permease
- Transacetylase.

MUTATION

Definition

Mutation is a random, undirected, heritable variation caused by an alteration in the nucleotide sequence at some point of the DNA of the cell. It may be due to addition, deletion or substitution of one or more bases.

The molecular mechanism of mutation is that during DNA replication, some error occurs while progeny strands are copied. Though mutation occurs spontaneously, its frequency is increased by several agents called mutagens such as UV rays, alkylating agents, acridine dyes, etc.

Mutation is a natural event, taking place all the time. Most mutations are either lethal or they affect some minor function that may not be expressed. Mutation is best expressed when it involves a function which can be readily observed. It is also of importance if it gives a survival advantage.

Mutation is influenced by the environment.

If a streptomycin resistant mutant develops in a patient under treatment with the drug, it multiplies selectively and replaces the original population. If the patient was not on treatment this would not happen.

Mutation occurs irrespective of the environment too. Mutation may affect any gene and hence may modify any character of the bacterium.

The practical importance of mutation lies in the drug resistance and development of live vaccines.

Types of Mutation

- Missense mutation—in which the triplet code is altered.
- Nonsense mutation—generates a nonsense codon.

- Transversion—subsitution of a purine for a pyramidine.
- Suppressor mutation—which suppresses the original mutation.
- Lethal mutation—which kills the bacteria.

Mutation rates of individual genes in bacteria are 10^{-2} to 10^{-10} per bacterium per cell division.

Mutation

1. *Frameshift mutation*: Caused by insertion on deletion of nucleotides that is not evenly divisible by three from a DNA sequence.

   Insertion: Mutations in which extra base pairs are inserted into a new place in the DNA.

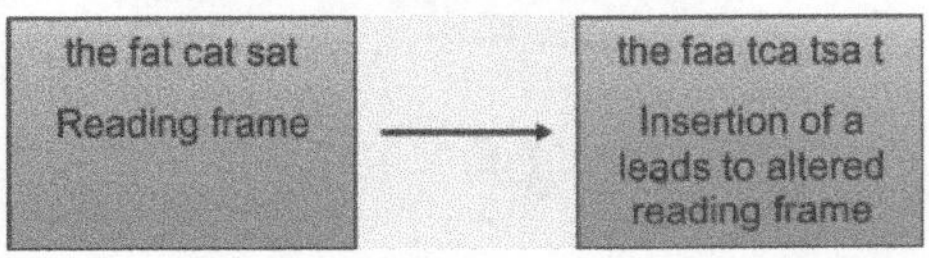

   Deletion: Mutation in which a section of DNA is lost or deleted.

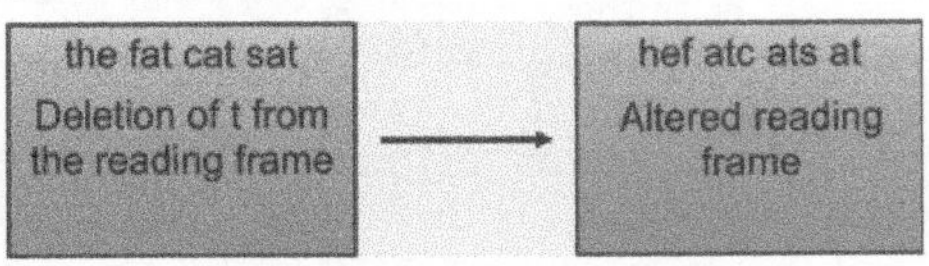

   Due to the triplet nature of gene expression by codons, the insertion or deletion can disrupt the reading frame, on the grouping of the codons, resulting in a completely different translation from the original. This usually generates truncated proteins that are useless and uninformative.

2. *Point mutation*: These are single-base substituions. Often caused by chemicals on malfunction of DNA replication, exchange a single nucleotide for another. There may be:
   - *Transitions*: A purine (A ↔ G) is replaced by a purine and a pyrimidine (C ↔ T) is replced by a pyrimidine.
   - *Transversion*: A purine (C/T↔A/G) is replaced by a pyrimidine and vice versa.

   Missense mutation: Point mutation where a single nucleotide is changed to cause substitution of a different amino acid.

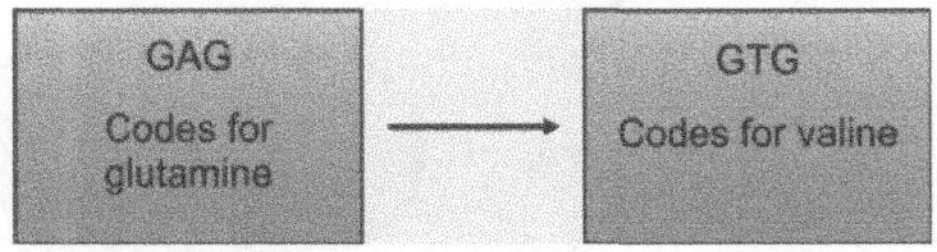

   Silent mutation: Occurs in an amino acid codon which results in the use of a similar amino acid.

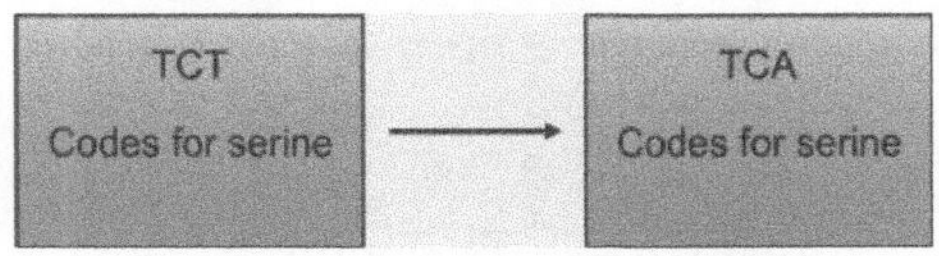

   Nonsense mutation: Point mutation in a sequence of DNA that results in a premature stop codon

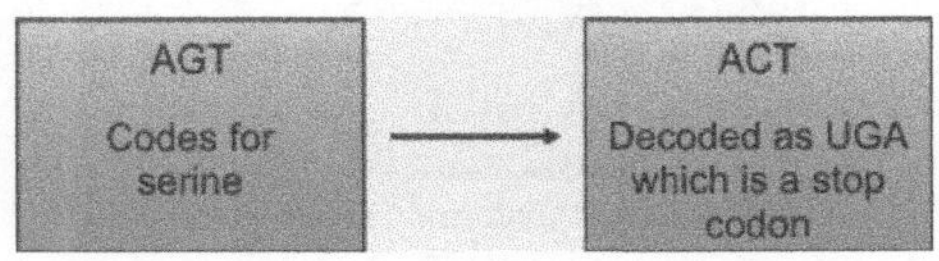

TRANSMISSION OF GENETIC MATERIAL

Mutation is the commonest source of genetic variation in bacteria, but in addition, the genome may be changed by acquisition of DNA from outside the cell.

Transformation

Transformation is the transfer of genetic information through the introduction of free DNA (Fig. 13.3).

In some species, free DNA either extracted artificially or released by lysis from the cells of one strain may be taken up directly by the cells of another strain.

It was the first example of genetic exchange in bacteria to be discovered. Griffith in 1928 found that mice died when injected with a mixture of live noncapsulated pneumococci and heat killed capsulated pneumococci. Neither of them was separately fatal.

Avery, Mcleod and McCarty in 1944 identified that DNA was the transforming factor.

Transformation has been studied in *Pneumococci, Bacillus* and *H. influenzae* though it may occur in other bacteria also. Pieces of DNA involved in transformation may carry 10 to 50 genes.

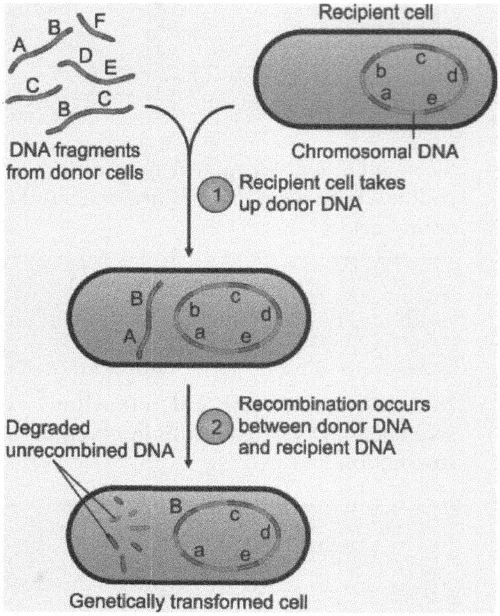

Fig. 13.3: Process of transformation

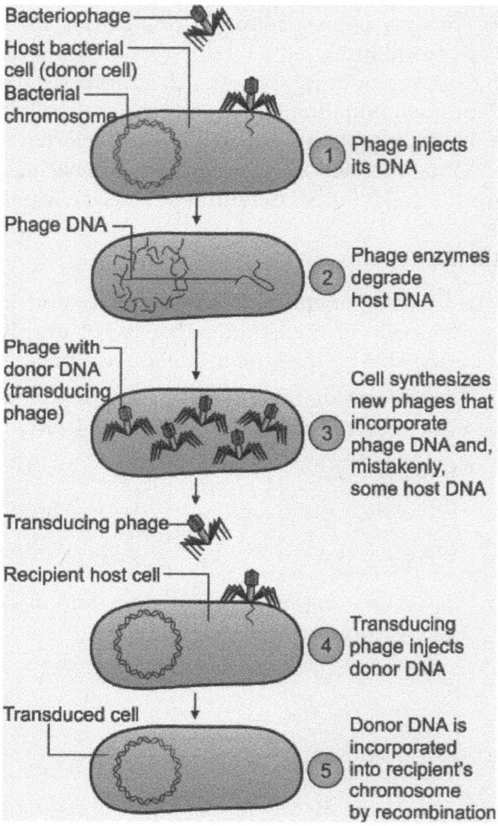

Fig. 13.4: Process of generalized transduction

Transduction

The transfer of a portion of the DNA from one bacterium to another by bacteriophages is known as transduction (Fig. 13.4).

Bacteriophages are viruses that parasitize bacteria and consist of a nucleic acid core and a protein coat. During assembly of bacteriophage progeny inside infected bacteria, packaging errors may happen occasionally. A phage particle may have at its core besides its own nucleic acid, a segment of the host DNA. When this particle infects another bacterium, it transfers the host DNA and the recipient cell acquires new characters coded by the donor DNA.

Transduction may be:

1. Generalized
2. Restricted

Generalized transduction: It involves any segment of the donor DNA. *Restricted transduction* may involve transfer of only a particular genetic tract.

Transduction may involve transfer of chromosomal DNA, episomes or plasmids. The plasmids determining penicillin resistance in staphylococci are transferred from cell to cell by transduction.

Transduction is the most widespread mechanism of gene transfer among *Prokaryotes* and also an excellent tool for the genetic mapping of bacteria.

Lysogenic Conversion

Bacteriophages have two types of life cycle. In the virulent or lytic cycle, large numbers of phages are built inside the host bacterium which ruptures to release them.

In the temperate or nonlytic cycle, the host bacterium is unharmed. The phage DNA becomes integrated with the bacterial chromosome as the prophage which multiples with the host DNA and is transferred to the daughter cells. This process is called lysogeny and the bacteria harbouring prophages are called lysogenic bacteria. Lysogeny is extremely frequent in nature.

This prophage codes for new characters. The process by which the prophage DNA confers genetic information to a bacterium is called lysogenic or phage conversion. In transduction the phage acts only as a vehicle carrying bacterial genes from one cell to another but in lysogenic conversion the phage DNA is the new genetic element. The lysogenic conversion in diphtheria bacilli helps acquire toxigenicity and therefore virulence by phage beta. Elimination of the phage from a toxigenic strain renders it nontoxigenic.

Conjugation

Definition

Conjugation in bacteria is equivalent of sexual mating in higher organisms.

It is the process by which a male or donor bacterium mates or makes physical contact with a female or recipient bacterium and transfers the genetic material into it. The female bacterium after mating is converted into a male bacterium.

History

Lederberg and Tatum in 1946 extensively studied conjugation in a strain of *E. coli* called K12.

Mechanism

Conjugation takes places between a male cell and female cell.

The plasmid DNA replicates and a copy of it passes from the donor to the recipient cell probably along the sex pilus (conjugation tube). As a result the recipient cell can now turn into a donor cell and can conjugate with other female cells. Thus, maleness is an infectious character. The plasmid responsible is called sex factor or fertility factor or the F factor. When other similar plasmids were discovered, the name transfer factor came to be used for all such plasmids which gave their host cells the ability to act as donors in conjugation.

Now, how does gene transfer take place by conjugation. We will study three ways.

1. *F factor*: The F factor can exist in two ways. If it is free in the cytoplasm of the cell it can only transfer the ability to form the sex pilus. The cells carrying the F factor have no distinguishing features other than their ability to mate with the F^- cells and render them F^+. The other way in which F factor can exist is as an episome, i.e. it has the ability to exist integrated into the host chromosome. Such cells are able to transfer chromosomal genes to recipient cells with high frequency are known as Hfr cells. This conversion of a F^+ cell into Hfr state is reversible. When the F factor reverts from the integrated to the free state it may carry with it some chromosomal genes from near to its site of attachment. Such a F factor incorporating some chromosomal genes is called an F′ prime (F′) factor.
When a F′ cell mates with a F^- cell it transfers along with the F factor the host genes incorporated with it. This process of transfer of host genes through the F factor resembles transduction and has therefore been called sexduction (Fig. 13.5).

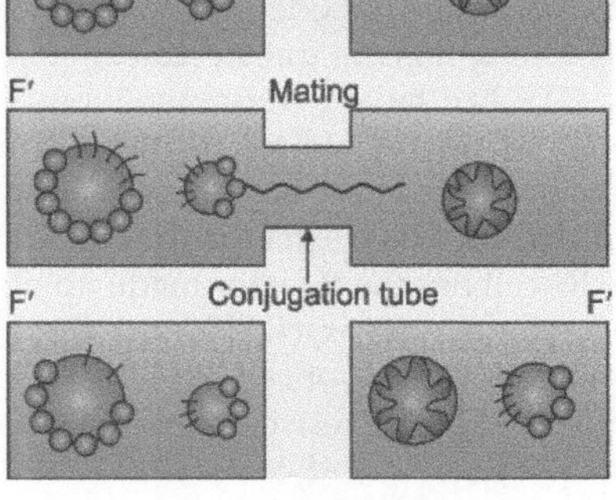

Fig. 13.5: Sexduction

2. *Col factor (Colicinogenic)*: Col factor is a plasmid which resembles the F factor in promoting conjugation leading to self-transfer and at times transfer of chromosomal segments. This col factor gives rise to formation of colicins which are antibiotic substances which will kill other bacteria. Many bacteria produce this and hence, the name bacteriocin is given to it, e.g. Pyocin by *Pseudomonas pyocyanea*, diphthericin by *Corynebacterium diphtheriae*, etc.

   Chemically they may be proteins to lipoprotein-polysaccharide complexes or a particle resembling defective phage.
3. *Resistance transfer factor*: This plasmid is responsible for transferring multiple drug resistance among bacteria. This was first discovered by Japanese workers in 1959 who reported a sudden increase in infections caused by *Shigella strains* resistant simultaneously to sulphonamides, streptomycin, chloramphenicol and tetracycline. This mechanism of drug resistance is known as transferable, episomal or infectious drug resistance.

This plasmid consists of two components—resistance transfer factor called (RTF) which is involved in conjugational transfer and the resistance determinant (r) for each of the several drugs. The whole plasmid (RTF + r determinants) = R factor.

An R factor can have many r determinants and resistance to as many as eight or more drugs can be transferred simultaneously.

Sometimes the R factor and the r determinants may dissociate and although the host cell remains drug resistant, it is not transferable.

The RTF can have determinants other than those for drug resistance. Enterotoxin and hemolysin production has been shown to be transmitted by the transfer factor (Fig. 13.6).

The R^+ cell has the R factor made up of resistance transfer factor (RTF) and resistance determinants to antibiotics 1, 2, 3, 4 and 5.

Transferable drug resistance is seen widely in various pathogenic and commensal bacteria of man and animals: *Enterobacteriaceae, Vibrio, Pseudomonas, Pasteurella.*

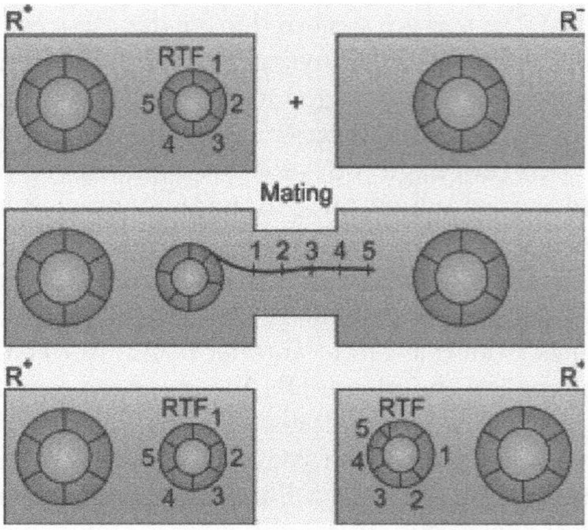

Fig. 13.6: Transferable drug resistance

Transferable drug resistance in the normal gut can be inhibited by many factors like:
- Anaerobic conditions
- Bite salts
- Alkaline pH
- Abundance of anaerobic gram-positive bacteria.

But in the intestines of persons on oral antibiotic therapy, transfer readily occurs due to destruction of the normal flora and the selective pressure produced by the drug.

Transferable drug resistance can involve all the commonly used antibiotics. It depends upon the frequency of use of antibiotics in that area.

Bacteria carrying R factors can spread from animals to man.

GENETIC MECHANISMS OF DRUG RESISTANCE IN BACTERIA

Bacteria may acquire drug resistance by:
1. Mutation.
2. One of the methods of genetic transfer.

Ultimately, the way in which the resistance mechanism develops is one of the following:
- Decreased permeability to the drug.
- Development of alternate metabolic pathways.
- Production of enzymes inactivating the drugs.

Mutational resistance—is mainly of two types:

1. The step-wise mutation as seen with penicillin where high levels of resistance are achieved only by a series of small step mutations.
2. The one step mutation—as seen with streptomycin.

In clinical practice mutational resistance is of importance in tuberculosis. If a patient is treated with streptomycin alone initially the bacteria die in large numbers but soon resistant mutants appear and multiply unchecked. If two or more antituberculous drugs are used for combined treatment, repopulation by resistant mutants does not occur, as a mutant resistant to one drug will be destroyed by others. This is the reason behind combined treatment in tuberculosis.

Transferable drug resistance by transformation is almost unknown.

Acquisition of resistance by transduction is common in *Staphylococci*.

Transferable drug resistance mediated by the R factor is the most important method of drug resistance. Acquisition of an R factor simultaneously confers resistance against several drugs.

The mechanism of resistance is by the production of degrading enzymes and the level of resistance is usually of a high order. The resistance of typhoid bacilli to multiple antibiotics is of this kind.

Table 13.1 shows the comparison of the two types of drug resistance.

Table 13.1: Comparison of mutational and transferable types of drug resistance in bacteria

Mutational drug resistance	*Transferable drug resistance*
1. Involves resistance to one drug at a time	Simultaneous resistance to multiple drugs. May involve all drugs used in clinical treatment
2. Degree of resistance usually low	Degree of resistance usually high
3. May be overcome by high drug dosage	High drug dosage ineffective
4. Resistance can be prevented by treatment with combination of drugs	Combination of drugs cannot prevent resistance
5. Resistance does not spread	Resistance spreads to other cells of same or different species of the genus
6. Resistant mutants are usually metabolically defective	Metabolically normal
7. Virulence of resistant mutants may be low	Virulence of resistant mutants not decreased

TRANSPOSABLE GENETIC ELEMENTS

Certain structurally and genetically discrete segments of DNA have been identified that have the ability to move around between chromosomal and extra chromosomal DNA molecules within cells. These DNA molecules are called transposons and this mode of genetic transfer as transposition.

A transposon is a segment of DNA with one or more genes in the center and the two ends carrying inverted repeat sequences of nucleotides (these are nucleotides complementary to each other but in the reverse order). Transposons get attached at certain regions of chromosomal, plasmid or phage DNA. Insertion of a transposon leads to acquisition of new characters by the recipient DNA molecule.

By transposition, a segment of DNA can be transferred from one molecule to another molecule that has no genetic homology. In this it differs from recombination.

Characters transferred by transposons may sometimes confer survival advantage. It has been suggested that the resistance determinant segments of the R factors may have evolved as a collection of transposons each carrying a gene that confers resistance to one or several antibiotics. Transposons appear to accomplish in nature, gene manipulations similar to lab manipulation that have been called genetic engineering (Fig. 13.7).

GENETIC ENGINEERING

Genetic engineering also known as recombinant DNA technology involves isolating a particular gene coding for a desired protein from a

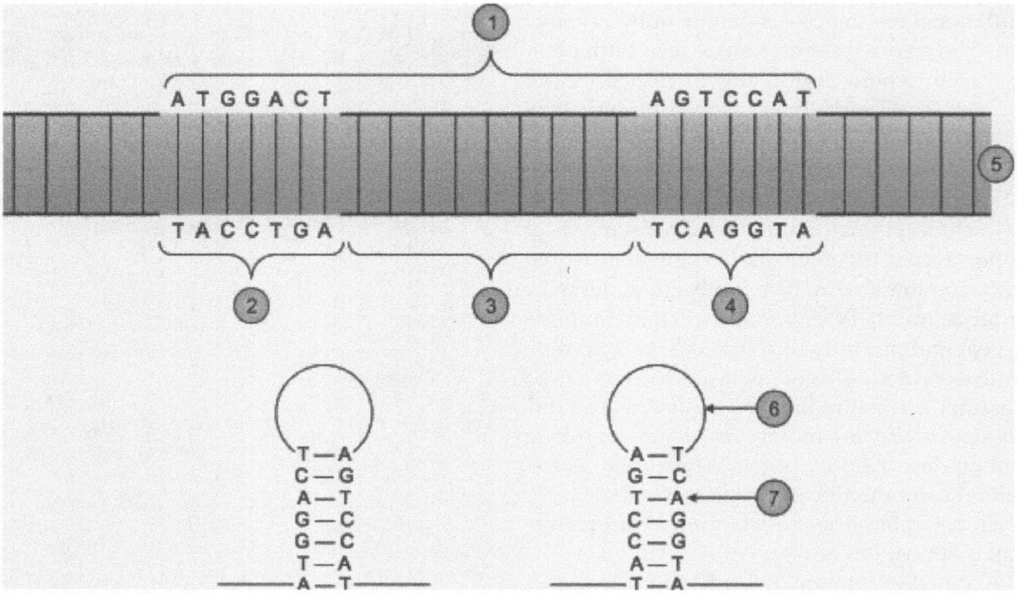

Fig. 13.7: (1) Transposon, (2) Inverted repeat sequences, (3) Gene, (4) Inverted repeat sequences, (5) Double-stranded DNA, (6) Single-stranded loop consisting of gene formed by a strand of transposon, (7) Double-stranded stem formed by hydrogen bonding between the terminal repeat sequences

microorganism or from cells of higher forms of life, introducing them into suitable microorganisms in which they would be functional directing the production of a specific proteins. This enables the production of any desired protein in pure form, in large quantities and at a reasonable cost.

Different ways have been desired for obtaining the desired genes.

- If the complete amino acid sequence is known, the gene can be synthesized in the lab. With larger proteins this is not possible.
- The DNA containing genes can be cut by specific enzymes called restriction endonucleases and the fragments containing the desired genes isolated.
- m-RNA isolated from cells producing desired protein. A DNA copy is made from m-RNA using enzyme reverse transcriptase. The double stranded DNA gene is then prepared using DNA polymerase. This is incorporated into temperate bacteriophages for insertion into microorganisms. The microorganism commonly employed is *E. coli* K 12 though many other bacteria and yeasts have also been used.

Use of genetic engineering:

- Production of:
  - Cloned human insulin
  - Interferons
  - Somatostatin
  - Growth hormones.

Section 2

Immunology

- Immunity
- Antigens
- Antibodies
- Antigen-Antibody Reactions
- Complement
- Structure and Function of the Immune System
- Hypersensitivity

IMMUNOLOGY

INTRODUCTION

Immunology is a very vast and upcoming field in microbiology which deals with the study of the immune response in the human body. The immune response involves the interaction between the antigens present on the microbes and the antibodies and killer lymphocytes produced in the human body against them. The basic function of the immune response is protective and serves to eliminate the foreign invader but sometimes it produces a harmful effect on the body too. This can happen in autoimmune diseases in which the body mounts a destructive immune response on its own self, or hypersensitivity in which the immune response is increased in certain sensitive individuals.

The interaction between antigens and antibodies forms the basis of serological diagnostic tests in which the level of antibodies in the blood against a particular antigen tells us of the presence and severity of infection and contributes greatly to diagnostic medicine.

The study of immunology helps us to understand various aspects of medicine such as transplantation and immunodeficiency diseases including the acquired immunodeficiency syndrome.

Immunotherapy (treatment with immune products) and immunoprophylaxis are branches of immunology that are rapidly advancing and help in patient care and treatment.

CHAPTER

14

Immunity

LESSON PLAN

- Definition
- Types
- Innate Immunity
  - Factors Determining Level of Innate Immunity
  - Mechanisms of Innate Immunity
- Acquired Immunity
  - Definition
  - Active Immunity
  - Passive Immunity
- Measurement of Immunity
- Local Immunity
- Herd Immunity

DEFINITION

Immunity is defined as the resistance of the host to infection by microbes or their products. Some people have good immunity and are able to fight diseases better than those who have poor immunity.

TYPES

1. Innate immunity
   a. Nonspecific
   b. Specific
2. Acquired immunity
   a. Active → Natural, Artificial
   b. Passive → Natural, Artificial

INNATE IMMUNITY

Innate immunity or native immunity is the resistance to infections which the person has because of his genetic make up. It does not depend on previous contact with the microorganisms or vaccination.

It may be nonspecific when resistance to infections in general is considered and specific when resistance to a particular pathogenic microorganism is concerned.

Innate immunity can be viewed at the level of the species, race or the individual.

At the level of the species, immunity refers to the resistance shown by all members of the species, e.g. all humans are totally resistant to pathogens that affect plants. Within a species, different races show different pattern of resistance to pathogens. But because of difference in environments and interracial marriage, this is not very clear. Genetic resistance to *Plasmodium falciparum* malaria seen in some parts of Africa is an example of racial resistance.

Within a race, there are differences in resistance shown between individuals. Many factors determine the level of innate immunity.

Factors Determining Level of Innate Immunity

Age

Immunity is low in the two extremes of life that is, in newborns and older people. This is because in newborns, the immune system is not very developed and in the older people it becomes weakened. The immune system is strongest in youth.

Hormonal Influence

Diseases such as diabetes mellitus, hypothyroidism and adrenal gland dysfunction are associated with an increased susceptibility to infections. Increase of steroids in the body decreases immunity. So, people under stress release more steroids and are more prone to developing infections. Also, pregnant women have high levels of steroids and more chances of infection.

Nutrition

Malnutrition depresses immunity. People who are malnourished are more prone to infections.

Mechanisms of Innate Immunity

There are certain mechanisms in our body which fight against invasion of the microorganisms. These are the body's natural defense mechanisms.

The Epithelial Surfaces

They form the first point of contact between the microorganism and the human body. The intact skin and mucous membrane covering the body give it good protection against microorganisms.

- The healthy skin has good bactericidal quality, because of high concentration of saline in the drying sweat and sebaceous secretions.
- Shape of the nose prevents entry of microorganisms. If they do enter, they are caught by the mucus lining and are swept back to the larynx where they are swallowed or coughed out. The cough reflex is an important defense mechanism of the respiratory tract. The cilia on the respiratory epithelial cells move particles upwards. Nasal and respiratory secretions contain mucopolysaccharides capable of neutralizing viruses. Particles that manage to reach the pulmonary alveoli are ingested by the phagocytic cells present there. The mouth is constantly bathed in saliva which has an inhibitory effect on many microorganisms. Particles deposited in the mouth are swallowed and are acted upon by digestive juices. The high acidity of the stomach contents destroys most microorganisms. The normal bacterial flora of the intestine exerts a protective effect by preventing colonization of bacteria that may gain entry. The intestinal epithelium is covered by a lace like network of mucus. Particles get caught up in the mucus and form small masses that are propelled by peristalsis.

The conjunctiva is made free of foreign particles by the flushing action of tears. Tears also contain an antibacterial lysozyme. Lysozyme is present in tissue fluids and in nearly all secretions except CSF, sweat and urine. It acts by splitting certain polysaccharide components of the cell walls of susceptible bacteria. Recently, it has also been found to occur in phagocytic cells.

The flushing action of the urine eliminates bacteria from the urethra. An antibacterial substance has been identified in semen. Acidity of the vagina also prevents the infection by pathogenic bacteria.

Antibacterial Substances in Blood and Tissues

The complement system possesses bactericidal activity and plays an important role in the destruction of pathogenic bacteria that invade the blood and tissues. There are many antibacterial substances present in the blood and tissues like properdin, beta lysin, basic polypeptide such as leukins, acidic substances such as lactic acid and an antibacterial substance called spermine isolated from the kidneys. A method of defence against virus infections is the production of interferon by cells stimulated by live or killed viruses and certain other inducers.

Cellular Factors in Innate Immunity

Phagocytic cells destroy bacteria through the process of phagocytosis (cell eating process). Phagocytic cells were discovered by Metchnikoff (1833), who classified them into microphages and macrophages.

Inflammation

Inflammation is an important nonspecific mechanism of defense. Because of chemicals released at the site of injury, polymorphonuclear leucocytes escape and accumulate in large numbers there. Numerous chemical mediators flood this area because of the inflammatory response. This causes polymorphonuclear cells to migrate to this site and destroy bacteria. Inflammation is characterized by increased redness, swelling, heat, induration (hardness) and pain at the site.

Fever

A rise of temperature sometimes actually destroys the infecting pathogens. Fever also stimulates the production of interferon and helps in recovery from viruses.

Fever can aid in host defense. There are certainly some important immunological reactions that speed up by temperature and some pathogens with strict temperature preferences could be hindered. Fevers may be useful to some extent since they allow the body to reach high temperatures, causing an unbreakable environment for some pathogens. White blood cells also rapidly proliferate due to the suitable environment and can also help fight off the harmful pathogens and microbes that invaded the body

See Table 14.1 for differences in innate and acquired immunity.

ACQUIRED IMMUNITY

Definition

The resistance that an individual acquires during life is known as acquired immunity or adaptive immunity. Acquired immunity is of two types—active and passive.

Active Immunity

Active immunity is the resistance developed by an individual as a result of antigenic stimulus from outside. It is produced actively by the host's immune system. Active immunity sets in only after a latent period which is required to set the immunological machinery into motion. Once developed, the active immunity is long lasting. If an individual who has been actively immunized against an antigen experiences the same antigen subsequently the immune response occurs more quickly and abundantly than during

Table 14.1: Differences between innate immunity and acquired immunity

S. No.	*Innate Immunity*	*Acquired Immunity*
1.	Response is nonspecific	Pathogen and antigen specific response
2.	Exposure leads to immediate maximal response	Lag period between exposure and maximal response.
3.	Cell-mediated components	Humoral components
4.	No immunological memory	Exposure leads to immunological memory
5.	No immunological recognition	Immunological recognition of the antigen
6.	Destroys all the infected cells	Self/nonself discrimination is followed
7.	Second exposure to same antigen requires equal time to generate the immune response.	Quicker response on second exposure
8.	Found in nearly all forms of life	Found only in jawed vertebrates

the first encounter. This is known as the secondary response. Also the immune system retains for long periods, the memory of a prior antigenic exposure and it produces a secondary type of response when it meets with the same antigen again. Active immunity can be natural or artificial.

Natural Active Immunity

This results from either a clinical or a subclinical infection with a parasite. The natural active immunity varies with the concerned pathogen. The immunity is lifelong following many viral infections such as smallpox or measles. In some viral diseases such as influenza or the common cold, the immunity appears to be short lived. The influenza virus regularly undergoes antigenic variation and the immunity following the first infection is not effective against the second infection due to a different virus. Common cold is caused by a large number of different viruses. Hence, immunity to one does not protect against the other.

The immunity following bacterial infection is generally less permanent than following viral infections.

Artificial Active Immunity

This is the resistance induced by vaccines. Vaccines are preparations of live or killed microorganisms or their products used for immunization.

Examples of vaccines are:

1. Bacterial vaccines
   a. Live—BCG for tuberculosis
   b. Killed—TAB for enteric fever
2. Viral vaccines
   a. Live—Smallpox vaccine
   b. Killed—Salk vaccine for polio
3. Bacterial products
   Toxoids for diphtheria and tetanus.

Live Vaccine

- Live vaccine causes an infection similar to the natural infection, although it is milder.
- The immunity lasts for several years but a booster may be necessary.
- Live vaccines may be administered orally or parenterally.
- Live vaccines are more immunogenic than killed vaccines.

Killed Vaccine

- They are generally less immunogenic than live vaccines.
- Protection lasts only for a short period.
- They have to be given repeatedly, at least two doses being required for the production of immunity.
- The first dose is known as the primary dose and the next as booster doses.

See Table 14.2 for the differences between active and passive immunity.

Table 14.2: Comparison of active and passive immunity

Active immunity	*Passive immunity*
• Produced actively by the hosts immune system	Received passively by the hosts. Immune system does not participate
• Induced by infection or vaccines	Produced by readymade antibodies
• Gives effective protection	Protection temporary and less effective
• There is a lag phase (time required for preparation of antibodies)	Immunity is effective immediately
• Immunological memory present	No immunological memory
• Further challenges more effective (booster effect)	Further administration of antibody is less effective due to immune elimination
• Negative phase may occur	No negative phase
• Not applicable to immunodeficient hosts	Applicable to immunodeficient hosts
• Used as prophylaxis	Used for the treatment of acute infection
• No inheritance	May be acquired from the mother
• Both humoral and cell mediated immunity participate	Only humoral immunity participates

Passive Immunity

The resistance that is transmitted to a recipient in a readymade form is known as passive immunity. Here the recipient's immune system plays no active role. There is no antigenic stimulus and preformed antibodies are administered. There is no latent period in passive immunity. The protection is effective immediately following passive immunization. There is no negative phase. The immunity is short lived and lasts for days or weeks or only till the passively transmitted antibodies are metabolized or eliminated. No secondary response occurs in passive immunity. Passive immunity has another disadvantage. When we inject the antibodies once into the body antibodies are formed against them. Next time when the antibodies are injected it results in elimination of the antibodies. This process is called immune elimination.

Passive immunization is less effective and provides immunity inferior to that produced by active immunization. The main advantage of passive immunization is that it is immediate in action and can be employed when instant immunity is desired.

Natural Passive Immunity

It is the resistance passively transferred from the mother to the baby. This transfer is basically through the placenta. Human colostrum which is rich in IgA antibodies gives protection to the neonate. Maternal antibodies give passive protection against the infectious diseases to the infant till then. After the age of 3 months the infant starts making its own antibodies. By immunizing women in pregnancy, we can improve the quality of passive immunity.

Artificial Passive Immunity

It is the resistance passively transferred to a recipient by administration of antibodies. We either use sera of animal or human for this purpose. The serum used is either hyperimmune sera or convalescent sera or pooled human gamma globulin. The oldest and the most common method is to use hyperimmune horse sera. This is prepared by hyperimmunization in horses using the appropriate antigen, e.g. ATS (antitetanus serum). This is used for passive immunization against tetanus and is prepared by giving a series of doses of tetanus toxoids to horses, bleeding them and separating the serum.

As horse ATS is a foreign protein and causes serious and fatal hypersensitivity reactions it should be given only after testing. To avoid this complication of hypersensitivity, human ATS is employed. This is prepared by hyperimmunization of human volunteers with tetanus toxoid. With human ATS the protection lasts longer, there being no immune elimination of the human globulins.

Sera collected from patients recovering from an illness contain high levels of specific antibody and are called convalescent sera. This is especially used in measles and rubella.

Sera collected from healthy adults in the community have gamma globulin. The antibody fraction (gamma globulin) from pooled sera is used for passive immunization against common infectious diseases. The placenta is the convenient source for the preparation of human gamma globulin.

When is Passive Immunization Useful?

Passive immunization is given for immediate and temporary protection in a nonimmune host when there is:

1. Insufficient time for active immunization to take place.
2. Passive immunization may be employed for the suppression of active immunity when it is injurious, e.g. the use of Rh-immune globulin during delivery to prevent immune response in Rh negative women with Rh positive babies.

Sometimes, a combination of active and passive methods of immunization is employed simultaneously. This is known as combined immunization. This is given in case of tetanus. We inject ATS in one arm and the first dose of tetanus toxoid in the other. Antitetanus serum provides the necessary protection till active immunity is able to take effect.

MEASUREMENT OF IMMUNITY

To measure immunity we test the resistance of an individual to a challenge by the pathogen. But this is not a measure of the true immunity because it alters the state of immunity.

To test immunity we usually measure the specific antibody. The antibodies may be demonstrated by many techniques such as agglutination, precipitation, complement fixation, neutralization, etc. In some cases the protection is associated with cell mediated immunity. Here skin tests give an indication of immunity.

LOCAL IMMUNITY

Local immunity means the immunity of a local area. It is useful in the treatment of infections which are either localized or in treating infection at the site of entry of the pathogen. A special class of immunoglobulins (IgA) forms the major component of local immunity. One type of IgA antibodies called secretory IgA is produced locally by plasma cells present on the mucosal surfaces or in secretory glands.

HERD IMMUNITY

This is the overall level of immunity in a community and it is important in the control of epidemic diseases. When a large proportion of individuals in a community are immune to a pathogen the herd immunity to the pathogen is satisfactory. When herd immunity is low epidemics are likely to occur on the introduction of a suitable pathogen due to a large number of susceptible individuals in the community. If we want to eradicate communicable diseases we would have to raise the herd immunity.

CHAPTER

15

Antigens

LESSON PLAN

- Definition
- Types of Antigens
- What is an Antigenic Determinant?
- What Determines Antigenicity?
  - Size
  - Chemical Nature
  - Susceptibility to Tissue Enzymes
  - Foreignness
- Specificity of Antigens
  - Species Specificity
  - Isospecificity
  - Autospecificity
  - Organ Specificity
  - Heterogenetic Specificity

DEFINITION

An antigen is defined as a substance which when introduced into the body, stimulates the production of an antibody with which it reacts in a specific manner. The two requirements for antigenicity are therefore.

a. Induction of an immune response.
b. A specific reaction with antibodies.

TYPES OF ANTIGENS

Based on the ability of antigens to induce antibody formation and then specifically react with them, antigens can be of various types:

a. *Complete antigen*—A complete antigen is able to induce antibody formation and produce a specific and observable reaction with the antibody produced.
b. *Haptens*—Haptens are antigens that are incapable of inducing antibody formation by themselves but can react specifically with antibodies. Haptens when combined with a carrier particle become immunogenic or capable of producing antibodies.
c. *Proantigen*—Proantigen is a low molecular weight substance such as picryl chloride and dinitrochlorobenzene which do not induce antibody formation but cause delayed hypersensitivity (cell mediated immunity) when applied on the skin.
d. *Cryptantigens*—Crypt means hidden. Those antigens which have hidden antigenic determinants which are not available for antigenic antibody reactions are called cryptantigens.

WHAT IS AN ANTIGENIC DETERMINANT?

The smallest unit of antigenicity is known as an antigenic determinant. This is a small area on the antigen possessing a specific chemical structure and configuration which determines the specificity of the antibody produced. This determinant group has a size of 25 to 35Å and a molecular weight of about 400 to 1000. Large antigens carry many different types of antigenic determinants, each type inducing the formation of a specific antibody.

WHAT DETERMINES ANTIGENICITY?

The exact basis of antigenicity is not yet clear but a number of common properties of antigens have been observed.

Size

The higher the molecular weight, the more antigenic a substance is. If the molecular weight is less than 10,000 the substance is less antigenic. Low molecular weight substances may be made antigenic by adsorbing them on inert particles such as bentonite or kaolin.

Chemical Nature

Most naturally occurring antigens are proteins and polysaccharides. Lipids and nucleic acids are less antigenic. The presence of an aromatic radical is necessary for antigenicity.

Susceptibility to Tissue Enzymes

Only substances which are metabolized by tissue enzymes behave as antigens. Antigens introduced into the body are degraded by the host into fragments of appropriate size containing the antigenic determinants.

Those substances which are not broken down are not antigenic.

Foreignness

Only those antigens that are foreign to the individual (nonself) induce an immune response. An individual does not normally mount an immune response against his own normal constituent antigens because tolerance to self-antigens exists due to contact with them during development of the immune apparatus. Breakdown of this mechanism results in autoimmune diseases.

SPECIFICITY OF ANTIGENS

Antigens are specific; reacting only against their own antibody, but this specificity is not absolute. Cross reactions may occur between antigens which share antigenic determinants. Specificity can be of five kinds—species specificity, isospecificity, organ specificity, autospecificity and heterogenetic specificity.

Species Specificity

Specificity may be at the level of the species. Tissues of all individuals in a species contain species specific antigens. There is some degree of cross reaction between antigens from related species.

Isospecificity

Isoantigens are antigens found in some but not all members of a species. For example, isoantigens of the human erythrocyte antigens based on which individuals can be classified into different blood groups. These are genetically determined and are of importance in blood transfusion and disputed paternity cases. Histocompatibility antigens are very specific to an individual of a species. These antigens are associated with the plasma membrane of the tissue cells. The major histocompatibility antigens determining homograft rejection in man are antigens of the HLA (Human Leucocyte Antigen) system.

Autospecificity

Self antigens are not normally antigenic but there are exceptions.

Those antigens that are not found in free circulation or tissue fluids such as lens protein are not recognized as self antigens. Antigens that are absent in embryonic life and develop later (such as sperms) are also not recognized as self antigens. When these antigens are released into the tissues due to injury to the lens or damage to the testis, antibodies are produced against them. Sometimes, antigenic specificity of self antigens undergoes modification as a result of infections or irradiation and the body cannot recognize them as self. Autoimmune processes may also occur because of failure of homeostatic control of immune function.

Organ Specificity

Some organs such as brain, kidney and lens protein of different species share the same antigen. Such antigens characteristic for an organ or tissue are called organ specific antigens.

For example—Neuroparalytic complications following antirabic vaccination because the sheep and human brain share common antigens.

Heterogenetic Specificity

The same or closely related antigens sometimes occur in different biological species, classes and kingdoms. These are known as heterogenetic or heterophile antigens. The examples are:

- *Forssman antigen*—which is a lipid carbohydrate complex widely distributed in man, animals, birds, plants and bacteria.
- *Weil*—Felix reaction in typhus fevers.
- *Paul*—Bunnell reaction in infectious mononucleosis.
- Cold agglutinin test in primary atypical pneumonia.

For example—The Weil-Felix reaction for the serodiagnosis of typhus fevers is a heterophile agglutination test and is based on the sharing of a common antigen between typhus rickettsiae and some strains of proteus bacilli.

CHAPTER

16

Antibodies

LESSON PLAN

- Definition
- What are Immunoglobulins?
- Structure of Immunoglobulin
- Classes of Immunoglobulins
  - IgG
  - IgA
  - IgM
  - IgD
  - IgE

DEFINITION

Antibodies are substances that appear in serum and tissue fluids in response to an antigenic stimulus and react with the antigen specifically and in some observable manner.

WHAT ARE IMMUNOGLOBULINS?

The serum proteins are of two types—albumin and globulins. The globulins are further divided into alpha, beta and gamma globulins. Antibodies are mostly gamma globulins and hence, they are also called immunoglobulins. In 1964, the WHO introduced the term immunoglobulin which was defined as a protein of animal origin which had antibody activity. Besides antibodies it also includes the abnormal proteins found in myeloma, macroglobulinemia, etc. Immunoglobulins are synthesized by plasma cells and lymphocytes.

Immunoglobulins denote the structural concept while the term antibody is a biological concept. All antibodies are immunoglobulins but all immunoglobulins may not be antibodies. Immunoglobulins are written in written in short form as IgA, IgG, IgE, etc.

STRUCTURE OF IMMUNOGLOBULIN

Based on physicochemical and antigenic differences, five classes of immunoglobulins have been recognized—IgG, IgA, IgM, IgD and IgE. One molecule of immunoglobulin is split into three parts (by papain an enzyme)—one Fc and two Fab pieces. Immunoglobulins are glycoproteins, each molecule consisting of two pairs of polypeptide chains of different sizes held together by disulfide bonds (Fig. 16.1).

The smaller chains are called light (L) chains and the larger ones heavy (H) chains. The light chain has a molecular weight of 25,000 and the heavy chain of 50,000. The L chain is attached to the H chain by a disulfide bond. The 2 H chains are bound together by one to five disulfide bonds depending on the class of immunoglobulins.

The H chains are different structurally and antigenically for each class and are designated by Greek letters.

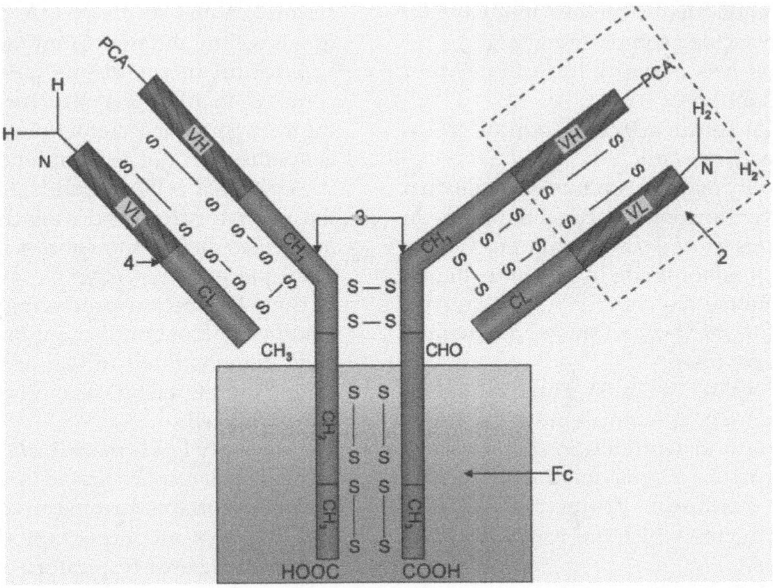

Fig. 16.1: Structure of IgG molecule. (1) Fc portion, (2) Antigen combining site at the variable end, (3) Heavy chain, (4) Light chain. VH and VL (variable portions of the heavy and light chains). CH_1 CH_2 CH_3 (Constant regions of heavy chains). CL-constant portion of light chain. S-S (disulphide linkages) (Reproduced from Textbook of Microbiology by Paniker and Ananthanarayan)

Immunoglobulin class	*Designation of H chain*
IgG	γ (gamma)
IgA	α (alpha)
IgM	μ (mu)
IgD	δ (delta)
IgE	ε (epsilon)

The L chains are similar in all classes of immunoglobulins. They occur in two varieties (kappa (K) and lambda (λ). A molecule of immunoglobulin may either have kappa or lambda chain but never both together.

Both the heavy and light chains have a constant and a variable region. In light chains the two regions are of equal length but in heavy chains the variable region constitutes 1/5 of the chain. The infinite range of immunoglobulins depends on the variability of the amino acid sequences at the variable regions of the H and L chains which form the antigen combining sites.

Rabbit IgG antibody when digested by papain in the presence of cysteine was split into two fractions an insoluble fraction which crystallized in the cold called Fc for crystallizable and a soluble fragment which did not precipitate with egg albumin but combined with it. This fragment is called the Fab (antigen binding) fragment.

The constant regions of the heavy chains are CH_1, CH_2, CH_3, whereas the constant part of the light chain is CL. The Fc fragment is composed of the carboxy terminal portion of the H chains. It does not possess antigen combining activity but determines the biological properties of the immunoglobulin molecule such as complement fixation, placental transfer, skin fixation and catabolic rate.

The area of the H chain in the C region between the first and second C region domains (CH_1 and CH_2) is the hinge region. It is more flexible and is more exposed to chemicals and enzymes.

CLASSES OF IMMUNOGLOBULINS

Human sera contain IgG, IgA, IgM, IgD and IgE.

IgG

- It is the major serum immunoglobulin constituting about 75 percent of the total. It has a molecular weight of 150,000.

- It is distributed equally between intravascular and extravascular compartments.
- It contains less carbohydrate than other immunoglobulins.
- The normal serum concentration of IgG is about 8 to 16 mg/mL.
- IgG is the only maternal immunoglobulin that is normally transported across the placenta and provides natural passive immunity in the newborn. It is not made by the fetus in any large amounts.
- IgG binds to microorganisms and enhances their phagocytosis.
- IgG participates in most immunological reactions such as complement fixation, precipitation and neutralization of toxins and viruses. It may be considered as a general purpose antibody protective against infectious agents which are active in blood and tissues.
- Passively administered IgG suppresses the similar antibody synthesis by a feedback process. This property is utilized in the isoimmunization of women by the administration of anti Rh (D) IgG during delivery
- IgG is a late antibody and makes its appearance after the initial immune response which is IgM in nature. Four subclasses of IgG have been recognized, each having a distinct type of gamma chain, IgG_1, IgG_2, IgG_3, and IgG_4.

They are distributed in human serum in the approximate proportions of 65 percent, 23 percent, 8 percent and 4 percent, respectively. Table 16.1 shows the comparison between the properties of immunoglobulins.

IgA

- IgA is found second in abundance after IgG. It constitutes 10 percent of serum immunoglobulins.
- The normal serum concentration is 0.6 to 4.2 mg per ml.
- It has a half-life of 6 to 8 days.
- It is the major immunoglobulin in colostrum, saliva and tears. It is found in two forms-serum IgA and secretory IgA. The secretory IgA is a little different from the serum IgA. IgA found in secretions (secretory IgA) contains an additional structural unit called the transport T or secretory piece. The T piece is synthesized not in lymphoid cells but in the epithelial cells of glands, intestines and the respiratory tract and is attached to the IgA molecules during transport across the cells. The T piece links together two IgA molecules at their Fc portion producing 11s dimers. Another polypeptide chain, the J chain has been demonstrated in IgA and IgM. The J chain (Joining chain) is synthesized by the lymphoid cells.
- The secretory IgA is more in amount than the serum IgA. It is concentrated in secretions and on mucus surfaces forming an antibody paste and it plays an important role in local immunity against respiratory and intestinal pathogens.
- IgA antibodies function by inhibiting the adherence of microorganisms to the surface of mucosal cells by covering the organisms and thereby preventing their entry into body tissues. IgA antibody helps in phagocytosis and intracellular killing of microorganisms. Two IgA subclasses have been described, IgA_1 and IgA_2. IgA_2 is a minor component of serum IgA but it is the dominant form in secretions (Fig. 16.2).

IgM

- IgM constitutes 5 to 10 percent of serum immunoglobulins (Fig. 16.3).

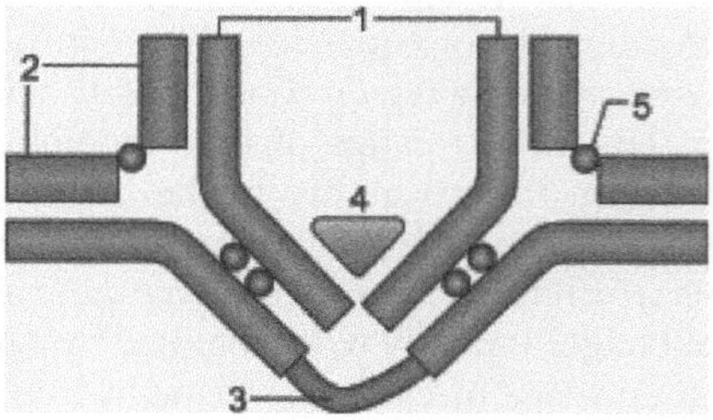

Fig. 16.2: Secretory IgA molecule showing 2 subunits; (1) Heavy chain, (2) Light chain, (3) J chain, (4) Secretory component (5) Disulfide bond

Table 16.1: Some properties of immunoglobulin classes

	IgG	*IgA*	*IgM*	*IgD*	*IgE*
Sedementation coefficient (S)	7	7	19	7	8
Molecular weight	150,000	160,000	900,000	180,000	190,000
Serum concentration mg/mL	12	2	1.2	0.03	0.00004
Half-life (days)	23	6	10	2.8	2.3
Daily production mg/kg	34	24	3.3	0.4	0.0023
Carbohydrate %	3	11	10	13	2
Intravascular distribution%	45	42	80	75	50
Complement fixation					
Clasical	++	–	+++	–	–
Alternative	–	+	–	–	–
Placental transport	+	–	–	–	–
Present in milk	+	+	–	–	–
Selective secretion by sero-mucus glands	–	+	–	–	–
Heat stability (56°C)	+	+	+	+	–
Examples	Many antibodies to toxins bacteria and viruses	Secretory antibody in mucous membrane	Antipolysaccharide antibody and cold agglutination	It is the immunoglobulin on the surface of beta lymphocytes in newborn	Antiallergic and antiparasitic antibodies

- Normal level is 0.5 to 2 mg/mL.
- IgM molecules are polymers of five subunits; it is therefore a heavy molecule.
- Most of the IgM is intravascular in distribution It is the earliest immunoglobulin to be synthesized by the fetus at about 20 weeks of age.
- It is not transported across the placenta, therefore if IgM is present in the fetus or newborn it indicates congenital infection like congenital syphilis, rubella and toxoplasmosis.
- IgM antibodies are relatively short lived, disappearing earlier than IgG. Hence, they indicate recent infection.
- The anti A, anti B and many other natural antibodies to microorganisms are usually IgM. Antibodies to typhoid O antigen and antibodies in syphilis are of this class.
- IgM antibody is found mainly in the intravascular compartment and is mainly responsible for protection against blood invasion by microorganisms.
- It is more effective than IgG in agglutination, and bactericidal action but less than IgG in neutralization of toxins and viruses.
- IgM deficiency is associated with septicemias.

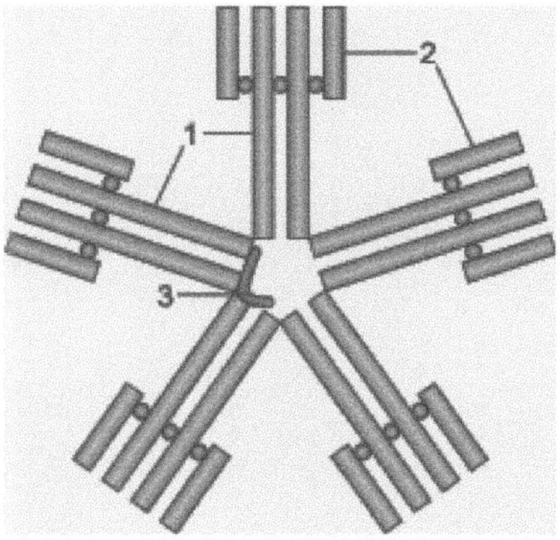

Fig. 16.3: IgM molecule: (1) Heavy chain, (2) Light chain, (3) J chain IgM

IgD

- It is present in a concentration of about 3 mg/ 100 ml of serum and it is mostly intravascular.
- Though the role of IgD is not very well understood, it is known that IgD and IgM occur on the surface of unstimulated lymphocytes and serve as recognition receptors for antigens.
- Two subclasses IgD_1 and IgD_2 are described.

IgE

- This antibody was discovered in 1966 by Ishizaka.
- It resembles IgG structurally.
- It is heat labile (inactivated at 56° in one hour) and has affinity for the surface of tissue cells (particularly mast cell).
- IgE does not pass the placental barrier. It is mostly extra vascular in distribution.
- Normal serum contains only traces (a few nanograms per ml) but greatly elevated levels are seen in atopic conditions such as asthma, hay fever and eczema.
- Children who have a high load of intestinal parasites have high serum levels of IgE.
- IgE mediates—Type 1-hypersensitivity reaction. It has been suggested that it may play some unidentified role in defense against intestinal parasitic infection.

In a nutshell we can say that:

- IgG—protects body fluids.
- IgA—protects mucous lining of respiratory and digestive tract.
- IgM—protects blood stream.
- IgE—mediates reaginic hypersensitivity.
- Role of IgD is unknown.

CHAPTER 17

Antigen-Antibody Reactions

LESSON PLAN

- Introduction
- General Features of Antigen-Antibody Reactions
- Measurement of Antigen and Antibody
  - Titer
  - Sensitivity
  - Specificity
- Types of Antigen-Antibody Reactions
  - Precipitation
  - Agglutination Reactions
  - Complement Fixation Tests
  - Neutralization Tests
  - Immunofluorescence
  - Enzyme-Linked Immunosorbent Assay
  - Radioimmunoassay

INTRODUCTION

When molecules of an antigen and an antibody are brought together in a solution they interact with each other by the formation of a link between the immunoglobulin molecule and the antigen molecule. These observable and specific reactions are called antigen antibody reactions. In the body they are responsible for antibody mediated immunity and protection against infectious diseases. Sometimes an exaggerated reaction results in tissue injury as in hypersensitivity and autoimmune disorders.

Outside the body that is in the laboratory the antigen and antibody reactions are called serological reactions. These help in the detection and quantitation of either antigens or antibodies and therefore help in the diagnosis of infectious agents, or quantitation of non-infectious agents such as enzymes.

The reaction between antigens and antibodies occur in three stages. The primary stage is the initial interaction between the two without any visible effects. The reaction is reversible and there are weak intermolecular forces between them. The primary stage is followed by the secondary stage leading to events we can see like precipitation, agglutination, lysis of cells, killing of live antigens, neutralization of motile organisms and phagocytosis. Some antigen antibody reactions occurring in vivo initiate chain reactions that lead to neutralization or destruction of injurious antigens or to tissue damage. These are tertiary reactions and include humoral immunity against infectious diseases as well as clinical allergy and other immunological diseases.

GENERAL FEATURES OF ANTIGEN-ANTIBODY REACTIONS

1. An antigen can give rise to more than one type of antibody. Also the same antibody can give rise to different type of reactions like precipitation, agglutination, etc. depending upon the nature of the antigen and the conditions of the reaction (Table 17.1).

2. The reaction is specific, an antigen combining only with its homologous antibody.
3. Entire molecules react and not fragments.
4. There is no denaturation of the antigen or the antibody during the reaction.
5. The combination occurs at the surface. Therefore, it is the surface antigens that are immunologically relevant. Antibodies to the surface antigens are generally protective.
6. The combination is firm but reversible.
7. Antigens and antibodies can combine in different proportions. Antibodies are generally bivalent but antigens are multivalent. IgM antibody has about 5 to 10 combining sites.

Table 17.1: Comparative efficiency of immunoglobulin classes in serological reactions

Reactions	*IgG*	*IgM*	*IgA*
Precipitation	Strong	Weak	Variable
Agglutination	Weak	Strong	Moderate
Complement fixation	Weak	Strong	Negative
Lysis	Weak	Strong	Negative

MEASUREMENT OF ANTIGEN AND ANTIBODY

How to measure how much antibody? For this we use the term titer.

Titer

The antibody titer of a serum is the highest dilution of the serum which gives an observable reaction with the antigen in the particular test.

Two important parameters of serological tests are sensitivity and specificity.

Sensitivity

This refers to the ability of the test to detect very minute quantities of antigen or antibody. When a test is highly sensitive, false negative tests will be highly minimal.

Specificity

Specificity refers to the ability of the test to detect reactions between homologous antigens and antibodies only and with no other. In a highly specific test, false positive reactions will be absent or minimal. In general, sensitivity and specificity of a test will be in inverse proportion.

TYPES OF ANTIGEN-ANTIBODY REACTION

There are many kinds of antigen antibody reactions:

- Precipitation reaction
- Agglutination
- Radioimmunoassay
- Complement fixation
- Neutralization
- Immunofluorescence
- ELISA (Enzyme-linked immunosorbent assay).

Precipitation

Definition

When a soluble antigen combines with its antibody in the presence of electrolytes (NaCl) at a suitable temperature and pH, the antigen antibody complex forms an insoluble precipitate. When instead of sedimenting, the precipitate remains suspended as floccules, the reaction is known as flocculation. Precipitation can take place in liquid media or in gels such as agar, agarose and polyacrylamide.

Mechanism of Precipitation

Antigens and antibodies can combine in different proportions. If we add increasing quantities of antigens to the same amount of antiserum in different tubes, precipitation will occur most rapidly and abundantly in one of the middle tubes in which the antigen and antibody are present in optimal or equivalent proportions. In the preceding tubes the antibody is in excess and in the later tubes the antigen is in excess. The precipitation in these tubes will be weak or even absent. The zone of antibody excess is called prozone. The peak is the zone of equivalence where maximum precipitation occurs. The later part is the zone of antigen excess (Fig. 17.1).

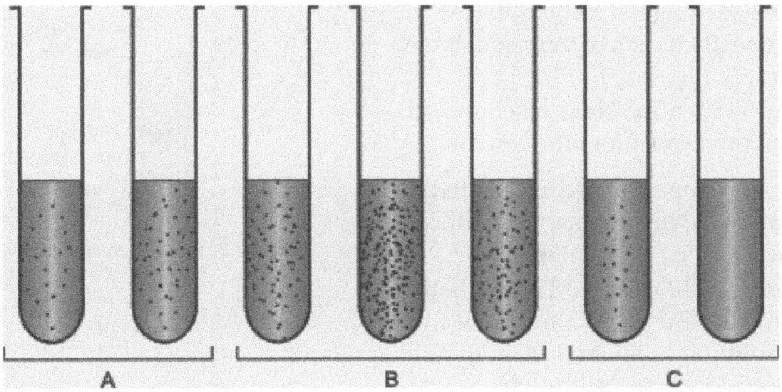

Fig. 17.1: A quantitative precipitation test showing: (A) Prozone (zone of antibody excess), (B) Zone of equivalence, (C) Zone of antigen excess

Marrack in 1934 proposed the lattice hypothesis for explaining the mechanism of precipitation. Precipitation results when a large lattice is formed consisting of alternating antigen and antibody molecules. This happens in the zone of equivalence. In the zones of antigen or antibody excess, the lattice does not enlarge, as the valencies of antibody and antigen are fully satisfied (Fig. 17.2). This can occur in agglutination also.

The prozone is of importance because sometimes in clinical serology, sera rich in antibody may give a false negative precipitation or agglutination result unless several dilutions are tested.

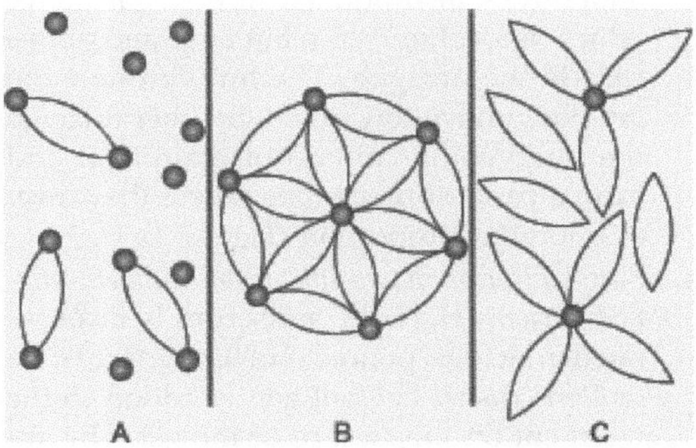

Fig. 17.2: Mechanism of precipitation by lattice formation. In A (antigen excess) and C (antibody excess) lattice formation does not occur. In B (zone of equivalence), lattice formation and precipitation occurs optimally

Applications of Precipitation Reaction

- Precipitation tests are more sensitive for the detection of antigens; very little amounts can be detected by precipitation test. Precipitation is less sensitive for the detection of antibodies.
- It finds forensic application in the identification of blood and seminal stains.
- It tests for food adulterants.

Types of Precipitation Tests

Ring test: This is the simplest of precipitation test consisting of layering the antigen solution over the column of antiserum in a narrow tube. A precipitate forms at the junction of the two liquids. Examples are the C reactive protein test and the grouping of streptococci by the Lancefield technique.

Slide test: When a drop each of the antigen and antiserum are placed on a slide and mixed by shaking, floccules appear. VDRL test for syphilis is an example of slide flocculation.

Immunodiffusion (precipitation in gel): As we had discussed earlier, precipitation can occur in a gel rather than in a liquid medium. There are many advantages in allowing precipitation to occur in a gel rather than in a liquid medium.

a. The reaction is visible as a distinct band of precipitation which is stable and can be stained for preservation if necessary.

b. If the number of antigens to be detected is greater than one, then each of them will have a different line.
c. It can also detect identity, cross reaction and non identity between different antigens.

Immunodiffusion is performed in a soft 1% agar gel/1% agarose. There are many modifications of this test:

a. *Single diffusion in one dimension*: The antibody is incorporated in agar gel in a test tube and the antigen solution is layered over it. The antigen diffuses downwards through the agar gel forming a line of precipitation (Fig. 17.3).
b. *Double diffusion in one dimension*: Here the antibody is incorporated in the agar above which is a column of plain agar and above that is the antigen. The antigen and the antibody move towards each other through the intervening column of plain agar and form a band of precipitate where they meet at optimum proportion (Fig. 17.4).
c. *Single diffusion in two dimensions (Radialimmunodiffusion)*: Here the antiserum is incorporated in agar gel poured on a flat surface (slide or Petri dish). The antigen is added to the wells cut on the surface of the gel. The antigen diffuses radially from the well and forms ring shaped bands of precipitation. The diameter of the halo is proportional to the concentration of the antigen. It is used for estimation of the immunoglobulin classes (Fig. 17.5)
d. *Double diffusion in two dimensions*: (Ouchterlony procedure) (Fig. 17.6).
   - This is used most widely and helps to compare antigens and antisera directly.
   - Agar gel is poured on a slide and wells are cut using a template.
   - The antiserum is placed in the central well and different antigens in the surrounding well.
   - If two adjacent antigens are identical, the lines of precipitate formed by them will fuse. If they are unrelated, the lines will cross each other.

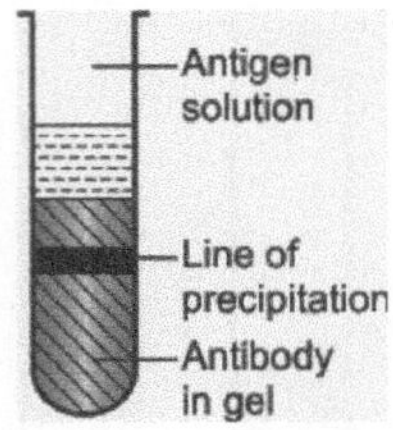

Fig. 17.3: Single diffusion in one dimension

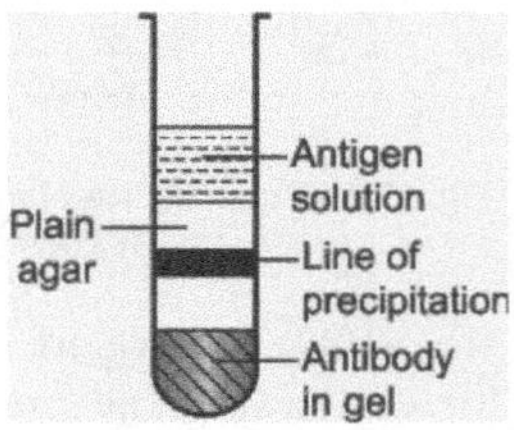

Fig. 17.4: Double diffusion in one dimension

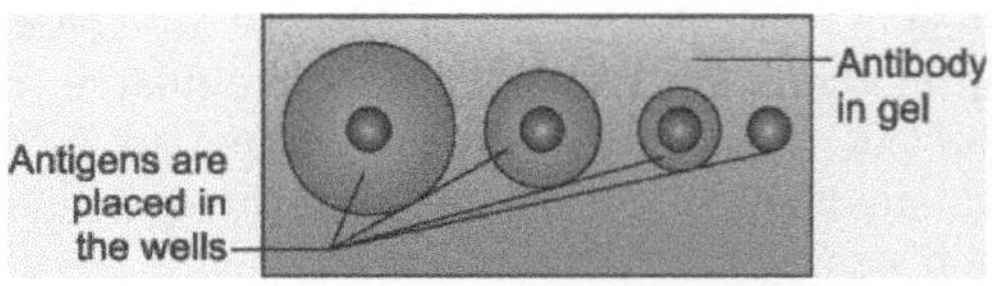

Fig. 17.5: Single diffusion in two dimensions

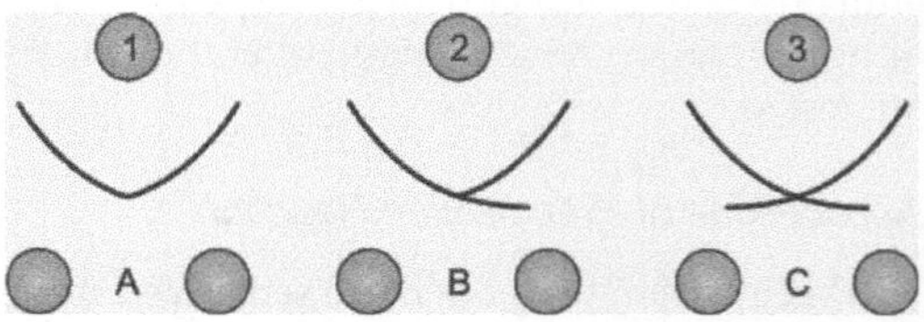

Fig. 17.6: Double diffusion in two dimensions. Wells 1,2,3 contain antibody. Unmarked wells contain antigen, (A) Shows identical antigens, (B) Shows partial identity and (C) Shows lack of relatedness

Immunoelectrophoresis: Electrophoresis means to break up the protein antigen into its component parts. If we allow the antigen and antibody to react with each other after electrophoresis, the process is called immunoelectrophoresis. This consists of two steps:

1. Agar electrophoresis of the antigen.
2. Reaction with antiserum.

Diagrammatic sequence of steps (Fig. 17.7).

1. Semisolid agar is layered on a glass slide. A well for antigen and a trough for antiserum is cut out of the agar.
2. The antigen well is filled with human serum.
3. Serum separated by electrophoresis.
4. Antiserum trough filled with antiserum to whole human serum.
5. Serum and antiserum allowed to diffuse into agar.
6. Precipitin lines form for individual serum proteins. By immunoelectrophoresis over 30 different antigens can be identified in human serum.

This technique is particularly useful in testing for normal and abnormal serum proteins.

Electroimmunodiffusion: If we apply electric current to the above, i.e. we drive the antigen and antibody towards each other, then the development of precipitin lines can be speeded up. One of the examples of electroimmunodiffusion is counterimmuno-electrophoresis. In this test we simultaneously perform electrophoresis of antigen and antibody in gel in opposite directions resulting in precipitation at a point between them. This method produces visible precipitation lines within thirty minutes (Figs 17.8 and 17.9).

Rocket electrophoresis: One of the simplest and most widespread methods of quantitative determination of antigens is the rocket electrophoresis. In this method the test antigen is subjected to electrophoresis in a plate of agarose gel (1%) mixed with the corresponding antiserum. Thus, the rocket-shaped peak of the precipitation is formed upon electrophoresis which has an area that is proportional to the quantity of antigen in the sample or, more accurately, to the ratio between the antigen concentration in the sample and the antibody concentration in the gel. It can be used as a very effective tool for qualitative and quantitative analysis and in preformulation studies of antigens.

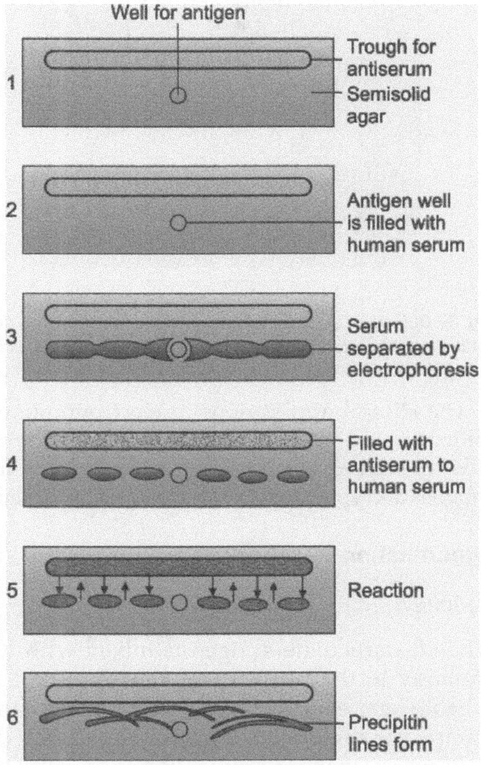

Fig. 17.7: Immunoelectrophoresis: 4 steps (1) Semisolid agar layered on the glass slide. A well for antigen and a trough for antiserum cut out of agar, (2) Antigen well filled with human serum, (3) Serum separated by electrophoresis, (4) Antiserum trough filled with antiserum to whole human serum, (5) Serum and antiserum allowed to diffuse into agar, (6) Precipitin lines form for individual serum proteins

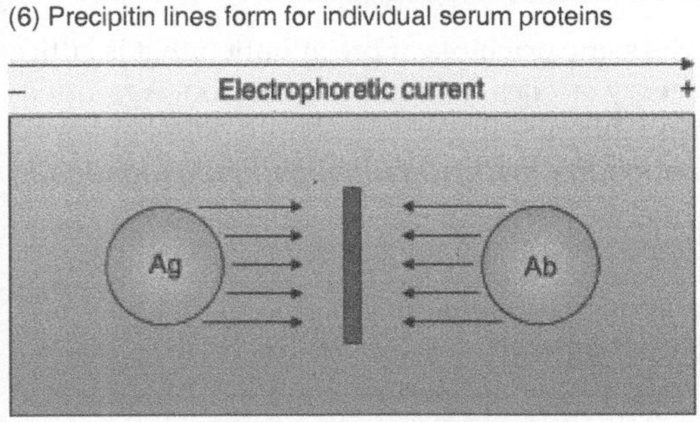

Fig. 17.8: One-dimensional double electroimmunodiffusion. Antigen and antibody are driven together by an electric current and a precipitin line forms

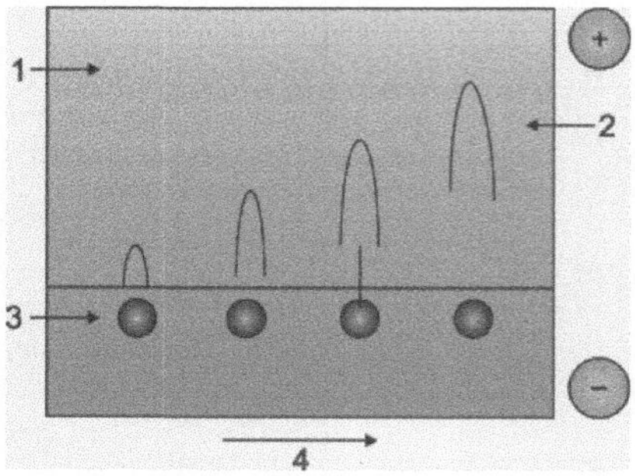

Fig. 17.9: Rocket electrophoresis. Antigen is driven into gel containing antibody. (1) Antibody in agarose gel, (2) Precipitin arcs, (3) Antigen wells, (4) Increasing antigen concentration

The clinical applications of electroimmunodiffusion are to detect various antigens such as HBsAg, Alpha-1 feto protein in serum and specific antigens of cryptococcus in the cerebrospinal fluid.

Agglutination Reactions

Definition

When a particulate antigen is mixed with its antibody in the presence of electrolytes at a suitable temperature and pH, the particles are clumped or agglutinated.

As we see that in agglutination as opposed to precipitation the antigen is particulate and agglutination is more sensitive than precipitation for the detection of an antibody.

Mechanism of Agglutination

The same principle of precipitation that is lattice theory applies for agglutination too. Agglutination occurs optimally when antigens and antibodies react in equivalent proportions.

Applications of Agglutination Reaction

Direct Aggutination Test:

Slide agglutination: When a drop of the appropriate antiserum is added to a smooth uniform suspension of a particulate antigen in a drop of saline on a slide or a tile, agglutination takes place. A positive result is indicated by clumping of the particles. Mixing the antigen and antiserum with a loop or by gently rocking the slide helps the reaction. Depending upon the titer of the serum, agglutination may occur instantly or within seconds. Clumping occurring after a minute may be due to drying of the fluid and should be disregarded. It is essential to have on the same slide a control too. Slide agglutination is a routine procedure for the identification of many bacterial isolates from clinical specimens. It is also the method used for blood grouping or crossmatching.

Tube agglutination: This is the standard quantitative method for the measurement of antibodies. When a fixed volume of a particulate antigen suspension is added to an equal volume of serial dilutions of an antiserum in test tubes, the agglutination titer of the serum can be estimated. Tube agglutination is routinely used for serological diagnosis of typhoid fever known as the Widal test. In this, two types of antigens are used the H or the flagellar antigen and the O or the somatic antigen. When fixed particulate antigens H and O are added to antibody (serum) dilutions, the titer of the antibodies can be detected by the highest dilution of serum showing agglutination. Other examples are Weil-Felix reaction for serodiagnosis of typhus fevers and Paul-Bunnell Test for diagnosis of infectious mononucleosis. The Weil-Felix reaction for serodiagnosis of typhus fevers is a heterophile agglutination test and is based on the sharing of a common antigen between typhus rickettsiae and some strains of proteus bacilli. Paul-Bunnell test is based on the appearance in the sera of infectious mononucleosis patients agglutinins to sheep erythrocytes which are adsorbed by ox red cells but not by guinea pig kidney extract.

Passive or Indirect Agglutination Test: Agglutination tests are more convenient and more sensitive for the detection of antibodies. If we have soluble antigens and we want to perform agglutination test we can attach the soluble antigens to the surface of the carrier particles and perform agglutination. The carrier particles used are red cells, latex particles, or bentonite. Human or sheep erythrocytes adsorb a variety of antigens.

Latex agglutination tests are commonly used these days.

Polystyrene latex can be manufactured as uniform spherical particles. 0.8 to 1 μ in diameter and can adsorb several types of antigens. The latex agglutination test for rheumatoid arthritis uses latex particles coated with gamma globulin. In Rheumatoid Arthritis, an autoantibody (RA factor) appears in the serum, which acts as an antibody to gamma globulin. When the patient's serum is mixed with the antigen suspension, agglutination should occur.

Passive agglutination tests are very sensitive and yield high titers. We can also adsorb the antibody to the carrier particle instead of the antigen.

Complement Fixation Tests

Introduction

We shall study about complement in detail in the next chapter but here we shall introduce complement. It refers to a system of factors occurring in normal serum that are activated by antigen antibody interaction and carry out a number of biologically significant functions.

Components of Complement

Complement is not a single substance but a complex of 9 different protein fractions. They are named from C1 to C9. C1 is made up of 3 protein subunits. So a total of 11 different proteins have been identified.

Complement fixation test is a complex procedure consisting of two steps and five reagents.

1. Antigen
2. Antibody
3. Complement
4. Sheep erythrocytes
5. Amboceptor (rabbit antibody to sheep red cells).

Each of these reagents has to be separately standardized.

Antigen may be soluble or particulate. The antiserum should be heated at 56°C (inactivated) for half an hour before the test to destroy any complement activity the serum may have and also to remove some nonspecific inhibitors of complement present in some sera.

Antibody is to be detected in the patient's serum. Complement is normally present in the body in an inactive form but when its activity is initiated by antigen antibody complexes, the complement components react in a specific sequence or a cascade. During the stages in the cascade several biologically active fragments are released as by products. These fragments help to amplify the defense mechanism by enhancing the inflammatory process.

Complement as a whole mediates immunological membrane damage (cytolysis, bacteriolysis), amplifies the inflammatory response and participates in the pathogenesis of certain hypersensitivity reactions. It also exhibits antiviral activity and promotes phagocytosis.

The ability of antigen and antibody complexes to fix complement is made use of in complement fixation test.

Source of complement is guinea pig serum. The guinea pig serum should be titrated for complement activity.

A good example of complement fixation test is the Wassermann reaction used for the serodiagnosis of syphilis.

The test has two steps.

1. The inactivated serum of the patient is incubated at 37°C for one hour with the Wassermann antigen and fixed amount of units of guinea pig complement, i.e. Ag + (Ab) in test serum) + Complement

   If the serum contains syphilitic antibody the complement will be utilized during the antigen antibody interaction. In other words, the complement will be fixed. If the serum does not contain the antibody, no antigen antibody reaction occurs and therefore complement is left intact.
2. Now, we have to test for complement. This is the second step in the test and consists of adding sensitized cells (sheep erythrocytes

coated with antibody to sheep RBC) or amboceptor and incubating at 37° for 30 minutes. Here the sheep erythrocytes are the antigen and the amboceptor is the antibody.

- If the complement was fixed in the 1st step then it will not be available for hemolysing the second stage and hence we will see no hemolysis.
- If the test serum did not have antibody, then the complement was not utilized in the 1st stage and it was free to interact with the hemolytic system causing hemolysis.

Appropriate controls should be put up for the proper performance of the tests.

In short

Antigen + Test serum (contains antibody) } Complement fixed
+ Complement
+ Hemolytic system Result—no hemolysis

Positive Complement Fixation Test

Antigen + Test serum (contains no antibody) } Complement not fixed
+ Complement Result-Hemolysis
+ Hemolytic system

Negative Complement Fixation Test

Neutralization Tests

Specific antibodies neutralize the biological effects of viruses, toxins and enzymes.

Virus Neutralization

Neutralization of viruses by their antibodies can be demonstrated in various systems. Neutralization of bacteriophages can be demonstrated by the plaque inhibition test. When bacteriophages are applied on lawn cultures of susceptible bacteria plaques of lysis are produced. Specific antiphage serum inhibits plaque formation. Neutralization of animal viruses can be demonstrated in 3 systems—animals, eggs and tissue culture.

Toxin Neutralization

Bacterial exotoxins are good antigens and induce the formation of neutralizing antibodies (antitoxins), e.g. diseases like diphtheria and tetanus.

Toxin neutralization tests can be tested *in vivo* or in vitro.

In vivo: This is carried out in animals who are injected with toxin antitoxin mixtures and the least amount of antitoxin that prevents death or disease in the animal is estimated.

In vitro: Toxin neutralization in vitro depends on the inhibition of some demonstrable toxic effect. For example, in anti-streptolysin O test the antitoxin present in patient's sera neutralizes the hemolytic activity of the streptococcal O hemolysin .

Immunofluorescence

Fluorescence is the property of absorbing light rays of one particular wavelength and emitting rays with a different wavelength. Fluorescent dyes show up brightly under ultraviolet light as they convert ultraviolet into visible light. Fluorescent dyes can be conjugated to antibodies and labelled antibodies can be used to locate and identify antigens in tissues. This fluorescent antibody or immunofluorescence technique has many diagnostic and research applications.

There are two types of fluorescence:

- Direct immunofluorescence
- Indirect immunofluorescence

Direct Immunofluorescence

It is used for the identification of bacteria, viruses or other antigens using the specific antiserum labelled with a fluorescent dye. For example, direct immunofluorescence is used as a sensitive method of diagnosing rabies. But the disadvantage of this method is that separate fluorescent conjugates have to be prepared against each antigen to be tested.

Indirect Immunofluorescence

The indirect immunofluorescence test overcomes this problem by using an antiglobulin fluorescent conjugate (Fig. 17.10).

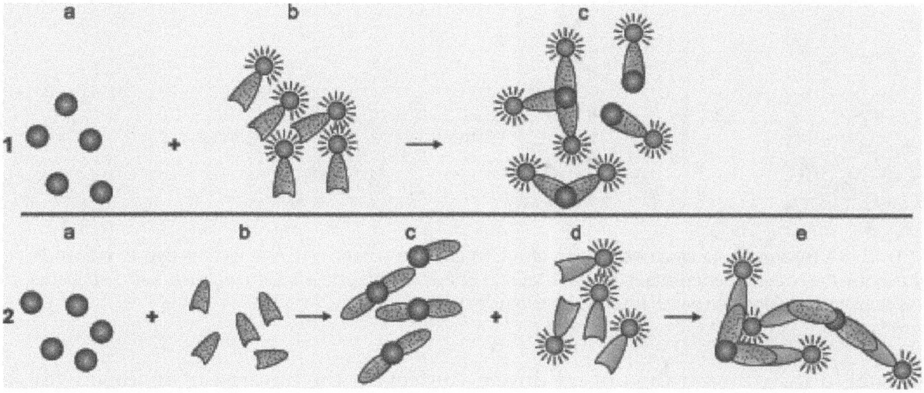

Fig. 17.10: Immunofluorescence (1) Direct test: Antigen (a) is mixed with fluorescent-conjugated antibody (b). The antigen antibody complex is fluorescent (c). (2) Indirect test: (a) antigen is mixed with antibody (b). The antigen antibody complex, (c) is treated with fluorescent conjugated antiglobulin serum (d). The final product is fluorescent (e)

For example, fluorescent treponemal antibody test for the diagnosis of syphilis. A single antihuman globulin fluorescent conjugate can be employed for detecting human antibody to any antigen. Fluorescent dyes may also be conjugated with complement. Labeled complement is a versatile tool and can be used for detection of antigen or antibody. Antigens also take fluorescent labeling but not as well as antibodies do.

The fluorescent dyes commonly used are fluorescein isothiocyanate and lissamine rhodamine exhibiting blue green and orange red fluorescence respectively.

Enzyme-Linked Immunosorbent Assay (ELISA)

ELISA test is a simple and sensitive technique. It needs only microliter quantities of test reagent.

ELISA has found application for the detection of a variety of antibodies and antigens such as hormones, toxins and viruses (Fig. 17.11).

The test may be done in polystyrene tubes (macro-ELISA) or polyvinyl microtiter plates (micro-ELISA).

Principle of the Test

The basic principle of the ELISA is that we bind to the wells, antigens or antibodies specific to our test specimen. Then we add the patients serum. After the antigen or antibody has bound to its counterpart, we provide an anti-antibody attached to an enzyme. This is called an enzyme conjugate. In the last step a substrate is added on which the enzyme acts to give color. The intensity of color developed is proportional to the original concentration of antigen or antibody in the serum.

For an understanding of the ELISA technique, we shall study an example. The estimation of total IgE levels in the patient's serum is done by a solid phase enzyme linked immunosorbent assay (micro-ELISA). The wells are coated with anti-IgE antibodies. The samples, standards and controls are allowed to incubate in the wells. The IgE present in the patients sample gets attached to the anti IgE. After washing, the enzyme conjugate is added (this means an enzyme bound with anti-IgE antibodies. This enzyme here is horseradish peroxidase).

A sandwich complex is formed (Anti-IgE-IgE-anti IgE + E). The unbound conjugate is again washed off with water. The amount of bound enzyme (horseradish peroxidase) is proportional to the concentration of the IgE present in the samples. Upon the addition of the substrate, it is broken down by the enzyme present to give a color. The intensity of the color developed is

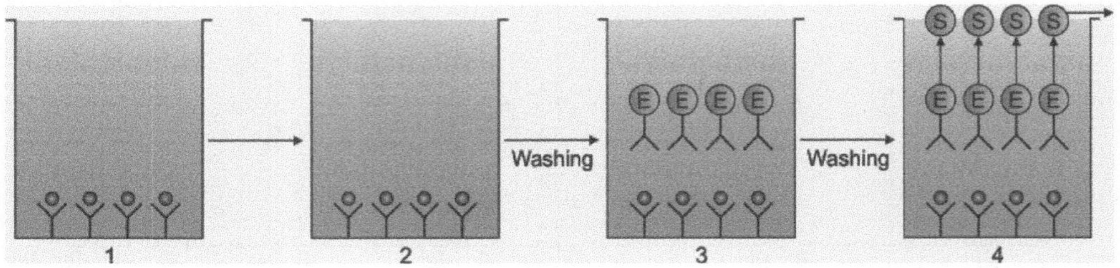

Fig. 17.11: ELISA (example—to show estimation of IgE in patients serum). (1) Anti IgE antibodies coated to the wells, (2) IgE present in the patients serum attaches to anti IgE, (3) Enzyme conjugate is added (enzyme + Anti-antibody), (antibody to IgE) (4) Substrate is added on which enzyme acts to give color

proportional to the concentration of IgE in the serum.

Radioimmunoassay

Radioimmunoassay (RIA) was introduced into clinical medicine by Berson and Yalow (1960). It is a sensitive and specific method for the assay of various substances such as hormones, drugs such as digoxin and antigens such as hepatitis antigen.

RIA is based on the principle of competition between a radioactively labeled and unlabeled antigen to bind to a specific antibody. We keep the unknown as unlabeled antigen. In order that competition occurs, the number of binding sites of the antibody must be less than the total amounts of labeled and unlabeled antigen. The quantity of unlabeled antigen is measured by its effect on the binding of labeled antigen and by comparing the effect with that of a known amount of unlabeled antigen. Either the amount of free labeled antigen or the amount of antibody labeled antigen or both can be measured after separation.

It is a general method employing the reaction of an antigen with its specific antibody, permitting measurement of the concentration of virtually any substance of biological interest, often with unparalleled sensitivity. The basis of the method is summarized in the competing reactions shown in the illustration. The unknown concentration of the antigenic substance in a sample is obtained by comparing its inhibitory effect on the binding of radioactively labeled antigen to a limited amount of specific antibody with the inhibitory effect of known standards.

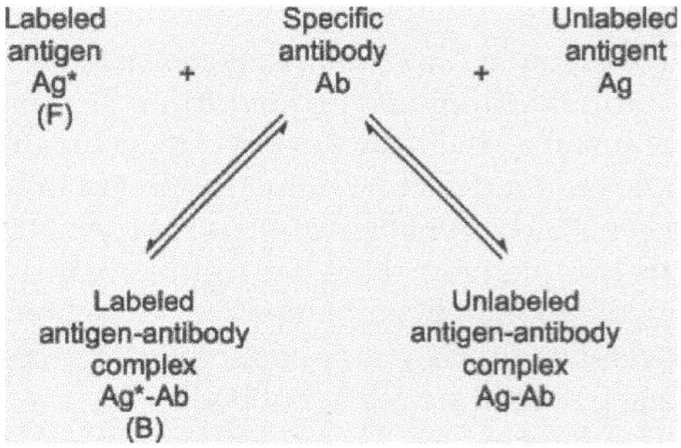

Competing reactions that form basis of radioimmunoassay; * indicates the labeled antigen, and † "in known standard solutions or unknown samples

A typical radioimmunoassay is performed by the simultaneous preparation of a series of standard and unknown mixtures in test tubes, each containing identical concentrations of labelled antigen and specific antibody. After an appropriate reaction time the antibody-bound (B) and free (F) fractions of the labeled antigen are separated by one of a variety of techniques. The B/F ratios in the standards are plotted as a function of the concentration of unlabeled antigen (standard curve), and the unknown concentration of antigen is determined by comparing the observed B/F ratio with the standard curve.

The radioimmunoassay principle has found wide application in the measurement of a large and diverse group of substances in a variety of problems of clinical and biological interest. It is therefore not unexpected that there are differences in the specific methods employed for the assay of a particular substance. The full potential of the method has yet to be exploited. It seems that virtually any substance of biologic interest can be measured, the method being modified according to the characteristics of the particular substance.

CHAPTER 18

Complement

LESSON PLAN

- Definition
- Components of Complement
- Functions
- Classical and Alternative Pathway of Complement Activation
- Biological Effects of Complement
- Deficiencies of the Complement System

DEFINITION

The term complement refers to a system of factors occurring in normal serum that are activated by antigen antibody interaction and then carry out some biologically significant actions. This term was given by Ehrlich because it complemented the action of antibody. It is heat labile.

COMPONENTS OF COMPLEMENT

Complement is not a single substance but a complex of nine different protein fractions. They are named from C_1 to C_9. The fraction labeled C_1 is made up of three protein subunits. So, a total of 11 different proteins have been identified.

FUNCTIONS

Table 18.1 shows the complement cascade.

The complement makes up approximately 10 percent of the human serum globulins. Though some of the components are heat stable, complement as a whole is heat labile, undergoing spontaneous denaturation slowly at room temperature and in 30 minutes at 56°C. When the serum is deprived of its complement activity it is said to be inactivated. Complement does not combine with either antigen or antibody alone but with the antigen antibody complexes. Complement is normally present in the body in an inactive form but when it is stimulated, the complement components react in a specific sequence or cascade. During successive stages in the cascade several biologically active fragments are released from the complement components as by-products. These components amplify the defence mechanism by enhancing the inflammatory process, increasing vascular permeability, causing smooth muscle contraction, causing chemotaxis of leucocytes, promoting virus neutralization, detoxifying endocrines and affecting the release of histamine from mast cells.

CLASSICAL AND ALTERNATIVE PATHWAY OF COMPLEMENT ACTIVATION

The central process in the complement cascade is the activation of C_3 which is the major component of C. In the classical pathway, activation of C_3 is achieved by C_3 convertase. The activation of C_3 without the prior participation of C_3 convertase is called alternative pathway.

Table 18.1: The complement cascade

Components	*Reaction sequence*	*Biological effects*
C1	EA + Clqrs →(Ca) EAC1a ↓ → C_{4a} + C_{4bi}	
C4	→ EAC1a, 4b	→ Virus Neutralization
C2	→ Mg^{++} → C_{2i}, C_2	Kinins-increase vascular permeability
	EAC1a, 4b, 2a	
C3	→ C_{3a}	Anaphylatoxins; Chemotaxis
	EAC1a, 4b, 2a, 3b	Enhances phagocytosis; Virus neutralization; Immune adherence
C5	→ C5a	Anaphylatoxin II; Chemotaxis
	EAC1a, 4b, 2a, 3b, 5b	Initiates membrane damage
C6,7	→ C567	Chemotaxis; Sensitization of 'Bystander cells'; detoxifies endotoxin
	EAC1a, 4b, 2a, 3b, 5b, 6,7	Prepares cells for lysis; Increases cell susceptibility; Killer lymphocytes
C8,9	→ EAC1a, 4b, 2a, 3b, 5b 6,7,8,9	→ Lysis of cell

Table 18.2: Clinical syndromes associated with genetic deficiencies of complement components

Group	*Deficiency*	*Syndrome*
I	C1 inhibitor	Hereditory angioneurotic oedema
II	Early components of classical pathway C1, C2, C4	SLE and other collagen-vascular diseases
III	C3 and its regulatory protein C3 b inactivator	Severe recurrent pyogenic infections
IV	C5 to C8	Bacteraemia, mainly with Gram-negative diplococci, toxoplasmosis.
V	C9	No particular disease

Table 18.3 shows the biosynthesis of complement component.

Table 18.3: Biosynthesis of complement

C_1 is synthesized in intestinal epithelium
C_2,4 is synthesized in macrophages
$C_{5,8}$ is synthesized in spleen
$C_{3,6,9}$ is synthesized in liver
C_7 → site is unknown

BIOLOGICAL EFFECTS OF COMPLEMENT

Complement mediates immunological membrane damage (cytolysis, bacteriolysis), amplifies the inflammatory response and participates in the pathogenesis of certain hypersensitivity reactions. It shows antiviral activity and promotes phagocytosis.

The classical C pathway results in bacteriolysis and cytolysis. Cells vary in their susceptibility to complement mediated lysis. Gram-negative bacteria are sensitive to lysis while gram-positive cells are killed without lysis. Complement participates in the type II and III hypersensitivity reactions.

DEFICIENCIES OF THE COMPLEMENT SYSTEM

Complete or partial deficiencies of all the classical complement components and several of the complement inhibitors have been described in man or animals. Some are associated with severe disease while in others clinical manifestations are sporadic. Complement deficiencies result in the host being unable to efficiently eliminate microbial antigens or circulating immune complexes. Recurrent bacterial and fungal infections and collagen diseases occur (Table 18.2).

CHAPTER

19

Structure and Function of the Immune System

LESSON PLAN

- Introduction
- Structure of the Lymphoid System
  - Central Lymphoid Organs
  - Peripheral Lymphoid Organs
  - Cells of the Lymphoreticular System
- Immune Response
- Humoral Immune Response
  - Primary and Secondary Responses
  - Presentation of Antigens and Production of Antibodies
  - Monoclonal Antibodies
- Cellular Immune Response

INTRODUCTION

The lymphoreticular system or the immune system is a complex organization of various cells with different morphology distributed widely in the organs and tissues of the body. This system consists of lymphoid cells and the reticuloendothelial cells. The lymphoid cells are lymphocytes and plasma cells which are concerned with the specific immune response. The reticuloendothelial cells includes the phagocytic cells which are concerned with the function of destroying foreign particles.

The immune response to an antigen can be of two broad types:

a. Humoral or antibody mediated immunity
b. Cellular or cell mediated immunity

Humoral immunity is mediated by antibodies produced by plasma cells while cellular immunity is mediated directly by sensitized lymphocytes.

STRUCTURE OF THE LYMPHOID SYSTEM

The lymphoid system consists of lymphoid organs and lymphoid cells.

Lymphoid organs—The lymphoid organs can be classified into:

a. Central (primary)
b. Peripheral lymphoid organs

Central lymphoid organs are those in which precursor lymphocytes proliferate, develop and acquire immunological capability. The thymus gland and the bursa of Fabricius in birds, are primary lymphoid organs responsible for cell mediated immunity and humoral immunity respectively. The equivalent of the avian bursa in mammals has not been identified but it may be the bone marrow. After acquiring immunocompetence, the lymphocytes migrate through blood and lymph streams, accumulate in the peripheral lymphoid organs and following antigenic stimulus, effect the appropriate immune response. The spleen and the lymph nodes constitute the major peripheral lymphoid organs and the lymphoid tissues in the gut, lungs, liver, bone marrow and the lymphoid collections in other organs are a part of the minor peripheral lymphoid system.

Central Lymphoid Organs

Thymus

The thymus is the first organ in all animal species to become predominantly lymphoid. In man the thymus reaches its maximum relative size just before birth. It continues to grow till about the 12th year. After puberty, it undergoes spontaneous involution. It functions best in early life. The thymus is located behind the upper part of the sternum. The primary function of the thymus is the production of thymic lymphocytes. It is the major site for lymphocyte proliferation in the body. But of the lymphocytes produced only one percent leave the thymus. The rest are destroyed locally. In the thymus the lymphocytes acquire new surface antigens and become immunocompetent. They are educated so that they become capable of mounting cell mediated immune response against appropriate antigens. These lymphocytes are called T lymphocytes. They are selectively seeded into certain sites of the peripheral lymphatic tissue.

Bursa of Fabricius

This is a lymphoepithelial organ arising as a pouch from the dorsal part of the cloaca in birds. Its development, structure and function parallel those of the thymus. The bursal equivalent in mammals is not known. It has been suggested that the gut associated lymphoid tissue may carry out this function. These consists of the tonsils, (lingual, palatine and pharyngeal) the Peyer's patches and the solitary follicles of the small intestine and appendix. The bone marrow has also been proposed as the possible bursal equivalent in mammals.

Peripheral Lymphoid Organs

Lymph Nodes

The lymph nodes are small, round or ovoid bodies placed along the course of lymphatic vessels. It contains both T and B lymphocytes. Lymph nodes act as filters for the lymph, each group of nodes draining a specific part of the body. They phagocytose foreign materials including microorganisms. They help the proliferation and circulation of T and B cells. They enlarge following local antigenic stimulation (Fig. 19.1).

Spleen

The spleen is the largest of the lymphoid organs. The spleen is the graveyard for dead red blood cells and filters the circulating blood borne foreign antigens. It has both T and B lymphocyte areas.

Cells of the Lymphoreticular System

The cells of the lymphoreticular system consist of structural cells (reticulum cells, endothelial cells and fibroblasts) and those that perform specialized immunological functions (lymphocytes, plasma cells and macrophages).

Lymphocytes

Lymphocytes are small round cells found in the peripheral blood, lymph, lymphoid organs and in many other tissues. In peripheral blood, they constitute 20 to 45 percent of the leukocyte population while in lymph and lymphoid organs they are the predominant cell type. According to their size, lymphocytes can be classified into small (5 to 8 μ), medium (8 to 12 μ) and large (12 to 15 μ) lymphocytes. Lymphopoiesis takes place in the bone marrow, central lymphoid organs and peripheral lymphoid tissues. These populations of lymphocytes do not remain distinct but mix together in the process known as lymphocyte recirculation. There is a constant traffic of lymphocytes in the blood, lymph, lymphatic organs and tissues. Recirculating lymphocytes are mainly T cells. Circulating T and B lymphocytes can be differentiated by many ways. T lymphocytes are about 55 to 75 percent and B cells 15 to 30 percent. Table 19.1 shows some of the differences between T cells, B cells and macrophages.

T lymphocytes can be differentiated into various subsets based on antigenic determinants present on their surface.

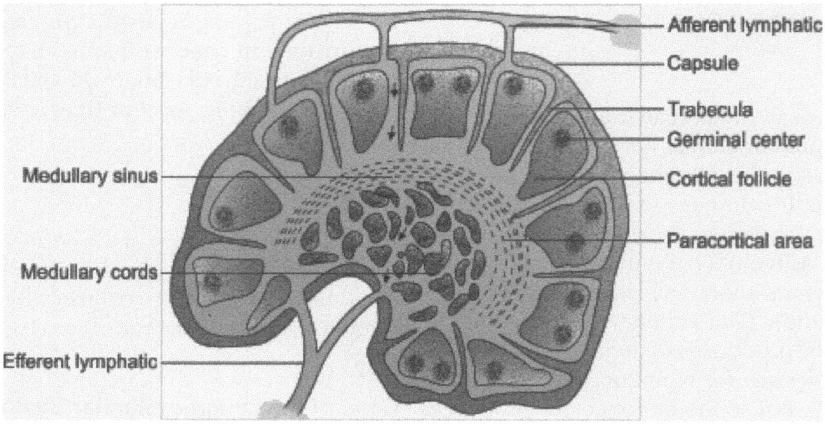

Fig. 19.1: Diagrammatic section of lymph node. Arrows indicate the path of lymph flow

Table 19.1: Some distinguishing characteristics of T cells, B cells, and macrophages

Property	*T cell*	*B cell*	*macrophage*
Surface immunoglobulins	–	+	–
Receptor for Fc piece of IgG	–	+	–
C_3 receptor	–	+	–
SRBC rosette	+	–	–
Thymus specific antigens	+	–	–
Numerous microvilli on surface	–	+	–
Blast transformation with-			
• PHA			
• Concanavalin A	+	–	–
• Endotoxins	–	+	–
Phagocytic action	–	–	+
Adherence to glass surface	–	–	+

- T cells bind to sheep erythrocytes at 37°C forming rosettes (SRBC or E rosette) while B cells do not
- B cells bind to sheep erythrocytes coated with antibody and complement forming EAC rosettes. T cells do not. EAC rosette formation is due to the presence of a C_3 receptor on B cell surface.

The Helpers cells (TH)	35 to 75 percent
Suppressor cells (TS)	25 to 40 percent

Apart from this there is a small proportion of lymphocytes which cannot be classified and these are known as null cells.

Earlier T cells were known as T1,T3, etc. They have been renamed as CD-1, CD-3, etc.

CD = cluster of differentiation. Table 19.2 shows the classification of T cells.

Table 19.2: T lymphocyte subsets

A. Regulatory T cells
   1. Helper cells (T_H) CD_4)
   2. Suppressor cells (T_S) (CD_8)

B. Effector cells
   1. Cytotoxic T lymphocytes (CTL)—CD_8
   2. Delayed type hypersensitivity (DTH)—CD_4
   3. Mixed lymphocyte reactivity (MLR)

Plasma Cells

Antigenically stimulated B cells undergo blast transformation and change into plasma cells. The mature plasma cell is the antibody secreting cell. It is an oval cell about twice the size of a small lymphocyte. It has an eccentrically placed oval nucleus containing large blocks of chromatin located peripherally (cartwheel or clock face appearance). Plasma cells are end cells and have a short life span of two or three days. A plasma cell makes an antibody of a single specificity.

Phagocytic Cells

Phagocytosis is the oldest defense mechanism in animals. It was discovered by Metchnikoff in 1882. The phagocytic cells of the body are the macrophages of blood and tissues and the microphages.

The primary function of macrophages is phagocytosis. The cells move slowly in a purposeful manner. They accumulate in areas of inflammation or of tissue damage by chemotaxis. Particles sensitized by antibodies are phagocytosed more readily. The phagocytosed particle is held inside a vacuole (phagosome), the membrane of which fuses with a lysosome forming a phagolysosome. Some bacteria like typhoid, brucellosis and tuberculosis resist digestion, may multiply inside cells and are transported in them to other locations.

The microphages are polymorphonuclear leukocytes—neutrophils, eosinophils and basophils. Neutrophils are actively phagocytic and are the predominant cell type in a acute inflammation.

IMMUNE RESPONSE

The specific reactivity induced in a host by an antigenic stimulus is known as the immune response. This is usually protective but can be dangerous as for example, in hypersensitivity or autoimmunity (destruction of self organs). The immune response can be of two types the humoral (antibody mediated) and the cellular (cell mediated). These two types may develop together though at times one or the other may be the predominant type.

Antibody mediated immunity provides defense against most extracellular bacterial pathogens, helps in defense against viruses that infect through the respiratory or intestinal tracts, prevents virus infections from occurring again and participates in the pathogenesis of immediate hypersensitivity and certain autoimmune diseases. Cell mediated immunity protects against fungi, viruses and intracellular bacterial pathogens, participates in rejection of grafts, provides immunological surveillance and immunity against cancer and mediates pathogenesis of delayed type IV hypersensitivity and certain autoimmune diseases.

HUMORAL IMMUNE RESPONSE

The production of antibodies involves three steps:

a. The entry of the antigen, its distribution and fate in the tissues and its contact with appropriate immunocompetent cells (the afferent limb).
b. The processing of antigen by cells and the control of the antibody forming process (central functions).
c. The secretion of antibody, its distribution in tissues and body fluids and the manifestations of it's effects (efferent limb).

Just like, the growth curve, antibody production follows a characteristic pattern consisting of:

a. Log phase: The immediate stage following antigenic stimulus during which no antibody is detected in circulation.
b. lag phase: There is a steady rise in titer of antibodies.
c. Plateau or steady state: There is equilibrium between antibody synthesis and catabolism.
d. Phase of decline: Catabolism exceeds production and the titer falls.

Primary and Secondary Responses

Primary response to an antigen means the first response to an antigen. Secondary response is the response of the immune system, the next time the antigen comes into contact. The primary response is slow, sluggish and short-lived with a long lag phase and low titer of antibodies that do not persist for long. In contrast the secondary response is prompt powerful and prolonged with a short lag phase and a much higher level of antibodies that lasts for long periods. The antibody formed in the primary response is predominantly IgM and in the secondary response IgG. The duration of the lag phase and the persistence of the antibody vary with the nature of the antigen. A single injection of an antigen helps more in sensitizing or priming the immunocompetent cells producing the particular antibody. Effective levels of antibody are usually induced by subsequent injections of the antigen. It is for this reason that nonliving vaccines are given in multiple doses for active immunization. The first injection is known as the priming dose and the other injections as booster doses. With live vaccines, a single dose is sufficient as multiplication of the organism in the body provides a continuing antigenic stimulus that acts both as priming and booster doses.

Presentation of Antigens and Production of Antibodies

When the antigen first enters the body it is broken down and engulfed by the macrophages and the antigens are presented to the lymphocytes for antibody formation or the initiation of cell mediated immunity. With the appearance of the specific antibody the phase of immune elimination begins during which antigen antibody complexes are formed which are rapidly phagocytosed resulting in a rapid disappearance of the antigen from circulation.

The cells that recognize antigens and initiate antibody synthesis are the immunocompetent B lymphocytes. When an antigen reactive cell is stimulated by contact with the appropriate antigenic determinant it undergoes clonal proliferation and blast transformation and gets converted to plasma cells which secrete antibodies. Some antigens do not require the help of T lymphocytes whereas others like erythrocytes, serum, proteins, etc. do. T lymphocytes first interact with the antigen, concentrate them on the cell surface and present them to B cells for antibody formation. Antibody formation by B cells is stimulated by helper T cells and inhibited by suppressor T cells. Optimal antibody response depends on balanced activity of T helper and suppressor cells.

Following antigenic stimulus, not all B cells get converted to plasma cells. A small proportion of them develop into memory cells which have a long-life-span and serve to recognize the same antigens when introduced subsequently. The increased antibody response during secondary antigenic stimulation is due to the presence of memory cells induced by primary contact with the antigen.

Monoclonal Antibodies

A single antibody forming cell produces antibodies specifically directed against a single antigen or antigenic determinant only. When a clone of lymphocytes or plasma cells undergoes selective multiplication as in multiple myeloma, antibodies with a single antigenic specificity accumulate. Such antibodies produced by a single clone and directed against a single antigenic determinant are called monoclonal antibodies. Monoclonal antibodies are very useful tools for diagnostic and research techniques.

A method for the production of monoclonal antibodies was described by Kohlerr and Milstein in 1975. In recognition of the great importance of this hybridoma technology, the nobel prize in medicine was awarded to them. This is the hybridoma technique. Hybridomas are somatic cell hybrids produced by fusing antibody forming spleen cells and the ability of the myeloma cells to multiply definitely. Monoclonal antibodies against several antigens are now available commercially.

Procedure for Making Monoclonal Antibodies

Lymphocytes from the spleen of mice immunized with the desired antigen are fused with mouse myeloma cells grown in culture and deficient in the enzyme hypoxanthine phosphoribosyl transferase (HPRT). The fused cells are placed in a basal culture medium which does not permit growth of the enzyme deficient myeloma cells. As normal lymphocytes cannot replicate indefinitely, only hybrid cells possessing properties of both the splenic lymphocytes and myeloma cells are grown in culture. These cultures called hybridomas are cloned and examined for the production of antibodies. Clones producing antibodies against the desired antigen are selected on continuous cultivation. Such hybridomas can be maintained indefinitely in culture and will continue to form monoclonal antibodies.

Table 19.3 shows the differences in between monoclonal and conventional antibodies.

CELLULAR IMMUNE RESPONSE

The term cell mediated immunity refers to the specific immune responses that do not involve

Table 19.3: Differences in monoclonal and conventional antibodies

Property	*Conventional antibody*	*Monoclonal antibody*
Useful antibody contents	Low	High
Composition	Multiple (variable from animal to animal)	Homogenous (defined and consistent)
Cross-reaction with other antigens	Partial with antigen bearing common antigenic determinants	Usually absent
Class and subclass of immunoglobulins	Mixture of many classes	Only one
Supply	Limited	Abundant

antibodies. Cell mediated immunity is as important as humoral immunity if not more for life. Cell mediated immunity (CMI) has the following functions:

a. Delayed hypersensitivity.
b. Immunity in infectious diseases caused by intracellular parasites. These include infections with bacteria like tuberculosis, leprosy, fungi, protozoa and viruses like smallpox, measles and mumps.
c. Transplantation immunity and graft versus host reaction.
d. Immunity against cancer.
e. Pathogenesis of certain autoimmune diseases like thyroiditis and encephalitis.

The nature of the antigenic stimulus is important in the induction of CMI. It is best developed following infections with intracellular parasites. Killed vaccines and other nonliving antigens do not induce CMI. When a sensitized cell comes into contact with the antigenic determinant it undergoes blast transformation and clonal proliferation in the para cortical areas of the lymph nodes. The activated lymphocytes release biologically active products (lymphokines) which are responsible for the manifestations of CMI. Macrophages and other mononuclear cells under the effect of lymphokines effect the destruction of micro-organisms.

CHAPTER

20

Hypersensitivity

LESSON PLAN

- Definition and Introduction
  - Sensitization
  - Allergy
- Classification of Hypersensitivity Reactions
  - Type I Hypersensitivity Reactions—Anaphylaxis
  - Atopy
  - Type II Reactions
  - Type III Immune Complex Diseases
  - Type IV Delayed Hypersensitivity Reaction
- Shwartzman Reaction

DEFINITION AND INTRODUCTION

We have studied that immunity is a protective process helping the body to fight against microbes. This is only one aspect of the immune response. Immune response may sometimes be harmful to the host. Hypersensitivity is an example of the harmful aspect of the immune response. The term hypersensitivity means an exaggerated, altered or excessive response usually injurious, in a sensitized host after contact with specific antigens. In the protective processes of immunity, the focus of attention is the antigen and what happens to it, for example killing of a bacterium or neutralization of a toxin. In hypersensitivity we are concerned with what happens to the host as a result of the immune reaction. The antigens are usually noninjurious and the nonsensitized individuals do not react to the antigen. However, the sensitized individuals overreact leading to tissue damage, disease and death.

Hypersensitivity is concerned with what happens to the host as a result of the immune reaction.

Sensitization

For induction of hypersensitivity reactions, the host should have had contact with the antigen (allergen). The initial contact sensitizes the immune system leading to priming of the appropriate B or T lymphocytes. This is known as the sensitizing or the priming dose. Subsequent contact with the allergen causes signs of hypersensitivity. This is known as the shocking dose.

Allergy

The term allergy is used very commonly in place of hypersensitivity. It is sometimes used for only one type of hypersensitivity namely atopy.

CLASSIFICATION OF HYPERSENSITIVITY REACTIONS

Hypersensitivity reactions have been classified into immediate and delayed types depending on the time required for a sensitized host to develop clinical reactions upon re-exposure to the antigen. The second contact with the allergen causes symptoms of hypersensitivity. This is known as the shocking dose.

There are many differences between features of immediate and delayed types of hypersensitivity (Table 20.1).

Immediate hypersensitivity includes:

1. Anaphylaxis.
2. Cytotoxic or cell stimulating.
3. Immune complex mediated.

Table 20.1: Differences between immediate and delayed hypersensitivity reactions

Immediate	*Delayed*
Appears and disappears fast	Appears slowly, lasts longer
Appears in 1 to 3 hours	Appears in 48 to 72 hours
Mediated by antibodies	Mediated by lymphocytes and transfer factor
Induced by antigens by any route	Induced by infection or by skin contact
Circulating antibodies are present and responsible for reaction	Circulating antibodies may be absent and not responsible for reaction. Cell mediated reaction present
Can be transferred with serum	Cannot be transferred with serum
Desensitization easy, but short lived	Desensitization difficult, but long lasting

Type I Hypersensitivity Reactions—Anaphylaxis

The term anaphylaxis (ana = without, phylaxis = protection) means a toxic reaction in a host who has been previously sensitized to that antigen. Sensitization is most effective when the antigen is introduced parenterally but may occur by any route including ingestion or inhalation. There is an interval of at least 2 to 3 weeks between the sensitizing and shocking doses. Once sensitized, the individual remains so for long periods. The main clinical effects are due to smooth muscle contraction and increased vascular permeability. The organs affected vary with the species. The tissues or organs predominantly involved in anaphylactic reaction are called target tissues or shock organs (cutaneous anaphylaxis—skin test for Type 1 hypersensitivity is useful in testing for hypersensitivity and in identifying the allergen responsible in atopic diseases).

Mechanism of Anaphylaxis

IgE molecules are bound to surface receptors on mast cells in tissues and basophils in circulation. Following exposure to the shocking dose, the antigen molecules combine with the cell bound IgE bridging the gap between adjacent antibody molecules. This cross linking increases the permeability of the cells to calcium ions and leads to degranulation with release of biologically active substances contained in the granules.

Other changes observed in anaphylaxis are edema, fall-in blood pressure, leukopenia and thrombocytopenia.

In man fatal anaphylaxis is rare. Symptoms and signs begin with itching of the scalp and tongue, flushing of the skin over the whole body and difficulty in breathing due to bronchial spasm. There may be nausea, vomiting, abdominal pain and diarrhea sometimes with blood in the stools. Acute hypotension, loss of consciousness and death follow.

Cutaneous Anaphylaxis

When a small shocking dose of an antigen is administered intradermally to a sensitized host, there is a local wheal and flare response (local anaphylaxis). The wheal is a pale central area of puffiness due to edema which is surrounded by a flare caused by hyperemia and subsequent erythema.

The manifestations of anaphylaxis are due to the pharmacological mediators which are of two types—primary and secondary.

Mediators: Primary mediators are preformed contents of mast cells and basophil granules (histamine, serotonin, eosinophil chemotactic factor of anaphylaxis, neutrophil chemotactic factor, heparin and various proteolytic enzymes and the secondary mediators are formed upon stimulation by mast cells, basophils and other leucocytes (slow reacting substance of anaphylaxis, prostaglandins and platelet activating factor) (Table 20.2).

Table 20.2: Pharmacological mediators of anaphylaxis

Mediator	*Source*	*Function*
Histamine	Preformed in mast cells, platelets and basophils	• Elevates cyclic AMP levels • Increases vascular permeability • Smooth muscle constriction • Increases gastric secretion • Stimulates suppressor lymphocytes
Heparin	Mast cell or basophils	Anticoagulant
Serotonin	Preformed in mast cell	Increases vascular permeability
Eosinophilic chemotactic factor	Preformed in mast cells	Attracts and deactivates eonsinophils
Platelet factor	Generated in macrophages, neutrophils, eosinophils	• Aggregates plate activating mast cells lets • Increases vascular permeability • Bronchoconstriction • Vasoconstriction
Prostaglandins	Generated in mast cells	• Increase cAMP • Smooth muscle constriction • Increase vascular permeability
Leukotrienes	Generated in mast cells, macrophages, neutrophils and eosinophils	• Smooth muscle constriction • Increase vascular permeability • Decrease peripheral blood flow. Generate prostaglandins • Decreases lymphocyte response
Neutrophil chemotactic factor	Preformed in mast cells	Attracts and deactivates lymphocytes

Atopy

Atopy means out of place or strangeness. It was introduced by Coca (1923) to refer to naturally occurring familial hypersensitivities of man, e.g. hay fever and asthma. The antigens commonly involved in atopy are inhalants (e.g. pollen, house dust) ingestants (eggs, milk), and contact allergens to which skin and conjunctiva may be exposed.

Atopic sensitization is developed spontaneously following natural contact with atopens inducing IgE antibodies. Its difficult to induce atopy artificially.

Predisposition to atopy is genetically determined. It therefore runs in families. What is inherited is not sensitivity to a particular antigen or a particular atopic syndrome but the tendency to produce antibody (IgE) in unusually large quantities. About 10 percent of people have this tendency to over produce reagin. Atopic sensitivity is associated with a deficiency of IgA. In normal individuals, the inhalant and the ingestant antigens are dealt with by the IgA lining the respiratory and intestinal mucosa and therefore do not come into contact with the potential IgE producing cells. When IgA is deficient, the antigens cause massive stimulation of IgE forming cells leading to overproduction of reagin (IgE).

Symptoms of atopy are caused by the release of pharmacologically active substances following combination between the antigen and the IgE attached to the mast cells. The clinical features of atopic reactions is dependent on the portal of entry of the antigen-conjunctivitis, rhinitis, gastrointestinal symptoms and dermatitis develop on exposure to eye, respiratory tract, intestine or skin respectively.

Specific desensitization (hyposensitization) is practiced in the treatment of atopy. This consists of a series of graded injections gradually increasing the amount of the atopen. The desensitization is thought to result from slow exhaustion of the store of intracellular histamine in mast cells by repeated injections of the allergens.

Type II Reactions

These reactions involve the combination of IgG or IgM antibodies with antigenic determinants on the surface of cells leading to cytotoxic or cytolytic effects. Examples are lysis of red cells caused by antierythrocyte antibodies in autoimmune anemias and hemolytic disease of the newborn. Sometimes the opposite happens. A free antigen or hapten may be adsorbed on the cell surface after being introduced. The presence of antigen leads to antibody formation. Subsequent reaction of the combined antigen or hapten with its corresponding antibody leads to cell damage. Many drugs act in this manner and cause complement mediated lysis of red cells, leukocytes and platelets.

Type III Immune Complex Diseases

Whenever, there is excess antigen over prolonged periods, as for example, in persistent infection, autoimmune disorders or by repeated contact with environmental agents, the antigen complexes combine with antibody and get deposited locally or in distant organs leading to clinical features of type III hypersensitivity reactions. The deposition depends on the nature of the complex.

If it is a large complex, the normal body mechanisms can handle it and it is destroyed. If it is very small it causes no harm and it can be filtered out. The intermediate complexes have a tendency to be deposited either locally or distantly. This depends on the relative proportion of the antigen or the antibody. If there is excess of antibody and mild antigen excess, it precipitates rapidly at the site of entry. If there is moderate or gross antigen excess, soluble complexes are formed which can be carried to different organs, like kidney, eye, etc. and lead to harmful effects based on target organs.

This usually causes problems and can be a generalized or localized phenomenon.

Generalized Serum Sickness

This is a systemic form of type III hypersensitivity. This appears 7 to 12 days following a single injection of a high concentration of foreign serum such as diphtheria antitoxin. The clinical syndrome consists of fever, lymphadenopathy, splenomegaly, arthritis, glomerulonephritis, endocarditis, vasculitis, urticarial rashes, abdominal pain, nausea and vomiting. The pathogenesis is the formation of immune complexes which get deposited on the endothelial lining of blood vessels in various parts of the body causing inflammatory infiltration. The plasma concentration of complement falls due to massive complement activation and fixation by antigen antibody complexes. The disease is self limited. With continued rise in antibody production, the immune complexes become larger in size and get phagocytosed and eliminated. When all foreign antigen is thus eliminated, free antibody appears and the symptoms clear without sequelae. With repeated infections, the disease manifests earlier than the latent period of 7 to 12 days. Serum sickness differs from other types of hypersensitivity reactions in that a single injection can serve both as the sensitizing and shocking dose. The syndrome is seen following injections of penicillin or other antibiotics.

Such immune complex syndromes occur in many diseases including bacterial, viral and parasitic infections (Poststreptococcal glomerulonephritis, hepatitis type B, malaria, disseminated malignancies and autoimmune conditions). The nephritis and arthritis seen in these conditions may be caused by deposition of immune complexes.

Local Type of Reaction: Arthus Reaction

Arthus observed that when rabbits were injected subcutaneously, repeatedly with horse serum, the initial injections were without any local effect but with later injections there occurred, intense local reaction consisting of edema, induration, and hemorrhagic necrosis. This is known as arthus reaction and is a local manifestation of generalized hypersensitivity. The tissue damage is due to the formation of antigen antibody precipitates which are deposited on the walls of blood vessels. This leads to increased vascular permeability and infiltration of the site with neutrophils. Leukocyte-platelet thrombi are formed that reduce the blood supply and lead to tissue necrosis.

Type IV Delayed Hypersensitivity Reaction

Delayed hypersensitivity reaction is an aspect of cell mediated immunity. These are provoked by specific antigens, evolve slowly and consist of a mixed cellular reaction involving lymphocytes and macrophages. The reaction is not induced by circulating antibody but by sensitized T cells which on contact with specific antigen release lymphokines that cause biological effects on leukocytes, macrophages and tissue cells. Delayed hypersensitivity cannot be passively transferred by serum but can be transferred by lymphocytes or by transfer factor. There are two types of delayed hypersensitivity reactions tuberculin type and contact dermatitis type.

Tuberculin Reaction

When a small dose of tuberculin is injected intradermally in an individual sensitized to tuberculoprotein by prior infection or immunization, an indurated inflammatory reaction occurs at the site within 48 to 72 hours. The tuberculin test differs from the skin test for type 1 hypersensitivity not only in the longer interval for appearance but also in its morphology and histology.

Tuberculin type of hypersensitivity is developed in many infections with bacteria, fungi, viruses and parasites especially when the infection is sub acute or chronic and the pathogen is intracellular. A similar hypersensitivity is developed in allograft reaction and in many autoimmune diseases.

Examples of tuberculin type of reaction

1. Bacterial hypersensitivity in diseases—Koch's phenomena (tuberculosis), psittacosis, trachoma, lymphogranuloma venerum, leprosy, syphilis, brucellosis, etc.
2. Viral hypersensitivity—mumps, and revaccination with vaccina virus.
3. Fungal hypersensitivity—coccidioides, sporotrichosis, blastomycosis and aspergillosis.
4. Parasitic hypersensitivity—hydatid cyst, filariasis, schistosomiasis, etc.

Contact Dermatitis

Delayed hypersensitivity results from skin contact with a variety of chemical-metals such as nickel and chromium, simple chemicals like dyes, picryl chloride, dinitrochlorobenzene, drugs such as penicillin and toileteries. Sensitization is particularly liable when contact is with an inflamed area of skin and when the chemical is applied in an oily base. Antibiotic ointments applied on patches of dermatitis frequently provoke sensitization. The substances involved are in themselves not antigenic but may acquire antigenicity on combination with skin proteins. Sensitization requires percutaneous absorption. As most of the substances involved are fat soluble passage along sebaceous glands may be the method of entry of the allergens.

Contact with the allergens in sensitized individuals leads to contact dermatitis, the lesions varying from macules to papules to vesicles that break down leaving behind raw weeping areas typical of acute eczematous dermatitis. Hypersensitivity is detected by the patch test. The allergen is applied to the skin under an adherent dressing. Sensitivity is indicated by itching appearing in 4 to 5 hours and local reaction which may vary from erythema to vesicle or blister formation in 24 to 48 hours.

SHWARTZMAN REACTION

This is not an immune reaction but is due to factors which affect intravascular coagulation. It is described here because it resembles hypersensitivity reactions.

Shwartzman (1928) observed that if a culture filtrate of S. typhi is injected intra dermally in a rabbit followed 24 hours later by the same filtrate intravenously, a hemorrhagic necrotic lesion develops at the site of intradermal injection. The intradermal and intravenous injections need not be of the same or even related endotoxins. Absence of specificity and the short interval between the two doses excludes any immunological basis for reaction.

The initial dose is of an endotoxin. The intravenous injection can be of a variety of substances—bacterial endotoxins, antigen antibody complexes, starch, serum, kaolin and others. The preparatory injection causes accumulation of white blood cells which condition the site by release of lysosomal enzymes damaging the capillary walls. Following the provocative dose, there occurs intravascular clotting, the thrombi leading to necrosis of vessel walls and hemorrhage.

For examples

Purpuric rashes of meningococcal septicemia and acute hemorrhagic adrenal necrosis found in overwhelming infections (Waterhouse-Friderichsen Syndrome).

Section 3

Systemic Bacteriology

- Gram-positive Cocci
  - *Staphylococcus aureus*
  - *Streptococcus pyogenes*
  - *Streptococcus pneumoniae*
- Gram-negative Cocci
  - *Neisseria meningitidis*
  - *Neisseria gonorrhoeae*
- Gram-positive Rods
  - Aerobic
    - *Corynebacterium diphtheriae*
    - *Mycobacterium leprae*
    - *Mycobacterium tuberculosis*
    - Atypical mycobacteria
  - Anaerobic
    - *Clostridium tetani*
- Gram-negative Rods
  - Enterobacteriaceae
    - *Escherichia coli*
    - *Klebsiella spp*
    - *Salmonella spp*
    - *Citrobacter spp*
    - *Proteus spp*
    - *Shigella spp*
  - Others
    - *Vibrio cholerae*
    - *Haemophilus spp*
    - *Pseudomonas spp*
    - *Moraxellaceae—Acinetobacter ssp*
- Miscellaneous Bacteria
  - Spirochaetes

Systemic Bacteriology

Introduction

In this section we will be dealing with the study of bacteria, its main groups or genus and one representative species. We shall also be studying about the diseases bacteria cause, their diagnosis and prevention. A similar pattern shall be followed in each chapter for easy understanding.

The details on antigenic structure of bacteria have been omitted and more relevant details of laboratory diagnosis have been introduced in this section.

Gram-positive Cocci

In this section we shall study the groups of bacteria which exist as Gram-positive cocci.

Gram-positive cocci

	Genus	Exist as	Representative species
1.	Staphylococcus	Gram-positive cocci in clusters	Staphylococcus aureus
2.	Streptococcus	Gram-positive cocci in chains	Streptococcus pyogenes
3.	Pneumococcus	Gram-positive cocci in pairs	Streptococcus pneumoniae
4.	Micrococcus	Gram-positive cocci in tetrads — groups of four	—
5.	Sarcina	Gram-positive cocci in groups of eight	—
6.	Peptostreptococcus	Anaerobic cocci	

The first three genera are pathogenic or disease producing. Others are harmless saprophytes that live in soil, water and other food stuffs. They also occur as harmless commensals in the throat, intestine and vagina. We shall be studying the representative species of the first three genera.

CHAPTER 21

Gram-positive Cocci: *Staphylococcus Aureus*

LESSON PLAN

- Introduction
- History
- *Staphylococcus Aureus*
  - Morphology
  - Culture
  - Biochemical Reactions
  - Resistance
  - Pathogenicity
  - Epidemiology
  - Modes of Infection
  - Transmission
  - Hospital Infections with *Staphylococcus*
  - Virulence
  - Laboratory Diagnosis
  - Serotyping
  - Phage Typing
- Coagulase Negative Staphylococci
- MRSA
  - What is MRSA?
  - Transmission of MRSA
  - Treatment of MRSA
  - Prevention of Spread of Hospital Acquired MRSA

Genus—Staphylococcus
Species—Staphylococcus aureus

INTRODUCTION

The genus Staphylococcus consists of gram-positive cocci that grow in grape like clusters, are aerobic and facultatively anaerobic; produce catalase and occur as parasites on the skin in man and other vertebrate animals.

There are two important species in Staphylococci—*Staphylococcus aureus* which is pathogenic and *Staphylococcus albus* which is nonpathogenic. *Staphylococcus aureus* is the commonest cause of localized pyogenic (pus producing) lesions in man and also causes hospital acquired infections. In 20 to 30 percent of healthy persons, however *Staphylococcus aureus* occurs as a harmless commensal in the anterior nares and on moist areas of the skin. Such individuals who only carry the bacteria and do not suffer from the disease are called carriers.

Staphylococcus albus is the nonpathogenic species and it occurs as a harmless commensal that grows on the whole surface of the skin and in the nostrils and mouth of all persons throughout their life but they can act as pathogens when the body defense mechanism is low. Thus, they are called opportunistic pathogens.

HISTORY

Staphylococcus was first seen in human pyogenic lesions by von Recklinghausen in 1871 but Sir Alexander Ogston, a surgeon from Scotland established the role of the coccus in an abscess and gave it the name Staphylococcus. Staphyle means a bunch of grapes and Kokkos means berry.

STAPHYLOCOCCUS AUREUS

Morphology

Staphylococcus aureus are gram-positive, spherical cocci, 1 μm in diameter, arranged in grape-like clusters due to cell division occurring in three planes with daughter cells tending to remain in close contact after cell division. They may be found singly, in pairs or in short chains of 3 or 4 cells. They are nonmotile, nonsporing and non-capsulated (Fig. 21.1).

Culture

- They are aerobic and facultatively anaerobic
- They grow readily on ordinary media
- The temperature range is 10°C to 42°C
- The optimum temperature for growth is 37°C
- The optimum pH for growth is 7.4 to 7.6.

The various culture media that can be used for the growth of staphylococci are:

1. *Nutrient agar*: After incubation for 24 hours, the colonies are large (2 to 4 mm) in diameter, circular, convex, smooth, shiny, opaque and produce golden yellow pigment.
2. *Nutrient agar slope*: There is confluent (the colonies are merged with each other) growth showing a characteristic oil paint appearance.
3. *Blood agar*: The colonies are similar to those on nutrient agar. Most strains are hemolytic especially when incubated under 20 to 25 percent CO_2. They produce beta hemolysis, especially marked on rabbit/sheep blood and weak on horse blood agar.

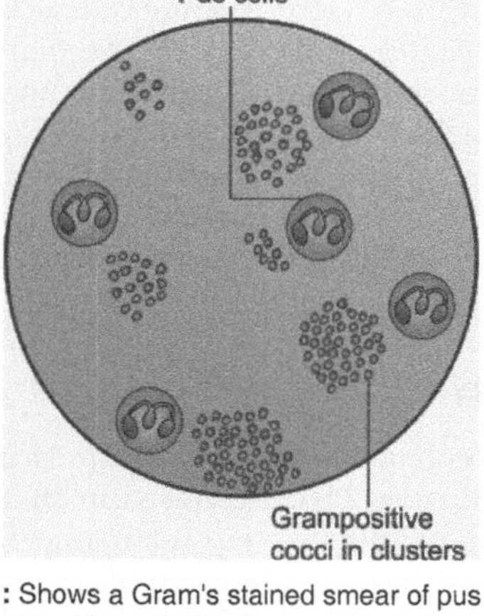

Fig. 21.1: Shows a Gram's stained smear of pus showing gram-positive cocci in clusters (Staphylococci)

4. *MacConkey's agar*: They grow on MacConkey's agar producing smaller colonies that are pink due to lactose fermentation.
5. *Peptone water*: Uniform turbidity is produced.
6. *Selective medium*: These are used for isolating *Staphylococcus aureus* from specimens such as feces.
   a. Media containing 8 to 10 percent NaCl (salt, milk, agar or salt broth).
   b. *Mannitol salt agar*: It is nutrient agar mixed with the following substances:
      1 percent mannitol
      7.5 percent NaCl
      0.0025 percent phenol red.
      Most strains ferment mannitol and so colonies are yellow due to acid production. Others are purple.
   c. *Ludlam's medium*: It has lithium chloride, tellurite and polymyxin.

Biochemical Reactions

Staphylococcus aureus ferments a number of sugars producing acid but no gas. This is not important except for mannitol which is fermented by *Staphylococcus aureus* but not by *Staphylococcus epidermidis*. The biochemical reactions are:

- Catalase +ve
- Oxidase -ve
- Urea +ve
- Liquefy gelatin
- MR + VP + ve
- Indole-negative
- Reduce nitrates to nitrites.

Phosphatase: It is useful for differentiating *Staphylococcus aureus* from *Staphylococcus epidermidis* as *Staphylococcus aureus* gives phosphatase test positive.

DNase: Also positive in *S. aureus*.

Resistance

- *Staphylococcus aureus* are quite resistant; they can even be isolated from dry pus after 2 to 3 months
- They can resist one percent phenol for fifteen minutes.
- Staphylococci were originally sensitive to sulphonamide, penicillin and other antibiotics but they developed resistance. Resistance to penicillin is due to the production of an enzyme pencillinase which inactivates penicillin. This gave them a survival advantage and penicillinase producing strains started increasing in the hospital.
- Staphylococci can grow in meat, milk and dirty water and can remain in the dormant state upto several months in pus, sputum, clothing or dust.

Pathogenicity

Staphylococcus aureus causes many infections.
- Cutaneous infections
- Deep infections
- Enterocolitis
- Food poisoning
- Exfoliative disease
- Toxic shock syndrome.

Cutaneous Infections

Cutaneous infections means the infections of the skin like pustules, furuncles, styes, boils, abscesses, carbuncles, impetigo, blepharitis, conjunctivitis, etc. It also causes sepsis in wounds and burns and the majority of hospital cross infections.

Deep Infections

The most common deep infection caused by *S. aureus* is acute osteomyelitis that is infection of the bones. Among the respiratory infections, tonsillitis, pharyngitis, sinusitis and pneumonia are common. Breast abscess is another common deep seated infections.

Staphylococcal septicemia can sometimes occur. From the blood it can spread to the meninges, kidney or heart. Tropical pyomyositis is a condition in young adults in which there are multiple staphylococcal abscesses in voluntary muscles.

Staphylococcal Enterocolitis

Staphylococcal enterocolitis usually develops after the administration of broad spectrum, antibiotics. Destruction of normal intestinal bacteria leads to the colonization of the gut by drug resistant staphylococci. Pseudomembranous enterocolitis that result is usually fatal. This usually follows abdominal surgery.

Staphylococcal Food Poisoning

When food contaminated with enterotoxin producing staphylococci is consumed, diarrhea and vomiting set in within about 6 hours of taking the contaminated food. The types of food responsible for this are meat, fish, milk and milk products.

Exfoliative Syndromes

Various exfoliative syndromes are caused by staphylococcus in which there is stripping of the superficial layers of the skin from the underlying tissues by the action of the exfoliative toxin.

Toxic Shock Syndrome

It is a multisystem illness in which there is onset of high fever, hypotension, vomiting, diarrhea and a rash. Severe cases progress to acute renal failure, peripheral gangrene and death. It is associated with the use of tampons.

Epidemiology

The sources of infection are the:
1. *Human patients or carriers*: Patients with superficial infections and respiratory infections throw large numbers of staphylococci into the environment.

Ten to thirty percent of healthy persons carry staphylococci in the nose. Ten percent have it in the perineum and also on the hair. Some carriers shed very large number of cocci for prolonged periods. The cocci shed by the patients and carriers contaminate handkerchiefs, bed linen and blankets and may persist on them for days and weeks.

2. Infected domestic animals such as cows can transmit infection through milk.

Modes of Infection

The way in which a person acquires the infection is called mode of infection. It may be:

1. *Exogenous,* i.e. from outside the body of the host. It could be from another human or animal.
2. *Endogenous* from inside the body of the host, e.g. a boil may be caused by cocci transferred on the fingers from the nose of the patient, himself.

Transmission

1. Contact—The most common method of spread is by direct contact (touching) with the contaminated hand or clothing of an infected person. Sometimes objects such as furniture, clothing, bedding, towels and baths are infected with staphylococci from patients or carriers and when we touch them we get infection.
2. Airborne dust Staphylococci can be carried in airborne dust shed from lesions of patients, or carriers, or from fomites (non-living objects which can carry the infection). These airborne staphylococci may fall on to the body surfaces or surgical wounds of patients or can be inhaled into the respiratory tract and can cause infection.
3. Droplet spray and airborne droplet nuclei—These are freely spread in speaking, coughing and sneezing by healthy nasal carriers or patients with respiratory tract lesions. But this is the least important method of spread since few of the droplets or droplet nuclei contain *Staphylococcus aureus.*

Hospital Infections with *Staphylococcus*

Hospital infections by staphylococci deserve special attention because they are very common and are caused by strains resistant to various antibiotics. The strains of staphylococcus causing hospital infections belong to a limited number of phage types and are commonly resistant to penicillin and other antibiotics routinely used in hospitals.

Prevention of staphylococcal infection in the hospital:

1. *Measures against the source of infection*:
   a. Patients with discharging lesions should be given antibiotic therapy, and their wounds should be dressed so as to allow no contact with the outside.
   b. Surgeons and other staff who have an infected lesion should not attend to patients.
   c. Carriers among patients and staff may be detected by nasal and perineal swabbing and treated.
2. *Measures against spread through the environment*:
   - Proper aseptic and antiseptic techniques in the operation theaters and post-operatively in wards
   - Early recognition and isolation of any infected case.
   - Taking adequate precautions against airborne infection.
3. *Antimicrobial prophylaxis*: It is generally not advisable as the antibiotic used will eliminate the sensitive members of the body's commensal flora and the patient can catch a resistant hospital strain.

   If at all antimicrobial treatment is required, a topical application of a drug is preferable since one can use a higher dosage and it will not lead to resistance. In those situations where systemic prophylaxis is required it is preferable to use a narrow spectrum antibiotic such as cloxacillin.
4. *Bacterial interference*: This method involves the introduction of a strain of staphylococcus, of known low virulence to avoid the infection by a virulent strain of staphylococcus later. This is usually done in newborns who have

not yet been colonized with *Staphylococcus*. It is not that successful in children already colonized with a staphylococcal strain.

Virulence

These mean those enzymes, toxins or cell wall components of the bacteria which help it to fight the body's defence mechanisms.

a. *Enzyme-coagulase*: This is a soluble enzyme like product of *Staphylococcus aureus* that converts the fibrinogen in citrated human or rabbit plasma into fibrin helped by an activator in the plasma. Inside the body, this enzyme contributes to pathogenicity by inactivating a bactericidal substance in normal serum or by protecting the cocci with a fibrin barrier against phagocytosis.
b. *The cell wall components of the coccus* include mucopeptide and different antigens that contribute to the virulence of bacteria.
c. *Toxins*: Exotoxins are secreted by the growing *S. aureus* cells. They are—toxin and the Panton Valentine (PV) leucoidin.

Enterotoxin is an intestinal toxin formed by 30 to 50 percent of the strains of *Staphylococcus aureus*. When ingested in food, the enterotoxin causes nausea, vomiting and diarrhea within six hours (Staphylococcal food poisoning).

Table 21.1 lists the differences between *S. aureus* and *S. albus*.

Laboratory Diagnosis

There is a standard format to be followed for the laboratory diagnosis of different bacterial infections as we shall see in the later chapters also. This is as follows:

a. Collection of samples.
b. Direct examination.
c. Culture examination.
d. Biochemical tests.
e. Antibiotic sensitivity test.
f. Confirmatory tests.
g. Treatment.

Table 21.1: Differences between *Staphylococcus aureus* and *albus*

Staphylococcus aureus	*Staphylococcus epidermidis or albus*
1. Forms golden yellow colonies on Nutrient agar	White colonies on Nutrient agar
2. Pathogenic	Nonpathogenic
3. Hemolytic on blood agar	Nonhemolytic on blood agar
4. Ferments mannitol	Does not ferment mannitol
5. Coagulase enzyme positive	Coagulase enzyme negative
6. Produces toxins	No toxins
Liquefies gelatin	Does not liquefy gelatin
Produces phosphatase	Does not produce phosphatase
• In a medium containing potassium tellurite reduces tellurite producing black colonies	Does not produce black colonies
• Production of DNase	Does not produce DNase enzyme

Collection of Samples

The type of sample collected depends upon the presenting complaint of the patient

a. *Pus sample*: This is taken in all boils, wounds, abscesses, burns, etc. either in a screw capped container or in a swab. It can also be collected by a sterile syringe and needle.
b. *Sputum sample and throat swab*: This is taken in cases of lower respiratory tract infections, e.g. pneumonia. It is coughed up from the bronchi into a wide mouthed jar. The sample should not consist of saliva.
c. *Feces/vomit*: This is taken if food poisoning is suspected. One to five ml is taken in a clean universal container.
d. *Remains of food:* Suspected of causing food poisoning is also taken into separate containers for testing.
e. *Blood:* The blood is taken from patients in suspected bacteriaemias, e.g. in osteomyelitis or endocarditis.

f. *Urine*: Urine is taken from patients with suspected urinary tract infection or kidney infection, a midstream sample is taken into a urine culture bottle.
g. *Anterior nasal and perineal swabs*: This is taken from suspected carriers. The swab should first be moistened with sterile water or broth and the nasal swabs should be rubbed over the anterior walls of both nostrils.

Direct Microscopy

The culture is put up first so that there is no contamination if a direct microscopic examination is done earlier. For direct microscopy, the sample is directly plated onto a slide and then a Gram's stain is done. We might observe Gram-positive cocci in clusters which has to be confirmed further. We might also see pus cells and mucus strands, etc.

Culture

As we have seen earlier, the sample needs to be plated on blood agar and nutrient agar. If staphylococci are scanty or out numbered by other bacteria, then we need to use selective media as described earlier. The characteristic appearance of the colonies gives us an idea about *Staphylococcus aureus* which is later confirmed by doing a Gram's stain.

Biochemical Reactions

Other confirmatory tests are:

Coagulase test: *Staphylococcus aureus* has the property of clotting citrated human or rabbit plasma. Human or rabbit plasma contains an activator, the coagulase reacting factor (CRF) which converts fibrinogen into fibrin. Clotting does not occur with the plasma of certain species (e.g. guinea pig) because they lack CRF. Seven antigenic types of coagulase exist, of which human strains produce coagulase A.

Method: When a saline suspension of *Staphylococcus aureus* is mixed on a slide with a drop of plasma, the cocci are clumped. This is due to the precipitation of fibrin on the cell surface by the bound coagulase.

There are two types of coagulase:

- *Free coagulase*: This is a heat labile enzyme secreted free into the medium, that requires the cooperation of coagulase reacting factor for its action. Tested by the tube test.
- *Bound coagulase*: This is a heat stable constituent of the cell wall and is independent of CRF. Tested by the slide test.

Tube test: This detects free coagulase. 0.1 mL of an overnight broth culture or an agar culture suspension of the organism is added to 0.5 mL of citrated, oxalated or heparinized human or rabbit plasma (diluted 1 in 5 with saline) in a narrow test tube. Diluted plasma alone in a similar tube serves as a control. The tubes are incubated in a water bath at 37°C for 3 to 6 hours. If positive, the plasma clots and does not flow when the tube is inverted.

Slide test: The slide test detects bound coagulase from an agar culture. The organism is emulsified in two drops of saline placed on a slide. After verifying that there is no spontaneous agglutination, a drop of undiluted plasma (human/rabbit) is added to one of the emulsions and mixed gently. Prompt clumping of the organism indicates the presence of bound coagulase. False positive results are caused by citrate utilising bacteria such as enterococci and pseudomonas. In doubtful cases the tube test should be done for confirmation.

Advantages of Coagulase

1. Promotes virulence of the organism by inhibiting phagocytosis.
2. It also protects the cells from the bactericidal substances present in tissue fluids.
3. By laying down a fibrin barrier around the cocci, it helps in walling off the lesion.

Antibiotic Sensitivity Test

Staphylococci are in general sensitive to many antibiotics such as benzyl penicillin, cloxacillin, cephalosporins, tetracycline, chloramphenicol, erythromycin, etc. At present, a lot of staphylococcal strains are resistant to benzyl penicillin. Many of the hospital strains are also resistant to several other antistaphylococcal antibiotics and these strains are often responsible for hospital cross infection.

Since different strains of *Staphylococcus aureus* differ in their sensitivity to different antibiotics, the choice of antibiotic in the treatment of a patient should be based on the results of sensitivity tests done on the strain of staphylococcus that he is harboring.

Serotyping

Strains of *Staphylococcus aureus* can be divided into a number of different types by a serological method. This method depends on their possessing different combinations of type specific surface antigens. These are demonstrable in slide agglutination tests with absorbed antisera. There are three main serotypes which are the same as the phage groups I–III.

Phage Typing

As we know, phages are viruses that kill bacteria. Different phages attack different strains of bacteria. Strains of *Staphylococcus aureus* can be differentiated into many phage types by observation of their pattern of susceptibility to lysis by a set of 24 different anti *Staphylococcus aureus* bacteriophages. Strains isolated from patients and carriers can be identified and their source and pattern of spread discovered.

Some of the phage types of *Staphylococcus aureus*, e.g. type 80 have been found to be more virulent than others.

COAGULASE NEGATIVE STAPHYLOCOCCI

There are two types of coagulase negative staphylococci—these are:

a. *Staphylococcus epidermidis*
b. *Staphylococcus saprophyticus*

Coagulase negative staphylococci are usually harmless commensals found on all areas of skin and in the nostrils, mouth, external ear and urethral meatus. They differ from *Staphylococcus aureus* in not forming toxins or other aggressive factors. When the skin squames are shed, large number of cocci go into the dust and air. For this reason, the organism is a common accidental contaminant of clinical specimens and has no clinical significance.

Sometimes *Staphylococcus albus* acts as an opportunistic pathogen and causes infection in persons with defective resistance. For example, cystitis (bladder infection) in persons with urinary tract abnormalities, septicemia or endocarditis in patients after cardiac surgery, meningitis with bacteremia in patients fitted with shunts and septicemia in immunosuppressed and immunodefective patients. These cases are recognized by the finding of large numbers of cocci in repeated specimens.

Staphylococcus saprophyticus is clinically important as a common cause of acute urinary tract infection particularly in young women. Infection is usually self limited. It may also cause urethritis.

METHICILLIN-RESISTANT *STAPHYLOCOCCUS AUREUS*

What is MRSA?

- *Methicillin-resistant Staphylococcus aureus* (MRSA) is any strain of *Staphylococcus aureus* that is resistant to the synthetic penicillins (methicillin, oxacillin, nafcillin). It is also resistant to cephalosporins and sometimes to other antibiotics (erythromycin, clindamycin, aminoglycosides, quinolone).
- Because of its resistance to antibiotics, management of MRSA infections requires more complicated, toxic, and expensive treatment.
- Methicillin-resistant *S. Aureus* is not a "super bug" and is not more likely to cause serious infection than antibiotic susceptible *S. aureus*. It is simply resistant to more antibiotics. The mechanisms of transmission of MRSA are virtually identical to those of the usual *S. aureus*, which is sensitive to methicillin.

Transmission of MRSA

- *S. aureus* is transmitted primarily through direct person-to-person contact, especially through the hands of health care workers. Nasal carriage of *S. aureus* is very common and may be due to hand to nose transmission. A nasal carrier often contaminates his/her own hands by hand to nose contact, then transmits the organism in the course of routine activities. Since skin to skin contract is the most significant mode of transmission, hand washing is of primary importance in preventing its spread.
- It can remain viable in the environment for long periods of time in linen, clothing, and dust. However, it is not thought that inanimate objects or environmental surfaces represent significant sources for transmission infection, if appropriately handled.
- Airborne spread usually plays little role in the transmission of *S. aureus* with the exception of burn wound infections in a burn unit, patients with *S. aureus* pneumonia, or patients with tracheotomies.

Treatment of MRSA

More serious MRSA infections, especially HA-MRSA (Hospital-acquired MRSA) infections, are becoming increasingly difficult to treat. Antibiotics that may still work include—clindamycin, daptomycin, doxycycline, linezolid minocycline, tetracycline, trimethoprim-sulfamethoxazole vancomycin.

Prevention of Spread of Hospital Acquired MRSA

The prevention of nosocomial spread of MRSA involves routine and terminal cleaning, use of disinfectants and antiseptics and maintenance of proper hand hygiene. Testing patients for MRSA upon admission, isolating MRSA-positive patients, decolonization of MRSA-positive patients, and terminal cleaning of patients' rooms and all other clinical areas they occupy is the current best practice protocol for prevention of nosocomial MRSA.

CHAPTER 22

Gram-positive Cocci: *Streptococcus Pyogenes*

LESSON PLAN

- Introduction
- History
- Classification
  - Alpha Hemolysis
  - Beta Hemolysis
  - Gamma or Nonhemolytic Streptococci
- Resistance of *Streptococcus*
- *Streptococcus Pyogenes*
  - Morphology
  - Culture
  - Biochemical Reactions
  - Antigenic Structure
  - Toxins and Other Virulence Factors
  - Pathogenicity
  - Epidemiology
  - Laboratory Diagnosis
  - Nonsuppurative Complications
- Group B Streptococci
  - Identification Features
- Alpha Hemolytic Streptococci
  - Properties of Alpha Hemolytic Streptococci (*Streptococcus Viridans*)
  - Pathogenicity
  - Laboratory Diagnosis
- Group D Streptococci
  - Fecal Streptococci
  - Nonfecal Species

Genus—Streptococcus
Representative species—Streptococcus pyogenes

INTRODUCTION

Streptococci are gram-positive, spherical or oval cells arranged in chains of different lengths, are nonmotile and nonsporing. They may be capsulated. The majority are facultative anaerobes but some species may be anaerobic. They are important human pathogens causing generalized pyogenic lesions with a characteristic tendency to spread (different from *Staphylococcus* infections which are localized). They are also responsible for non-suppurative conditions—acute rheumatic fever and glomerulonephritis.

HISTORY

They were first seen in wound infections by Billroth (1874) who called them streptococci meaning twisted or coiled.

CLASSIFICATION

Refer Flow chart 22.1.

Most of the pathogenic streptococci fall into the beta group and are called hemolytic streptococci. The hemolytic streptococci were classified by Rebecca Lancefield (1933) into groups based on the nature of the carbohydrate C antigen on the cell wall. These are known as Lancefield groups named A-V (without I and J). The majority of hemolytic streptococci producing

Flow chart 22.1: Streptococci based on O_2 requirements

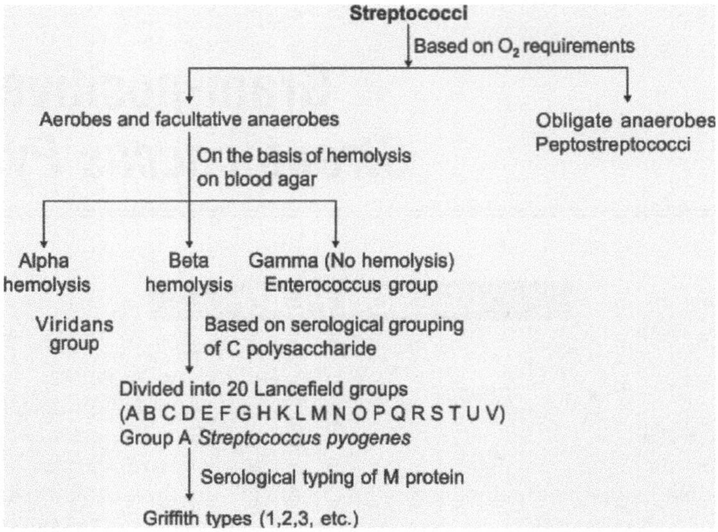

infections belong to group A. Group A is called Streptococcus pyogenes.

These are further divided into types based on proteins (M, T, R) which are antigens present on the cell surface. Eighty types of *Streptococcus pyogenes* have been recognized.

Alpha Hemolysis

This is a partial hemolysis around the colony along with a greenish discoloration. The zone of lysis is small, 1 to 2 mm wide. The margins are indefinite and unlysed erythrocytes can be made out microscopically in this zone.

Beta Hemolysis

This is a sharply defined clear zone of hemolysis which is 2 to 4 mm wide and completely colorless with fully lysed cells.

Gamma or Nonhemolytic Streptococci

- This produces no change in the medium and are called indifferent streptococci.

RESISTANCE OF *STREPTOCOCCUS*

Streptococcus is a delicate organism.

- It is easily destroyed by heat (54°C for 30 minutes)
- It dies in a few days in cultures unless stored at low temperature (4°C).
- It can survive in dust if protected from sunlight.
- It is more resistant to crystal violet than many bacteria and hence this dye is used in the preparation of selective media for streptococcus.
- Sensitivity to antibiotic bacitracin is employed as a good method for differentiating *Strept. pyogenes* from other hemolytic streptococci.

STREPTOCOCCUS PYOGENES

Morphology

They are spherical or oval cells, 0.5 to 1.0 in diameter, arranged in chains. The chain formation is due to the cocci dividing in one plane and the daughter cells failing to separate completely. They are nonmotile and nonsporing (Fig. 22.1).

Some strains have a capsule made up of hyaluronic acid. Capsules are best seen in very young cultures.

Culture

- *Streptococcus pyogenes* is an aerobe and a facultative anaerobe
- Grows best at temperatures of 37°C (22 to 42°C)
- It is fastidious

The culture media used for the growth of streptococcus are:

1. *Blood agar*—After incubation for 24 hours the colonies are small (0.5 to 1mm), circular, semitransparent, low convex discs with an area of clear hemolysis around them. Growth and hemolysis are promoted by 10 percent CO_2.
2. *Selective medium like crystal violet blood agar* and PNF horse blood agar (polymyxin, neomycin and fusidic acid) are used when we want to inhibit many throat commensal organisms.
   Crystal violet blood agar: The addition of a low concentration of crystal violet (1 in 500,000 or 0.002%) to blood agar inhibits the growth of some bacteria, e.g. staphylococci.

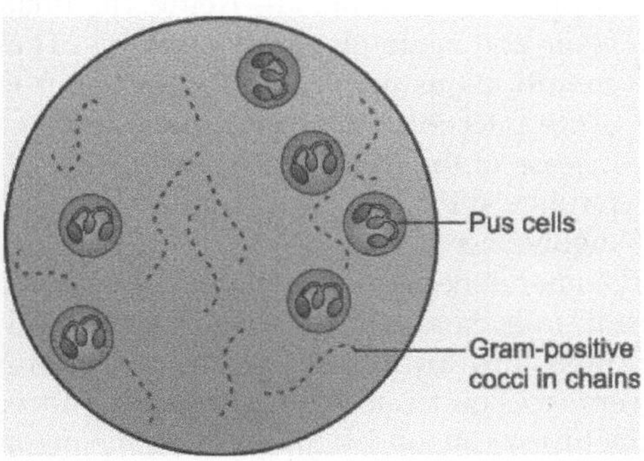

Fig. 22.1: Streptococci (Gram-positive cocci) in chains in a Gram's stained pus smear

   Constituents:
   - Sterile nutrient agar 90 mL
   - Sterile horse blood 10 mL
   - Crystal violet 1 in 1000 0.2 mL

   Melt agar, cool to 50°C, add the blood and crystal violet and pour plates.

   PNF medium—Horse blood agar (5%) with the following additives is selective for β hemolytic streptococci, but inhibits the growth of staphylococci and coliform species.

   Constituents:
   - Polymyxin B sulphate
   - Neomycin sulphate
   - Fusidic acid
3. *Liquid medium*—Glucose/serum broth. In both growth occurs as a granular turbidity and powdery deposit.

Biochemical Reactions

Streptococcus pyogenes is catalase negative and insoluble in bile.

It ferments several sugars producing acid but no gas.

Antigenic Structure

The capsule of *Streptococcus* pyogenes when present is composed of hyaluronic acid. It inhibits phagocytosis. It is not antigenic in man.

Cell wall is composed of an outer layer containing protein and lipotechoic acid, a middle layer of group specific carbohydrate and an inner layer of peptidoglycan. Serological grouping to streptococci depends on the group-specific C carbohydrate. As this antigen is an integral part of the cell wall, it has to be extracted for grouping by a precepitation test with group antisera (Fig. 22.2).

Many protein antigens have been identified in the outer part of the cell wall. *Streptococcus pyogenes* can be typed based on the surface proteins MTR. M is the most important of these. It acts as a virulence factor by inhibiting phagocytosis. About 80 M protein types have been recognized.

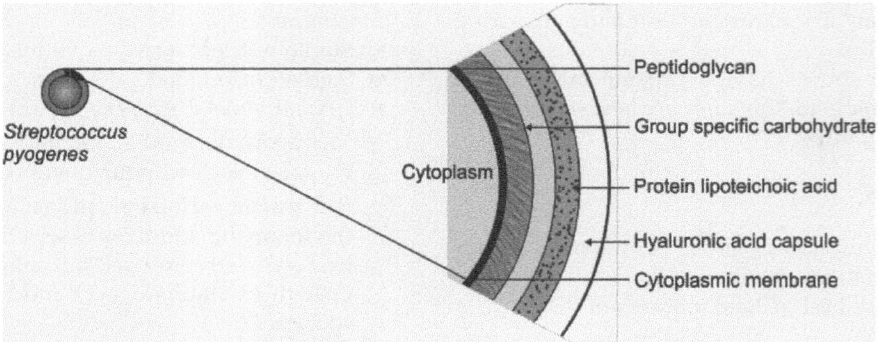

Fig. 22.2: Antigenic structure of *Streptococcus pyogenes*

The T protein is another antigen present in many serotypes of *Streptococcus pyogenes*. The T and R proteins have no relation to virulence.

Various structural components of *Streptococcus pyogenes* exhibit antigenic cross reaction with different tissues of the human body. This accounts for the nonsuppurative diseases produced by *Streptococcus pyogenes*.

Toxins and Other Virulence Factors

Streptococcus pyogenes forms many exotoxins and enzymes which contribute to virulence like hemolysins, deoxyribonucleases, hyaluronidases and proteinases.

Pathogenicity

Streptococcus pyogenes produces pyogenic infections with a tendency to spread locally, along lymphatics and through blood stream.

1. *Respiratory infections*: Sore throat is the commonest of streptococcal diseases. It may be localized as tonsillitis as in adults or may involve pharynx more (pharyngitis), as in children. Infection of the throat may result in complications like peritonsillar abscess, sinusitis, otitis media, mastoiditis or meningitis. Streptococcal bronchopneumonia may also develop.
2. *Skin infections*: It causes infection of the wounds or burns, lymphangitis or cellulitis. *Streptococcus pyogenes* also causes erysipelas or impetigo. Erysipelas is a spreading inflammation of the lymphatics of the dermis most commonly on the face or neck. Impetigo is found in younger children and characterized by vesiculopustular lesions on legs, arms or face. It is found mainly in young children.
3. *Genital infections*: *Both* aerobic and anaerobic streptococci are normal inhabitants of the female genitalia. But streptococci can cause puerperal sepsis, local inflammation of uterine tissues, pelvic cellulitis or septicemia.
4. *Other suppurative infections*: Abscesses in brain, lung, liver and kidney. It may also cause septicemia and pyemia.
5. *Nonsuppurative infections*: *Streptococcus pyogenes* leads to two important nonsuppurative sequelae—Acute rheumatic fever and acute glomerulonephritis. These complications occur 1 to 3 weeks after the acute infection. Acute rheumatic fever is a disease of the heart valves along with joint pains, skin and subcutaneous tissue involvement.

Glomerulonephritis is a kidney disease which results from cross reaction between a glomerular antigen and antibodies produced against streptococcus from previous skin or throat infections, caused by *Streptococcus pyogenes*. These strains of *Streptococcus* are called nephritogenic strains.

Epidemiology

- The major source of infection is the human upper respiratory tract—throat, nasopharynx, or nose of patients and carriers.
- The disease is transmitted by direct contact or through contaminated fomites.
- An important nonhuman source of infection is bovine mastitis, the organism being transmitted to man through milk.
- Streptococcal infections occur more frequently in children 5 to 8 years of age, and more in winters. Crowding predisposes to infection.
- Immunity is type specific and appears to be associated with antibody to M protein.
- Reinfections occur because of the multiplicity of serotypes.

Laboratory Diagnosis

Suppurative Infections

Samples to be Collected

1. *Throat swab*: The throat swab should be collected with a sterile swab from the tonsils, tonsillar fossa, posterior pharyngeal wall, uvula or any other suspected site. The patient should be well seated and lighting should be adequate. It is important that the patient should not have taken a course of antibiotics or gargled with normal saline before the throat swab is taken. Swabs are taken to diagnose acute infections, carrier state or to assess response to treatment.
2. Other swabs such as skin, pus or vaginal swabs.
3. Wound or skin curettings.
4. Pus aspirates.
5. Blood.
6. CSF.
7. Urine.
8. Sputum.

Transport

Drying of the swab should be avoided as it is sensitive to drying. If there is a delay, inoculate into a transport media. Pike's medium which is 10 percent blood agar with 1:1000000 crystal violet and 1:16000 sodium azide. We can also keep in the refrigerator if delay is too much. For the other samples we can use sterile screw capped bottles.

Direct Microscopy

Some information may be obtained by an examination of gram's stained films from pus and CSF. If we can see gram-positive cocci in chains it is indicative of streptococcal infection but smears are of no value in infections of the throat or genitalia where streptococci may form part of the resident flora.

Culture

Streptococcus is an aerobe and facultative anaerobe and grows best at 37°C. It is exacting in nutritive requirements and growth occurs only in enriched media. It does not grow on nutrient agar or MacConkey's agar.

Blood agar: After incubation for 24 hours at 37°C with 10 percent CO_2, the colonies are small (0.5 to 1 mm) circular, semitransparent, low convex, shiny discs with areas of clear hemolysis. Growth is improved by 5 to 10 percent CO_2. Based on the pattern of hemolysis, we do further differentiation.

Selective Media:

1. Crystal violet blood agar.
2. PNF medium.
3. *Liquid media*—Glucose broth, Todd Hewitt broth, brain heart infusion broth or thioglycollate broth. Liquid media show a granular turbidity with a powdery deposit. The granular deposit on the walls of the tube represents streptococci in long-chains.

Classification

The further processing depends on the type of hemolysis—α, β or γ.

If it is b hemolysis we can go in for Rebecca Lancefield's grouping. Serological grouping of streptococci depends upon the C carbohydrate present in the cell wall of bacteria. The antigen is extracted by special procedures and then tested by using antisera by an immunological procedure (precipitation, ELISA, immunoelectrophoresis, etc).

Streptococcus pyogenes belongs to group A, of the Lancefield's groups. *Streptococcus pyogenes* may be further subdivided into 80 types depending upon antigens present on the cell surface.

Rapid Diagnosis of Group A Streptococcal Antigen

1. Indirect fluorescent antibody test. Two to three hours old streptococcal broth cultures are stained with fluorescent group A specific antibody, for rapid detection of *Streptococcus* antigen.
2. ELISA.
3. Bacitracin sensitivity.

A filter paper disc dipped in a solution of bacitracin 1 unit/mL to give a concentration of 0.4 units/disc is applied on the surface of an inoculated blood agar. After incubation, a wide zone of inhibition is seen with *Streptococcus pyogenes* but not with other Streptococci. If a disc concentration of 0.7 units/disc is taken then > 14 mm inhibition is considered significant.

Biochemical Tests of Group A

1. Catalase-negative.
2. Not soluble in 10 percent bile unlike pneumococcus.
3. It ferments many sugars producing acid but no gas like—sorbitol, trehalose, lactose, maltose, dextrin, and mannitol.

Nonsuppurative Complications

Streptococcus pyogenes causes two important nonsuppurative sequelae:

1. Acute rheumatic fever.
2. Acute glomerulonephritis.

These complications usually occur 1 to 3 weeks after acute infection. Rheumatic fever follows a streptococcal throat infection where as glomerulonephritis usually occurs after a skin infection. These two diseases are called nonsuppurative because the organism itself and an inflammatory response are not present in the affected area.

Rheumatic Fever

Rheumatic fever is an inflammatory disease which occurs as a delayed response to pharyngeal infection with group A streptococci. It usually involves the heart, joints, CNS, skin and subcutaneous tissues. It causes cardiac involvement in which the acute stages may be fatal and in the chronic stages causes scaring and valvular deformities. The antibodies directed against the streptococcal cell membrane specifically bind to the heart muscle tissue forming immune complexes at that site which cause damage.

Not all streptococcal sore throats cause rheumatic fever. The attack rate of rheumatic fever following streptococcal pharyngitis is 3 percent. It is most common in the age group of 5 to 15 years.

Diagnosis is based on history and laboratory findings.

Diagnostic Criteria

There is no specific laboratory test that can establish a diagnosis of rheumatic fever. The diagnosis is therefore a clinical one but requires supporting evidence from the clinical microbiology and immunology laboratories. Jones in 1944 first proposed criteria to assist the clinician in standardizing the diagnosis of rheumatic fever. The most recent modification of the Jones criteria was published in 1992 by a special writing group of the American Heart Association (Table 22.1).

The five criteria termed major are so called because they are found commonly in patients with rheumatic fever.

The minor criteria are nonspecific and may be present in many clinical conditions. To fulfill the Jones criteria two major criteria or one major and

Table 22.1: The Jones criteria for rheumatic fever updated, 1992

Major criteria	*Minor criteria*
Carditis	Clinical fever
Migratory polyarthritis	Arthalgia (pain in joints)
Sydenham's chorea	Laboratory
Subcutaneous nodules	Elevated acute phase reactants
Erythema marginatum	Prolonged PR internal
	Plus
Supporting evidence of a recent gp A streptococcal (e.g. positive throat culture or rapid antigen detection test and/or elevated or increasing streptococcal antibody test)	

Source: Modified from the special writing group of the American Heart Association.

two minor criteria plus supporting evidence of an antecedent streptococcal infection are required. The latter may be provided by recovery of the organism on culture or by evidence of an immune response to one of the commonly measured group A Streptococcal antigens (e.g. antistreptolysin O, antideoxyribonuclease B, antihyaluronidase).

Criteria for diagnosis of rheumatic fever are:

1. Polyarthritis—It involves two or more big joints, and migrates from one joint to another. The joints involved are ankles wrists, knees and elbows over a period of days.
2. Carditis—Involvement of the valves leading to heart failure. Also involvement of pericardium and endocardium.
3. Subcutaneous nodules—These are small pea sized painless swellings on hands, feet and elbows. They are rare.
4. Sydenham's chorea—Sudden aimless irregular movements accompanied by muscle weakness.
5. Erythema marginatum—Pink rash on trunk and proximal part of extremities. This too is rare.

Serology

1. *Antistreptolysin O test*: In rheumatic fever a retrospective diagnosis of streptococcal infection may be demonstrated by showing high levels of antibodies to streptococcal toxins (hemolysins).

Streptococci produce two hemolysins—streptolysin O and streptolysin S. Streptolysin O is so called because it is oxygen labile. It is antigenic and antistreptolysin regularly appears in sera following streptococcal infection. ASO estimation is a standard serological test. It can be performed as a neutralization test by adding RBC suspension. If the antitoxin is present in the patients sera it neutralizes the hemolytic activity of the streptococcal O hemolysin and no hemolysis of the red blood cells is seen. If no antistreptolysin O is present, then the streptococcal O hemolysin is available for the hemolysis of RBC.

It can be done by latex agglutination also where latex particles are coated with antigen.

Interpretation of ASO

- A single titer of > 250 IU in adults is significant.
- A titer of > 333 IU in children is significant.
- A titer of 100 IU is significant in infants.
- In general titers > 200 IU are significant.
- Levels rise within 2 to 4 weeks of infection and fall after 2 months of infection.
- Titers may vary with the prevalence of streptococcus in normal healthy population and age.
- It is more useful with previous history of sore throat rather than skin infection (In skin infection, there is no production of SLO).

Other tests are:

2. *Anti DNase test*: Deoxyribonucleases are toxins produced by *Streptococcus pyogenes*. Demonstration of antibody against it is useful in retrospective diagnosis of skin infection.

   Antihyaluronidase antibodies can also be seen.

   Antistreptokinase

   AntiNADase
3. *Antistreptozyme test*: This is a passive haemagglutination test for diagnosing recent streptococcal infection. It uses erythrocytes sensitised with a crude preparation of extracellular antigens of streptococci. It becomes positive after all types of streptococcal infection.

Acute Glomerulonephritis

This is due to cutaneous infection with nephritogenic strains of β hemolytic streptococci which causes an acute inflammatory lesion of the glomerulus leading to abrupt onset of hematuria and proteinuria with salt and water retention. This is because the antibodies produced against previous streptococcal infection cross reacts with the antigens on the glomerular basement membrane. A retrospective diagnosis can be established by demonstrating high levels of antibody to streptococcal toxins. ASO levels are low. AntiDNase titers are high. They are greater than 350 IU. Other tests which can be done are:

- Antistreptokinase
- AntiNADase
- Antistreptozyme. Table 22.2 shows the comparison between rheumatic fever and glomerulonephritis.

GROUP B STREPTOCOCCI

Group B: These are important pathogens of cattle producing bovine mastitis. They have been implicated as a cause of neonatal meningitis and puerperal sepsis.

Table 22.2: Comparison of rheumatic fever and glomerulonephritis

	Acute rheumatic fever	*Acute glomerulonephritis*
Site of infection	Throat	Throat or skin
Serotype	Any	Nephritogenic strains (12, 4, 9, 2, 4, 52, 55, 57, 60)
Course	Progressive	Spontaneous cure
Prognosis	Variable	Good
Penicillin prophylaxis	Essential	Not indicated
Hereditary tendency	Present	Not known
Immune response	Marked	Moderate
Prior sensitisation	Essential	Not necessary
Complement levels	Unaffected	Lowered
Repeat attacks	Common	None

Identification Features

1. *Hippurate hydrolysis*: This is a biochemical test which is shown to be positive in group B bacteria and negative in others. Group B bacteria split hippurate and in the final reaction show a deep purple color.
2. *CAMP test* (Christie, Atkins, Munch, Peterson): A diffusable substance called, CAMP factor is produced by group B streptococci which completes the lysis of *Staphylococcus plazen* or enhances it. A staphylococcus strain called *Staphylococcus plazen* is streaked in the center of the plate (Fig. 22.3).

Perpendicular to that we streak strains of the unknown *Streptococcus*. If the strain is of group B, then at that junction we get an area of enhanced hemolysis or butterfly hemolysis. This is a confirmatory test for streptococci group B.

ALPHA HEMOLYTIC (*VIRIDANS STREPTOCOCCI*)

These include a group of streptococcal species which are present in large numbers as commensals in the bacterial flora of the mouth and oropharynx. Most strains produce partial hemolysis and green coloration. Some are non-hemolytic.

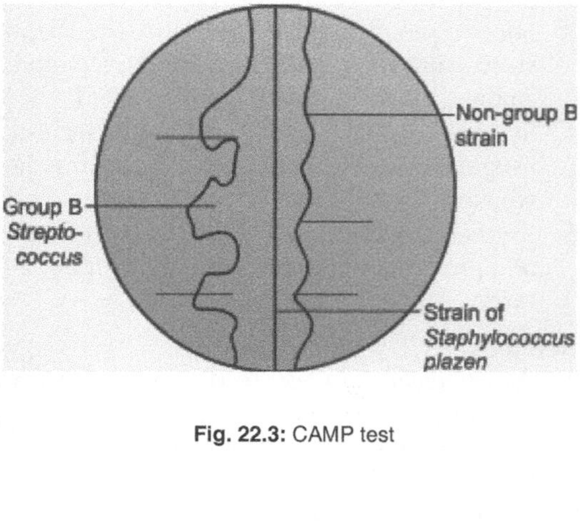

Fig. 22.3: CAMP test

Properties of Alpha Hemolytic Streptococci *(Streptococcus viridans)*

1. Morphologically they resemble *Streptococcus pyogenes*.
2. On culture the colonies resemble pneumococcal colonies but *Streptococcus viridans* can be distinguished from *Streptococcus pneumoniae* by being non-capsulated, non-bile soluble and resistant to optochin.

Streptococcus viridans is not a single species but is the name given to streptococci belonging to many species, e.g.

- *Streptococcus mitis*
- *Streptococcus milleri*
- *Streptococcus sanguis*
- *Streptococcus salivarius*
- *Streptococcus mutans*

Pathogenicity

Streptococcus viridans is a constant commensal of the mouth, being present in most people. It is not really pathogenic but it acts as an opportunistic pathogen and attacks tissues with lowered resistance. *Streptococcus viridans* plays a major role in the causation of dental caries, and periodontal infections. *Streptococcus viridans* can also cause subacute bacterial endocarditis. This infection occurs in damaged heart valves. With tooth extraction, bacteremia occurs throwing *Streptococcus viridans* into the circulation. They can settle on damaged heart valves resulting in subacute bacterial endocarditis. *S. milleri* is associated with deep sepsis including liver and brain abscess.

Laboratory Diagnosis

The viridans streptococci resemble. *S. pyogenes* morphologically but they are α hemolytic on blood agar. They should be differentiated from pneumococci. They grow well on nutrient agar and do not grow on MacConkey's agar.

We must remember that when isolated from the mouth, throat or any where else in the respiratory tract, *viridans streptococci* are generally regarded as harmless commensals. When found in the blood, or an abscess or a closed lesion, they are more likely to be pathogenic.

GROUP D STREPTOCOCCI

Streptococci belonging to group D streptococci are classified as the fecal streptococci (enterococci) and the nonfecal Streptococci- *Streptococcus bovis* and *Streptococcus equinus*.

Fecal Streptococci

Enterococci

Enterococci have some special properties:

1. They grow in the presence of:
   - 40 percent bile
   - 6.5 percent NaCl
   - pH 9.6
   - Temperature of 45°C
   - 1 percent methylene blue milk.
2. On MacConkey's medium they produce tiny deep pink colonies.
   - They are heat resistant surviving at 6°C for 30 minutes
   - They appear as pairs of oval cocci .The cocci in a pair arranged at an angle to each other (Fig. 22.4)
   - *Streptococcus fecalis* can be identified by its ability to ferment mannitol, sucrose, sorbitol and aesculin
   - It grows on tellurite blood agar producing black colonies.

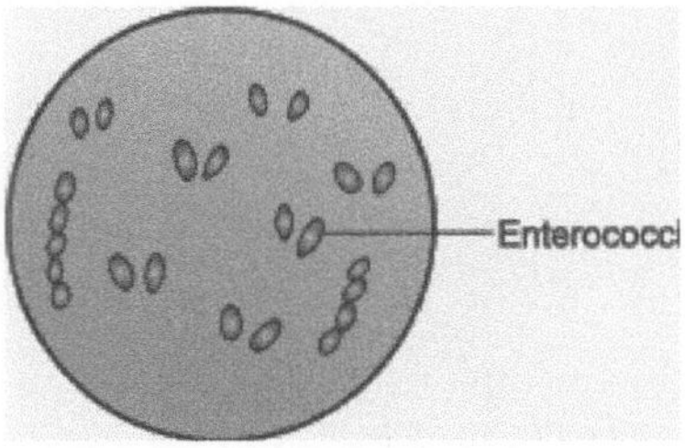

Fig. 22.4: Enterococci (oval cells arranged in pairs at an angle) or in short chains

Enterococci are present in the intestine, genital tract and saliva. They are isolated from cases of:

1. Urinary tract infection.
2. Wound infections.
3. Subacute bacterial endocarditis.
4. Infection of the biliary tract.
5. Septicemia.
6. Peritonitis.
7. Intra-abdominal abscess.

Strains resistant to penicillin occur frequently.

Nonfecal Species

(Streptococcus bovis, Streptococcus equinus)

- These species are generally susceptible to penicillin.
- These are inhibited by 6.5 percent sodium chloride or bile.
- They may cause urinary tract infection or endocarditis rarely.

CHAPTER

23

Gram-positive Cocci: *Streptococcus Pneumoniae*

LESSON PLAN

Genus—Pneumococcus
Species—Streptococcus pneumoniae

INTRODUCTION

Pneumococci are gram-positive cocci in pairs and are therefore called diplo (two) cocci. They resemble *alpha hemolytic streptococci* (*viridans streptococci*) and hence the pathogenic species is called *Streptococcus pneumoniae*. They differ from *Streptococcus* as we shall later find out. Pneumococci occur mainly in the human throat as commensals and are the most important cause of pneumonias.

HISTORICAL BACKGROUND

Pneumococci were first noticed in 1881 by Pasteur and Sternberg independently. The relationship between pneumococci and pneumonia was established only later by Fraenkel and Weichselbaum independently in 1886.

MORPHOLOGY

Pneumococci are small, slightly elongated cocci with one end broad or rounded and the other end pointed presenting a flame shape or a lanceolate appearance. They occur in pairs (diplococci) with the broad ends in apposition, the long axis of the coccus parallel to the line joining the two cocci in a pair.

Capsules are present with the capsule enclosing each pair. Capsules are best seen in fresh exudates. It can be demonstrated by India ink method. In cultures, the typical morphology may not be apparent and the cocci are more rounded and occur in short chains.

They are nonmotile and nonsporing (Fig. 23.1).

CULTURE

Pneumococci are fastidious microorgansims (with complex growth requirements).

Therefore, they grow only in enriched media. They are aerobes and facultative anaerobes.

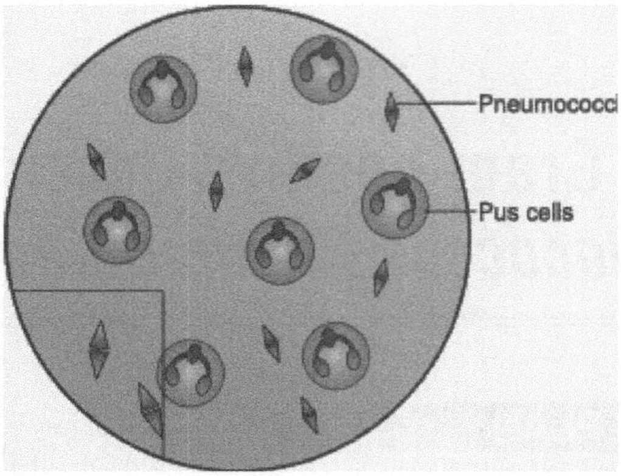

Fig. 23.1: Gram-positive cocci in paris seen in a sputum sample of a patient suffering from pneumonia

Optimum temperature for growth is 37°C (range 25°C to 42°C), pH = 7.8 (range 6.5 to 8.3) 5 to 10 percent CO_2 improves the growth.

The culture medium used are blood agar and chocolate agar.

Blood agar: On blood agar after incubation, colonies are small (0.5 to 1 mm), dome shaped, and shining with an area of greenish discoloration (alpha hemolysis) around them.

Chocolate agar: The colonies are similar to those on blood agar.

Glucose broth: In liquid medium such as glucose broth, the growth occurs as uniform turbidity. Pneumococci have one peculiar property that they readily undergo autolysis in culture due to the activity of intracellular enzymes. Autolysis is enhanced by bile salts and other surface active agents.

BIOCHEMICAL REACTIONS

1. Pneumococci ferment many sugars like glucose, lactose and sucrose forming acid only. Since, pneumococci require enriched culture medium, fermentation is tested in Hiss' serum water or serum agar slopes.
2. Fermentation of a sugar inulin by pneumococci is a useful test for differentiating them from streptococci as streptococci do not ferment inulin.
3. Pneumococci are bile soluble. If a few drops of 10 percent sodium deoxycholate solution are added to 1 mL of an overnight broth culture the culture clears due to lysis of the cocci in about 15 minutes at 37°C. The other method to check bile solubility is by adding a loopful of 10 percent sodium deoxycholate solution and placing it on a pneumococcus colony on blood agar. The colony lyses within a few minutes.

   Principle of bile solubility: The bile solubility test is based on the presence in the pneumococci of an autolytic amidase that breaks the bond between alanine and muramic acid in the peptidoglycan. This enzyme (amidase) is activated by surface active agents such as bile or bile salts resulting in lysis of organisms. The test should be carried out at neutral pH using deoxycholate and live young cells in saline suspension.
4. Pneumococci are catalase and oxidase negative.

RESISTANCE

Pneumococci are delicate organisms that are readily destroyed by heat and antiseptics. In culture too they die on prolonged incubation due to an accumulation of toxic peroxides.

Another important distinguishing feature of pneumococci is sensitivity to optochin (ethylhydrocuprein), a 5 g disc. When a disc with optochin is applied on a plate of blood agar inoculated with pneumococci, a wide zone of inhibition appears on incubation.

ANTIGENIC PROPERTIES

The most important antigen of the pneumococcus is the type specific capsular polysaccharide. This polysaccharide diffuses into the culture medium or the infective exudates and tissues, so it is called specific soluble substance (SSS). Pneumococci are classified into types based on the antigenic nature of the capsular polysaccharide. 85 serotypes of pneumococcus are now known. Typing may be carried out in three ways.

1. Agglutination of the cocci with type specific antiserum.
2. Precipitation of the specific soluble substance with specific serum.
3. By the capsule swelling reaction or the quellung reaction (quellung = swelling).

Quellung Reaction

Principle of the Quellung test: This was described by Neufeld (1902). In the presence of homologous antiserum to the capsular polysaccharide the capsule becomes sharply defined, apparently swollen and refractile. Hence the name-quellung (Quellung-swelling). The dye methylene blue is often added to the typing sera so that the bodies of cocci may stain and can be distinguished from unstained capsule.

Procedure: We can use either a pneumococcus culture suspension or directly the sputum, pus, CSF or peritoneal exudate from the mouse. Put a drop of antiserum and a drop of methylene blue on the pneumococcus suspension and see under oil immersion. If we see the margins of a capsule which is refractile and visibly separated from the cocci, we can call it positive (Fig. 23.2).

There are other minor antigens in pneumococci:

a. A nucleoprotein deep inside the cell.
b. A somatic C carbohydrate antigen.
c. A type specific protein antigen of the cell surface like the M protein of *Streptococcus pyogenes*.
d. A cell membrane antigen called Forssman antigen which is a lipotechoic acid.

An abnormal protein (beta globulin) that precipitates with the somatic C antigen of the pneumococci appears in the acute phase sera of cases of pneumonia but disappears during convalescence. It also occurs in some other pathological conditions. This is known as C-Reactive Protein (CRP). We must remember that it is not an antibody secreted as a result of pneumococcal infection. It is an acute phase substance produced in the hepatocytes. Its production is stimulated by bacterial infections, inflammation, malignancies and tissue destruction. It disappears when the inflammatory reaction subsides. CRP is used as an index of response to treatment with rheumatic fever.

Toxins of Pneumococcus: Pneumococcus has some minor toxins but the virulence of pneumococci is directly dependent on the production of the capsular polysaccharide. This substance protects the cocci from phagocytosis. Type 3 pneumococcus is very virulent due to the abundance of its capsular material. Non-capsulated strains are avirulent. The antibody to the capsular polysaccharide gives protection against infection.

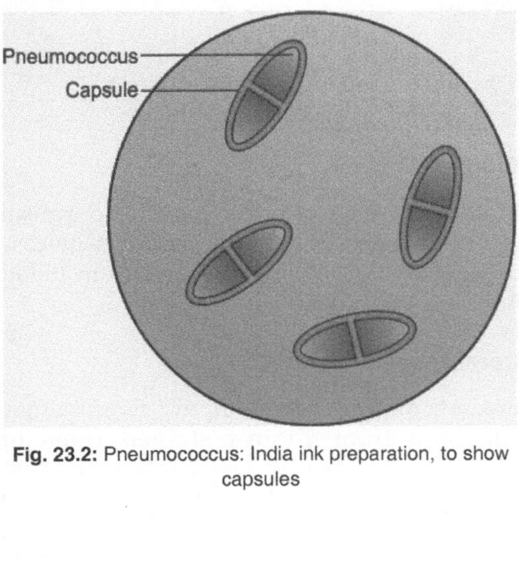

Fig. 23.2: Pneumococcus: India ink preparation, to show capsules

PATHOGENICITY

In man 80 percent of cases of lobar pneumonia and 60 percent cases of bronchopneumonia are caused by pneumococci. It also produces suppurative infections elsewhere in the body.

1. *Lobar pneumonia*: It can occur in two ways. It can result from external infection with a virulent pneumococcus or by symptomless infection with an avirulent pneumococcus. In this case pneumonia occurs when the general resistance is lowered.
2. Bronchopneumonia is a secondary infection and follows a viral infection of the respiratory tract. Pneumococcus is the most common causative agent.

3. Pneumococci are associated with the acute exacerbations in chronic bronchitis.
4. Meningitis is the most serious of pneumococcal infections. It usually follows other pneumococcal infections like pneumonia, otitis media, sinusitis or conjunctivitis.
5. Pneumococci may also produce suppurative lesions in other parts of the body like empyema, pericarditis, otitits media, sinusitis, conjunctivitis, arthritis, etc.

EPIDEMIOLOGY

The source of human infection is the respiratory tract of carriers and patients. Pneumococci occur in the throat of approximately half the population sampled at any one time. The mode of transmission from one person to another is by inhalation of droplet nuclei. Infection usually leads to temporary pharyngeal carriage. Disease occurs when the resistance of the body goes down by respiratory viral infections, malnutrition, cold, alcoholism or malnutrition.

Pneumococcal serotypes vary a lot in virulence. Ten percent serotypes account for 80 percent of all cases of pneumonia.

Type 3 is the most virulent with a case fatality rate of 40 to 60 percent.

Cases are more common in winters and affects two extreme age groups. The incidence of bronchopneumonia increases when an epidemic of influenza or other viral infections of the respiratory tract occur.

LABORATORY DIAGNOSIS

The clinical diagnosis of pneumonia is easy but the disease may be caused by several different microorganisms. The etiological diagnosis should be made by laboratory tests.

Samples to be collected:
1. Sputum
2. Blood
3. CSF in case of meningitis

Sputum

In the acute phase of lobar pneumonia, the rusty colored sputum contains pneumococci in large numbers along with a lot of pus cells and hardly any other bacterium. It can be demonstrated by Gram's stain and typed by quellung test in wet films. In later stages, pneumococci decrease in number. The sputum is inoculated on blood agar plates and incubated at 37°C under 5 to 10 percent CO_2. Growth occurs after overnight incubation. Pneumococci have to be differentiated from *Streptococcus viridans* which is present in the respiratory tract (Table 23.1). The isolates of pneumococcus may be typed with appropriate antisera.

Table 23.1: Differences between Pneumococcus and *Streptococcus viridans*

	Pneumococcus	*Strept. viridans*
Morphology	Capsulated, lanceolate diplococci	Noncapsulated, oval or round cells in chains
Quellung test	Positive	Negative
Colonies on blood agar	Dome shaped	Dome shaped
Growth in liquid media	Uniform turbidity	Granular turbidity
Bile solubility	Positive	Negative
Inulin fermentation	+	–
Optochin sensitivity	+	–
Intraperitoneal inoculation in mice	Fatal	Nonpathogenic
Effect on Blood agar	Narrow zones of α hemolysis	Wide or narrow zones

Blood

In the acute stage of pneumonia, the organism can be obtained from blood culture in glucose broth. Isolation of pneumococci from blood indicates bad prognosis.

Corebrospinal Fluid (CSF)

In case of meningitis, presumptive diagnosis may be made from Gram's stained films of cerebrospinal fluid. Gram-positive diplococci can be seen both inside polymorphs as well as extracellularly. Diagnosis is confirmed by culture. We can also demonstrate the SSS in CSF by precipitation with antisera. Capsular polysaccharide can be demonstrated in blood, urine and cerebrospinal fluid by counter-immunoelectrophoresis.

From specimens where pneumococci are less, isolation may be obtained by intraperitoneal inoculation in mice even if cultures are negative. Inoculated mice die in one to three days and pneumococci may be demonstrated in peritoneal exudate and heart blood. The test may be negative with occasional strains that are, avirulent for mice type 14 strains.

Prophylaxis

Immunity is type specific and it is associated with antibody to capsular polysaccharide. In India, we have a vaccine which contains 23 common serotypes.

Treatment

Most strains are still fully susceptible to penicillin but now 1 to 15 percent isolates show resistance to these antibiotics.

CHAPTER 24

Gram-negative Cocci: *Neisseria Meningitidis* and *Neisseria Gonorrhoeae*

LESSON PLAN

- Introduction
- *Neisseria Meningitidis*
  - Morphology
  - Culture
  - Biochemical Reactions
  - Pathogenicity
  - Antigenic Properties and Classification
  - Epidemiology
  - Laboratory Diagnosis
  - Treatment
  - Prophylaxis
- *Neisseria Gonorrhoeae*
  - Morphology
  - Culture
  - Biochemical Reactions
  - Antigenic Properties
  - Resistance
  - Pathogenicity
  - Epidemiology
  - Laboratory Diagnosis
  - Treatment

Genus—Neisseria
Species—Neisseria meningitidis, Neisseria gonorrhoeae

INTRODUCTION

The genus *Neisseria* consists of gram-negative, aerobic, nonsporulating, nonmotile, oxidase positive cocci arranged in pairs (diplococci). There are two important pathogenic species.

- *Neisseria meningitidis*
- *Neisseria gonorrhoeae*

It also consists of 30 other species that occur as commensals in the mouth or upper respiratory tract.

NEISSERIA MENINGITIDIS

Meningococcus or Diplococcus *intracellularis*.

N. meningitidis causes meningococcal meningitis or cerebrospinal fever. The meningococcus was first described and isolated in 1887 by Welchselbaum from the spinal fluid of a patient.

Morphology

They are gram-negative oval or spherical cocci with the following features:

- 0.6 to 0.8 μ in size arranged in pairs with adjacent sides flattened (Fig. 24.1).
- Nonmotile.
- Fresh isolates are capsulated.
- In smears from lesions the cocci are intracellular.

There may be variation in size, shape and staining properties in older cultures due to autolysis.

Culture

- Meningococci have complex growth requirements, i.e. they are fastidious.

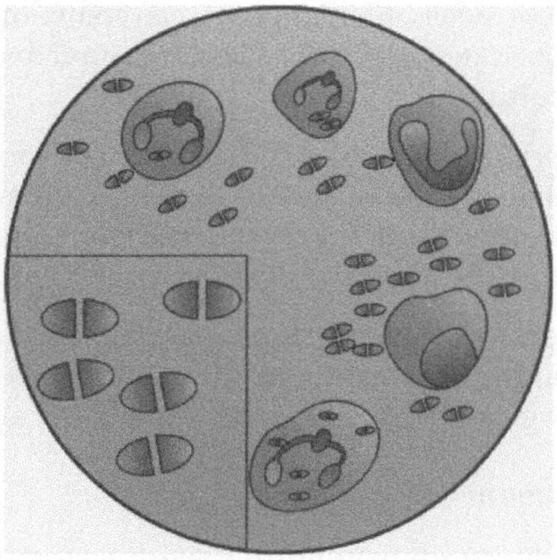

Fig. 24.1: Meningococci in cerebrospinal fluid—Inset show enlarged view of the meningococcus

- They do not grow on ordinary media.
- They are strict aerobes.
- Optimum temperature is 35° to 36°C.
- Optimum pH – 7.4 to 7.6.
- 5 to 10 percent CO_2 helps the growth.
- Require enriched media (blood, serum or ascitic fluid).

Culture media used are:

- Blood agar.
- Chocolate agar.
- Mueller-Hinton starch casein hydrolysate agar.
- There is no growth on MacConkey's agar or nutrient agar.

  On solid media after incubation for 24 hours the colonies are small (1 mm in diameter), translucent, round, convex, bluish gray, smooth shiny and easily emulsifiable. Show weak hemolysis on blood agar.
- Growth in liquid media is poor producing a granular turbidity with little or no surface growth.

Biochemical Reactions

They are catalase and oxidase positive:

Indole -ve

H_2S -ve

Fermentation of sugars is tested on peptone serum agar slopes containing sugar and an indicator. Glucose and maltose are fermented producing acid but no gas (Gonococci ferment glucose but not maltose).

Resistance

Meningococci are very delicate organisms, highly susceptible to heat and disinfectants. Penicillin resistance is now gradually being reported.

Pathogenicity

There are two disease syndromes produced by meningococcus.

- Cerebrospinal meningitis
- Meningococcal septicemia.

Cerebrospinal Meningitis

The cocci enter the body through nasopharynx. Usually there are no symptoms. The cocci then spread through the cribriform plate or through olfactory nerve, conjunctiva or bloodstream to reach the meninges where they setup an inflammatory reaction. The cocci are found in the spinal fluid both free and within the leukocytes.

Case fatality is very high up to 80 percent. Survivors develop complications of blindness or deafness.

Meningococcal Septicemia

Meningococcemia presents as fever with chills and hemorrhagic manifestations with metastatic involvement.

Antigenic Properties and Classification

The classification of meningococci is based on the capsular antigens. Meningococci possess carbohydrate and protein somatic antigens too but they have not been characterized. Meningococci have been classified into nine groups designated A, B, C, D, X, Y, Z and W135 and 29E (Z-). Groups A, B, C are responsible for the majority of infections. Meningococcal vaccine contains group A and C polysaccharides. B is a poor immunogen.

Epidemiology

The human nasopharynx is the only reservoir of meningococcus. Transmission from carriers is by airborne droplets. When there is no epidemic the carrier rate is about 5 to 10 percent. An increase in the carrier rate occurs during epidemics (up to 90%). Epidemic meningitis by group A has occurred in Delhi in 1985.

Laboratory Diagnosis

This is mainly done to rule out other bacteria.

Samples

The most important sample is cerebrospinal fluid. It is turbid with a large number of pus cells. We examine it microbiologically and biochemically. For bacteriological examination we divide the cerebrospinal fluid into three parts if it is present in sufficient quantity.

I. The first portion is centrifuged and Gram's stained smears are prepared from the deposit. Meningococci are seen inside polymorphs but extracellularly also. The supernatant has meningococcal antigen which may be demonstrated by precipitation test with polyvalent or monovalent antimeningococcal serum. It can also be detected by CIEP (Counterimmunoelectrophoresis).
II. The second portion of the CSF is inoculated onto blood agar or chocolate agar and incubated at 35°C to 36°C under 5 to 10 percent CO_2. Colonies are identified by morphology and biochemical reactions.
III. The third portion of CSF is incubated overnight either as such or after adding an equal volume of glucose broth and then subcultured on chocolate agar.

Blood culture: In meningococcemia and early cases of meningitis, blood culture is often positive. Cultures should be incubated for 4 to 7 days with daily subcultures.

Nasopharyngeal swab: This is useful for detection of carriers.

Petechial lesions: Meningococci can sometimes be demonstrated in petechial lesions by microscopy and culture.

Autopsy: Specimens may be collected from the meninges or the surface of the brain. Meningococci may die if specimens are not collected within 12 hours of the death of the patient.

Retrospective diagnosis: Retrospective evidence of meningococcal infection may be obtained by serological diagnosis.

Treatment

Meningococci are uniformly sensitive to penicillin. Early treatment reduces the case fatality rate to about 5 to 10 percent.

Prophylaxis

We can either prevent the disease by giving drugs that is called chemoprophylaxis or by vaccination.

Vaccine

Meningococcal vaccine contains gp A and C polysaccharide. A vaccine against W135 is being tried.

NEISSERIA GONORRHOEAE (GONOCOCCUS)

N. gonorrhoeae causes the veneral disease gonorrhea. The gonococcus was first described in gonorrheal pus by Neisser in 1879. Gonococci resemble meningococci very closely in many properties.

Morphology

In smears from urethral discharge in acute gonorrhea, the organism appears as a diplococcus with the adjacent sides concave. It is found mainly inside the polymorphs (Fig. 24.2). Gonococci contain pili.

Culture

- Gonococci are more difficult to grow than Meningococci.

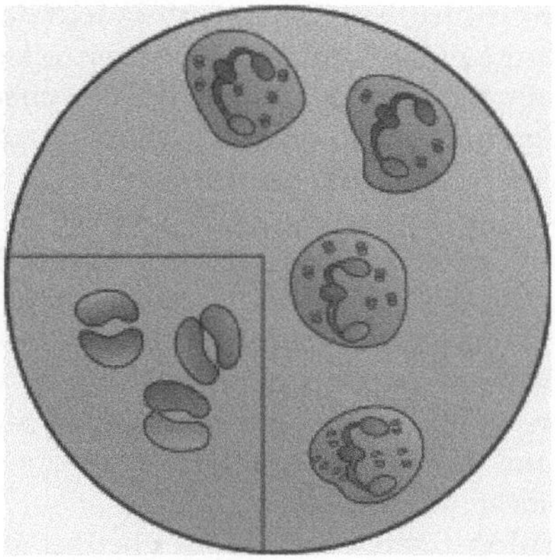

Fig. 24.2: Gonococci in urethral pus. Inset-entarged view to show kidney shaped gram-negative cocci with adjacent sides concave

- Growth occurs best at pH 7.2 to 7.6 at a temperature of 35°C.
- It is essential to provide 5 to 10 percent CO_2.
- Culture mediums used are:
  1. *Chocolate agar*
  2. *Thayer-Martin medium*: A popular selective medium is Thayer-Martin medium containing vancomycin, colistin and nystatin that inhibit most contaminants including nonpathogenic *Neisseria*.
  3. *The Chacko-nair egg* enriched medium although not as selective also supports good growth.
  4. *Modified New York City (MNYC) medium*: This is a special medium for *N. gonorrhoeae* and *N. meningitidis* containing yeast, blood, glucose and antibiotics. Colonies are similar to those on Thayer-Martin medium but are larger.

Colonies are small, round, translucent and convex with a finely granular surface. They are soft and easily emulsifiable.

Biochemical Reactions

Gonococci resemble meningococci except in the fermentation of maltose. Gonococci ferment only glucose and not maltose.

Antigenic Properties

Gonococci have many antigens. It shows cross reactions with meningococcus.

Resistance

The gonococcus is a very delicate organism. It is killed by heat, drying and antiseptics. It is a strict parasite and dies in 1 to 2 hours in exudates outside the body. In cultures, the coccus dies in 3 to 4 days.

Pathogenicity

Gonorrhea is a STD (sexually transmitted disease). The disease is acquired by sexual contact. The 1st step in infection is adhesion to urethra or other mucosal surfaces. Pili are involved in adhesion. The cocci then penetrate through the intercellular spaces and reach the subepithelial connective tissue by the 3rd day after infection.

Incubation period is 2 to 8 days.

In males: The disease starts as an acute urethritis with a mucopurulent discharge containing gonococci in large numbers. The infection extends along the urethra to the prostate, seminal vesicles and epididymis. Chronic urethritis leads to stricture formation.

In females: The initial infection involves the urethra and cervix. The infection may extend to the endometrium and fallopian tubes. Salpingitis may lead to sterility. Clinical disease is as a rule less severe in females. Proctitis (inflammation of the rectum) may develop in both sexes.

Epidemiology

Gonorrhea is an exclusively human disease. The only source of infection is a human patient or carrier. Since females can carry this organism and not suffer from any symptoms it makes them an ideal reservoir.

Laboratory Diagnosis

- In the acute stage, diagnosis can be established readily but in chronic cases it is difficult.
- In acute gonorrhea, the urethral discharge contains gonococci in large numbers. The meatus is cleaned and a sample of discharge is collected with a platinum loop for culture or placed directly on slides for smear preparation. In females besides urethral discharge cervical swab should also be collected.

In chronic infections, there may not be any urethral discharge. The morning drop of secretion may be examined or some exudate may be obtained after prostatic massage. Sometimes we can demonstrate gonococci in centrifuged deposits of urine in cases where no urethral discharge is available.

A direct microscopic examination in males will show intracellular gram-negative diplococci in stained smears. But in women diplococci exist as normal flora also and hence it becomes difficult to diagnose.

For culture, specimens are inoculated on prewarmed plates immediately after collection. The samples can be collected with charcoal impregnated swabs and sent to the laboratory in Stuart's transport medium. From acute gonorrhea cases, bacterial growth can be obtained on chocolate agar incubated at 35° to 36° under 5 to 10 percent CO_2. But in chronic cases, where mixed infection is usual and in lesions such as proctitis, it is better to use a selective medium such as Thayer-Martin medium. Growth is identified by morphology and biochemical reactions.

Serology can be used in chronic cases. Complement fixation test, immunofluorescence and radioimmunoassay are some of the tests that can be used.

Treatment

Large doses of penicillin injections (intramuscular) are used. Now strains resistant to penicillin are appearing.

CHAPTER

25

Gram-positive Rods: Aerobic—*Corynebacterium Diphtheriae*

LESSON PLAN

- Introduction
- *Corynebacterium Diphtheriae*
- History
- Morphology
- Culture
  - Loeffler's Serum Slope
  - Potassium Tellurite Blood Agar
- Biochemical Reactions
- Pathogenesis
- Laboratory Diagnosis
- Toxigenicity Demonstration
- Treatment
- Prophylaxis
- Other Pathogenic Corynebacteria
- Diphtheroids

Genus—Corynebacteria
Species—Corynebacterium diphtheriae

CORYNEBACTERIUM DIPHTHERIAE

INTRODUCTION

Corynebacteria are gram-positive, nonmotile and nonacid fast rods. They show club shaped swellings and irregular staining. Coryne means club shaped.

The representative species is called *Corynebacterium diphtheriae*. It causes the disease diphtheria. Diphtheria is a rare disease today but was quite common before adequate immunization practices. It involves a localized inflammation of the throat leading to the formation of a false membrane (pseudomembrane) and a generalized toxemia because of secretion of the toxin (exotoxin). The membrane that is formed is tough and leathery and hence the name diphtheros that means leather.

HISTORY

The diphtheria bacterium was first observed and described by Klebs and cultivated by Loeffler. It is known as Klebs-Loeffler's bacillus.

MORPHOLOGY

Corynebacterium diphtheriae are:

- *Gram-positive slender rods* but they get decolorized easily.
- They have a tendency to *clubbing* at one or both ends.
- They measure 3.6 μ × 0.6-0.8 μ.
- They are *nonsporing, noncapsulated* and *nonmotile.*
- These bacteria are arranged in a special way and are at obtuse angles to each other resembling the letter V or L (Fig. 25.1). This kind of arrangement is called *cuneiform arrangement*. This is because of incomplete separation of daughter cells after cell division (binary fission).

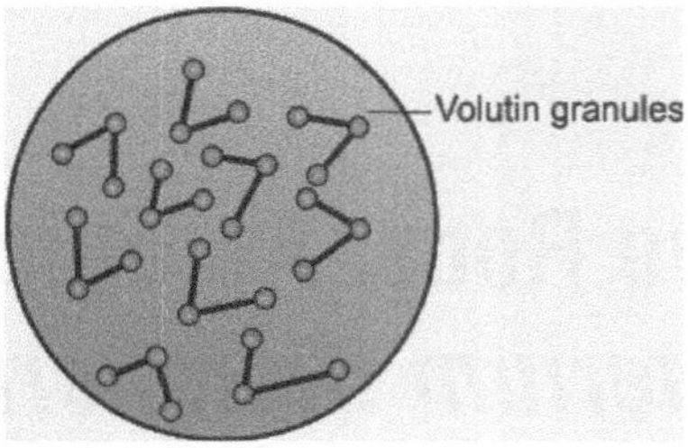

Fig. 25.1: *Corynebacterium diphtheriae* are arranged in the form of letter V or L with volutin granules

- The other special thing about *Corynebacterium diphtheriae* is the presence of metachromatic granules.

Metachromasia is the property of a part of the bacteria taking up a different color from the rest of the bacteria. These granules are also called volutin granules or **Babès-Ernst granules** or **polar bodies** because they are situated at the poles of bacteria in shorter bacilli. They are composed of *polymetaphosphate*. They are more strongly Gram-positive than the rest of the bacterial cell.

Stained with Albert's stain the granules take up a bluish purple color and are called meta-chromatic granules. Other stains used to demonstrate these bacteria are Neisser's and Ponder's.

Because of the presence of these granules the bacteria look beaded when stained with simple stains.

Some strains of *Corynebacterium diphtheriae* do not form granules and some fail to form them on certain media. They are best seen on a moist young culture of Loeffler's serum slope.

CULTURE

- Growth is less on ordinary media.
- *Corynebacterium diphtheriae* are erobes and facultative anerobes requiring enriched media (blood, serum or egg) for their growth.
- Optimum temp = 37°C.
- Optimum pH = 7.2.

The culture mediums used are:

1. Loeffler's serum slope.
2. Potassium tellurite blood agar.

Loeffler's Serum Slope

As the name suggests this culture media is set in a slope form in a small Bijou bottle. It is cream in color.

Composition

Serum of ox, sheep, horse-300 mL.
Nutrient broth, pH 7.6 to 100 mL.
Glucose 1 g.

It is solidified by inspissation. It is put into small 6 ml Bijou bottles and left at a slant at 80°C for 2 hours. 2.5 mL of medium is poured into 6 ml capacity bottles.

The growth is very fast on Loeffler's serum slope. The colonies can be seen in 6 to 8 hours. The colonies are small, circular, white and opaque.

Advantages of Loeffler's Medium

- Growth is very fast.
- Metachromatic granules are seen well.
- There is a small collection of fluid at the base of the medium that is called water of condensation. The water of condensation can be used for animal toxigenicity tests and biochemical reactions.
- We can check if the throat swab has been taken properly because the growth appears very fast, when the swab is plated on Loeffler's medium.

Potassium Tellurite Blood Agar

Composition: Potassium tellurite (0.04%) is used with blood agar. This is a selective medium and inhibits the growth of other bacteria. Diphtheria bacilli reduce tellurite to tellurium that makes the colonies appear black. There are three types of potassium tellurite medium that are used:

- *McLeod's potassium tellurite medium* in this lysed rabbit blood is used.
- *Hoyle's potassium tellurite medium in* which lysed horse blood is used.
- *CTBA (Cystine tellurite blood agar)*.

The growth on tellurite medium is slow and colonies may take 2 days to appear.

Based on the colony morphology on the tellurite medium, **McLeod** classified diphtheria bacilli into three types:

Gravis, Intermedius, Mitis.

These types differ in their morphology, colony characteristics, biochemical reactions and pathogenicity (Table 25.1).

The gravis and intermedius are more serious conditions and the mitis is a milder condition.

The advantage of tellurite medium:

- It is a selective medium
- It gives discrete colonies of *C. diphtheriae* when grown on it
- It can differentiate strains of *C. diphtheriae*.
- It can be used to isolate *C. diphtheriae* bacteria from contacts or carriers as even the presence of a small number of bacteria can be detected.

Special Media

Tinsdale's cystine-sodium thiosulphate tellurite serum agar. The colonies are grey black and are surrounded by a dark brown halo. The halo is due to the formation of H_2S from cystine by the action of cystinase, present in *C. diphtheriae*.

Blood Agar

There is slow growth but the colonies appear after two days and are greyish opaque discs. A small zone of hemolysis may be seen.

BIOCHEMICAL REACTIONS

Corynebacterium diphtheriae ferment, with the production of acid but no gas-glucose, galactose, maltose, dextrin but not lactose, mannitol or sucrose. We use Hiss' serum peptone water for doing sugar fermentation tests.

- It is catalase positive and oxidase negative
- Urease negative
- No proteolytic activity
- Gravis strains ferment starch and glycogen.

PATHOGENESIS

This disease was earlier an important childhood disease but now it is found only in developing countries because of immunization (DPT).

The incubation period is 3 to 4 days. It occurs in the age group of 2 to 5 years. It is common in crowded areas. The disease is transmitted by

Table 25.1: Differences between the three types of *Corynebacterium diphtheriae*

	Gravis	*Intermedius*	*Mitis*
Morphology	Short rods, uniform staining, few or no granules Some degree of pleomorphism	Long, barred forms with clubbed ends. Poor granules Resemble diphtheroids	Long, curved pleomorphic rods with prominent granules. Protoplasm stains evenly
Colony on Tellurite blood agar	Daisy head colony. In 2–3 days the colony has a raised dark center and crenated edge with radial striation	**Frogs egg colony**. In 4-8 hours, dull granular center with smoother more glistening periphery and a lighter ring near the edge	Poached egg colony. In 2–3 days, colony becomes flat with a central elevation
Consistency of colonies	Brittle, not easily emulsifiable	Intermediate	Soft buttery
Antigenic Str.	13 types	4 types	40 types
Hemolysis	Variable	Nonhemolytic	Hemolytic
Glycogen, Starch	Positive	Negative	Negative
Dextrin fermentation			
Animal pathogenicity	Virulent	Virulent	Often avirulent
Case fatality	High	High	Low
Toxigenicity	95–99% strains are toxigenic	95–99% are toxigenic	80–85% strains are toxigenic

carriers or patients by direct contact. Throat or nose carriers are themselves asymptomatic.

The site of infection may be in the throat, larynx, nose, ear, conjunctiva, genital or cutaneous (around mouth and nose) area.

Common complications of diphtheria are:

- *Asphyxia*: This is due to mechanical obstruction of the respiratory passage by the membrane.
- *Acute circulatory failure*: It can be peripheral or cardiac.
- Postdiphtheritic paralysis.
- Septic Pneumonia and otitis media.

Diphtheria is a toxemia. The bacteria remain at the site of entry where they multiply and form the toxin. The toxin causes local necrotic changes leading to fibrinous exudate, disintegrating epithelial cells, leukocytes, erythrocytes and bacteria. These together form the pseudomembrane. It is called pseudomembrane because it remains adherent to the area and is not a true membranous part of the underlying tissue. If we remove the membrane it leaves a raw bleeding surface.

It produces a powerful toxin that travels through the blood stream and has special affinity for heart muscle that causes heart failure. If the nerve endings are affected it causes paralysis. If the adrenal glands are affected it causes shock.

The gravis strains and intermedius strains produce more toxin.

Diphtheria toxin is a protein. It has 2 fragments A and B. All enzymatic activity is present in fragment A. Fragment B is responsible for binding the toxin to the cells. The toxigenicity of the diphtheria bacteria depends on the presence of a bacteriophage that controls toxin production.

LABORATORY DIAGNOSIS

- The laboratory diagnosis is not essential for treatment to be started. As soon as there is clinical suspicion, the treatment should be started.
- The laboratory diagnosis is important for control of epidemics and detection of carriers and contacts.
- Laboratory diagnosis involves the isolation of diphtheria bacteria and also demonstration of its toxicity.

Collection of Samples

The samples to be collected are:

1. Throat swab.
2. Swab from pseudomembrane.
3. Nasopharyngeal swab from carriers.

The sample should be processed within two hours of collection. If there is a delay we can use transport media (Amie's and Stuart's). Blood culture is not useful because there is no bacteremia.

Processing of Samples

Direct staining: To demonstrate morphology and metachromatic granules three smears should be made:

- Gram's stain
- Albert's stain
- Immunofluorescence stain.

A Gram's stain can also identify other gram-positive cocci like *Staphylococcus*, *Streptococcus*, *Candida* or other organisms.

Albert's stain is done to detect metachromatic granules.

Other organisms that have metachromatic granules are:

- *Neisseria*
- Diphtheroids
- Some *Rickettsia* species
- *Lactobacillus*
- *Spirillum volutans*. This bacteria was the first to be detected with volutin granules and the granules are named after them
- *Actinomyces*
- *Yersinia*
- *Bordetella*
- *Mycobacteria phlei*
- *Gardnerella vaginalis*

We should always remember that diphtheria bacilli may not always be demonstrated in smears from lesions nor can they be differentiated from commensal corynebacteria found in the throat. A smear alone is not enough.

TOXIGENICITY DEMONSTRATION

Virulent strains of *Corynebacterium diphtheriae* produce a very powerful exotoxin. The pathogenic effects are due to the toxin. Almost all strains of gravis and intermedius (95 to 99%) are toxigenic. 80 to 85 percent of mitis strains are toxigenic. Convalescents, contacts and carriers are nontoxigenic.

Testing for Toxins

Toxin testing can be done < In vivo / In vitro

In vivo

A subcutaneous or intracutaneous injection of the culture filtrate is done in a control and a test animal. The control animal is protected with antitoxin. Toxigenicity is indicated by death or inflammatory reaction at the site of injection progressing to necrosis in 48 to 72 hours.

In vitro

Elek's gel precipitation test: In this test, a rectangular strip of filter paper 6 × 1 cm is impregnated with diphtheria antitoxin 1000 units/mL and placed on the surface of a 20 percent normal horse serum agar in a Petri dish while the medium is still fluid. When the agar has set the surface is dried and narrow streaks of the test strains are made at right angles to the filter paper strip. A positive and negative control should be put. The plate is incubated at 37°C for 24 to 48 hours. The toxin produced by the bacterial growth will diffuse in the agar and where it meets the antitoxin at optimum concentration will produce a line of precipitation. The presence of such arrow head lines of precipitation will indicate that the strain is toxigenic. No precipitate will form in the case of nontoxigenic strains (Fig. 25.2).

Tissue culture tests: The toxigenicity of diphtheria bacilli can be demonstrated by incorporating the test strains into the agar overlay of cell culture monolayers. The toxin produced diffuses into the cells and kills them.

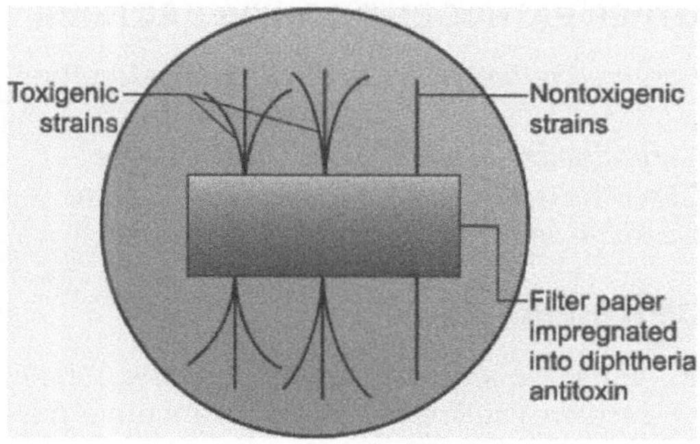

Fig. 25.2: Elek's gel precipitation test

TREATMENT

Specific treatment:	Antitoxin and antibiotic therapy.
Antitoxin:	20,000 units I/M for moderate cases. 50,000 to 100 000 units for serious cases.
Antibiotics:	Erythromycin, Penicillin.

PROPHYLAXIS

The susceptibility or immunity to diphtheria can be tested by Schick test.

Principle of Schick Test

When the diphtheria toxin is injected intradermally into a susceptible person it causes a local reaction but in an immune individual, no reaction is seen, as toxin is neutralized by the antitoxin in circulation.

Immunization

A course of immunization consists of 3 doses at monthly intervals. The antitoxin response is better when formal toxoid is administered with an adjuvant or when given with tetanus toxoid and pertussis vaccine (DPT). This is given in the 3rd, 4th and 5th month of life followed by a booster at school going age.

Formal toxoid is a toxin that is converted to toxoid by incubation with formaldehyde at pH 7.4 to 7.6 for 3 to 4 weeks at 37°C.

OTHER PATHOGENIC CORYNEBACTERIA

Corynebacterium ulcerans	Causes ulceration of the throat
Corynebacterium acnes	Causes acne
Corynebacterium haemolyticum	Causes severe sore throat

DIPHTHEROIDS

- These are corynebacteria resembling *Corynebacterium diphtheriae* that are sometimes mistaken for diphtheria bacilli and are called diphtheria like or diphtheroids.
- Diphtheroids stain more uniformly than diphtheria bacilli and are more gram-positive.
- Possess few or no metachromatic granules.
- They are arranged in parallel rows or palisades rather than chinese letter pattern.
- Pleomorphism is absent.
- Biochemically they are different.
- No toxin produced.

Examples:
- *Corynebacterium pseudodiphtheriticum.*
- *Corynebacterium hofmanni.*

The above two bacteria are found in the throat.

Corynebacterium xerosis is found in the conjunctival sac.

Table 25.2: Differences between *C. diphtheriae* and diphtheroids

C. diphtheriae	*Diphtheroids*
1. *Morphology*	
– They are gram-positive and thin	They are gram-positive, short and thick
– Metachromatic granules are more	– Metachromatic granules are less/absent
– Pleomorphism present	Absent
– Chinese letter arrangement	Parallel arrangement
2. *Culture*	
They grow on enriched media	They grown on ordinary media
3. *Fermentation*	
It ferments glucose only	It ferments glucose and sucrose
4. *Toxicity*	
It is toxic	It is nontoxic

These are harmless commensals that include members of the normal flora of the human skin, throat and conjunctiva. Some diphtheroid bacilli now called the JK group of corynebacteria have been thought of in the causation of opportunistic infections in immunocompromized hosts.

Table 25.2 shows the differences between *C. diphtheriae* and diphtheroids.

CHAPTER 26 Gram-positive Rods: Aerobic—*Mycobacterium Tuberculosis*, *Mycobacterium Leprae* and Atypical Mycobacteria

Genus—Mycobacteria
Species—Mycobacterium tuberculosis, Mycobacterium leprae, Atypical mycobacteria

INTRODUCTION

Mycobacteria mean fungus like bacteria. This is because mycobacteria are slender rods that sometimes show branching filamentous forms resembling fungal mycelium. *Mycobacterium tuberculosis* is one important member of this genus. This causes tuberculosis. We will study many other members. These bacteria are called acid fast bacilli or AFB also because once stained, they resist decolorization with dilute mineral acids. They are aerobic, nonmotile, non-capsulated and non-sporing. Growth is generally slow.

HISTORY

The first member of this genus is the lepra bacillus discovered by Hansen in 1868. Koch (1882) isolated the mammalian tuberculosis bacillus and proved its causative role in tuberculosis by satisfying Koch's postulates.

CLASSIFICATION OF MYCOBACTERIA (TABLE 26.1)

Table 26.1: Classification of mycobacteria
A. Tubercle bacilli
1. Human—*M. tuberculosis*
2. Bovine—*M. bovis*
3. Murine—*M. microti*
4. Avian—*M. avium*
5. Cold blooded—*M. marinum*
B. Lepra bacilli
1. Human—*M. leprae*
2. Rat—*M. leprae murium*
C. Mycobacteria causing skin ulcers
1. *M. ulcerans*
2. *M. balnei*
D. Atypical mycobacteria
1. Photochromogens
2. Scotochromogens
3. Nonphotochromogens
4. Rapid growers
E. Johne's bacillus
M. paratuberculosis
F. Saprophytic mycobacteria
M. butyricum, M. phlei, M. stercoris, M. smegmatis and others

Johne in 1895 described *M. paratuberculosis* (Johne's bacillus) as the agent causing specific enteritis in cattle. Stefansky (1905) described *M. leprae murium* as the bacillus causing rat leprosy. Saprophytic mycobacteria are isolated from a number of sources:

- *M. butyricum from butter.*
- *M. phlei from grass.*
- *M. stercoris from cow dung.*
- *M. smegmatis from smegma.*

Several mycobacteria which are different from human or bovine tubercle bacilli and have been associated with human pathological material are classified as atypical mycobacteria.

MYCOBACTERIUM TUBERCULOSIS

Morphology

- *M. tuberculosis* is a straight or slightly curved rod, 1–4 μ × 0.2–0.8 μ occurring singly or in clumps
- They are nonmotile, nonsporing and non-capsulated
- The bacilli are gram-positive though they do not take the stain readily
- When stained by Ziehl-Neelsen method or by fluorescent dyes (auramine O, rhodamine) they resist decolorization by 20 percent sulphuric acid and absolute alcohol for 10 minutes (acid and alcohol fast). Acid fastness is due to an unsaponifiable wax (mycolic acid) or a semipermeable membrane around the cell or related to the integrity of the cell wall. Beaded or barred forms may be seen in *M. tuberculosis* while *M. bovis* stains more uniformly.

Culture

- The bacteria grow slowly; the generation time is 14 to 15 hours. Colonies may sometimes appear in 2 weeks or take 6 to 8 weeks.
- Optimum temperature is 37°C.
- Growth does not occur when temperature is less than 25°C or greater than 40°C.
- Optimum pH is 6.4–7.0
- *M. tuberculosis* is an obligate aerobe.
- *M. bovis* is microaerophilic, gradually becoming aerobic on subculture.
  Growth is stimulated by 5 to 10 percent CO_2
- *M. tuberculosis* grows well in culture but *M. bovis* grows sparsely. They are therefore called eugonic or dysgonic respectively. Sodium pyruvate improves the growth of both types of bacilli, but glycerol (0.5%) improves the growth of human strains while it either does not have any effect or may inhibit bovine strains.

Solid Media

There are many *solid* media like:

- Loeffler's serum slope
- Pawlowsky's medium (Potato containing)
- Egg containing—Dorset, Petragnini or Löwenstein-Jensen media
- Blood (Tarshis medium).

Tubercle bacilli do not have exacting growth requirements but are highly susceptible to even traces of toxic substances like fatty acids in culture media. The toxicity is neutralized by serum albumin or charcoal.

The most widely used solid media is Löwenstein-Jensen media.

Löwenstein-Jensen Media

Constituents

1. Coagulated hens egg—This enriches the medium, solidifies it and neutralizes the toxic fatty acids.
2. The mineral salt solution includes potassium dihydrogen phosphate, magnesium sulfate, magnesium citrate, etc. These provide essential growth factors and maintain the isotonicity of the medium.
3. Asparagine is a source of nitrogen.
4. Malachite green. This dye has an inhibitory effect on the growth of organisms other than mycobacteria and provides a color contrast that can help in the identification of bacterial colonies.
5. Glycerol (0.5% glycerol). This encourages the growth of *Mycobacterium tuberculosis*.

Preparation of LJ Medium

- Mineral salt solution

Potassium dihydrogen phosphate, (KH_2PO_4) anhydrous	– 2.4 g
Magnesium sulphate $MgSO_4$	– 0.24 g
Magnesium citrate	– 0.6 g
Asparagine	– 3.6 g
Glycerol	– 12 mL
Water	– 600 mL

Dissolve the ingredients with heating. Autoclave at 121°C for 15 minutes to sterilize. The solution keeps indefinitely. Prepare separately a 2 percent solution of malachite green in sterile water. Allow the dye to dissolve by holding at 37°C in the incubator for 1 to 2 hours.

To prepare egg solution—The eggs must be fresh. All utensils used to prepare the medium must be sterile. About 20 to 22 eggs will be required. Wash them thoroughly with warm water and a brush and plain alkaline soap. Then rinse them in running water for 30 minutes. Crack the eggs with a sterile knife into a sterile beaker and beat them till a uniform mixture is obtained. Add the mineral salt solution and malachite green to the mixed egg fluid.

Complete Medium

• Mineral salt solution	600 mL
• Malachite green solution	20 mL
• Egg fluid	1 liter

Mix the complete medium and distribute it in 5 mL amounts into McCartney bottles.

Lay the bottles horizontally in the inspissator and heat at 80°C for 1 hour to coagulate and solidify the medium.

The original medium prepared by Jensen in 1954 has been modified by the omission of starch.

Note: The details of this medium need not be memorized.

Löwenstein-Jensen Pyruvate Medium: This medium is used for primary isolation of *M. bovis*.

It is also used to isolate some drug resistant strains of *M. tuberculosis* but it interferes with the action of INH.

This medium is made by substituting 7 g sodium pyruvate for the 12 mL glycerol in the standard medium.

Stonebrinks Medium: Stonebrinks medium contains 4.2 g of sodium pyruvate in the medium.

Dorset's Egg Medium: This is actually used for maintenance of lab strains of tubercle bacilli but in an emergency it may be used for isolations too.

Mixed egg fluid (2 to 3 hen's egg)	75 mL
Sterile nutrient broth	25 mL

Prepare the mixed white and yolk egg fluid. Mix in the broth and dispense into bottles with sterile precautions for inspissation as for LJ medium.

Liquid Media

Liquid media are not generally used for routine cultivation but are used for sensitivity tests, chemical tests and preparation of antigens and vaccines.

The liquid media can be:

- Dubo's and Davis
- Middlebrook's—$7H_9$
- Proskauer and Beck's
- Sula's and Sauton's Media
- Selective Kirchner's medium.

Dubos and Davis Media: This liquid media is used to give uniformly dispersed cultures which can serve as inocula for drug sensitivity and identification tests. It has bovine albumin solution 9 percent, salts like potassium dihydrogen phosphate, disodium hydrogen phosphate, sodium citrate, magnesium sulfate, Tween 80 (10% solution), casein hydrolysate (20% solution) and distilled water.

This media without the help of any dispersing agent, the growth begins at the bottom, creeps up the sides and forms a prominent surface pellicle. Diffuse growth is obtained in Dubo's medium containing a detergent Tween-80 (sorbitan monooleate) which disperses the growth.

Selective Kirchner Medium: For specimens other than sputum, this liquid selective medium is used in addition to culture on Löwenstein-Jensen slopes.

Tubercle bacilli many also be grown in chick embryos and in tissue culture too.

Cord factor: Virulent strains of *M. tuberculosis* tend to form long serpentine cords in liquid media while avirulent strains grow in a more dispersed fashion. The cord factor by itself is not responsible for virulence. The cord factor consists of 2 mycolic acids linked to a molecule of trehalose. It is present in some nonpathogenic species of mycobacteria as well.

Resistance

Mycobacteria are killed at 60°C in 15 to 20 minutes. Cultures may be killed by exposure to direct sunlight for 2 hours but bacilli in sputum may remain alive for 20 to 30 hours. Eighty percent ethanol has been recommended as a disinfectant for skin.

Biochemical Tests

The important biochemical tests are:

1. *Niacin test*: Human tubercle bacilli form niacin when grown on egg medium.
   10 percent cyanogen bromide +4 percent aniline in 96 percent ethanol are added to a suspension of the culture—a canary yellow color shows a positive reaction.
   Mycobacterium tuberculosis is positive.
   Mycobacterium bovis is negative.
2. *Arylsulfatase test*: This enzyme is formed by atypical mycobacteria only. The organisms are grown in a medium containing 0.0001 M tripotassium phenolphthalein disulphate. To test for this 0.2N NaOH is added drop wise to the culture. A pink color indicates a positive reaction.
3. *Neutral red test*: Virulent strains of tubercle bacilli are able to bind neutral red in alkaline buffer solution while avirulent strains are unable to do so.
4. *Catalase-peroxidase*: Atypical mycobacteria are strongly catalase positive while tubercle bacilli are weakly positive in comparison. Tubercle bacilli but not atypical mycobacteria are peroxidase positive. A mixture of equal volumes of hydrogen peroxide and 0.2 percent catechol in distilled water is added to 5 mL of a test culture and allowed to stand a few minutes. Effervescence indicates catalase production and browning of colonies indicates peroxidase activity.
5. *Amidase activity*: The ability to split amides has been used to differentiate atypical mycobacteria. 5 amides are used:
   - Acetamide
   - Benzamide
   - Carbamide
   - Nicotinamide
   - Pyrazinamide
6. *Nitrate reduction*: *M. tuberculosis* reduce nitrate but *M. bovis* does not.

See Table 26.2 for the differences between *M. tuberculosis* and *M. bovis*.

Antigenic Properties

There are two main antigens in *Mycobacterium tuberculosis*. Group specificity is due to polysaccharide and type specificity due to the protein antigen (tuberculin). There is some antigenic relationship between lepra and tubercle antigens and also between protein antigens of tubercle bacilli, *M. bovis* and certain atypical mycobacteria.

In those patients infected with mycobacteria antibodies are present against polysaccharide protein and phosphatide antigens of the tubercle bacilli but they are not very relevant in immunity.

Pathogenesis

Tuberculosis is a chronic bacterial infection caused by *Mycobacterium tuberculosis* or *M. bovis* characterized pathologically by the formation of tubercles and a tendency to fibrosis and caseation. The usual site of the disease is the lung but other organs may be involved.

M. avium and *M. microti* may rarely infect man. *M. microti* is antigenically almost identical with the human or bovine type and its properties fall between the two of them. *M. tuberculosis* has 2 variants. The African type called *M. africanum* shows properties intermediate between human and bovine types, and the Asian type is a variant of the human type, isolated in South India and is of low virulence for guinea pigs.

M. tuberculosis causes natural infection in man, other primates, dogs and other animals which have close contact with man. Experimentally it is highly infectious for guinea pigs but not for rabbits, cats, goats or fowls.

M. bovis is generally more pathogenic for animals. It produces tuberculosis in cattle, man and other primates. Experimentally, it is highly pathogenic for rabbits, guinea pigs and calves.

The tubercle is the characteristic pathological lesion in tuberculosis. This is an avascular granuloma composed of a central zone containing giant cells with or without caseation, necrosis surrounded by epitheloid cells and a peripheral zone of lymphocytes and fibroblasts. The tubercle bacillus does not appear to contain or produce a toxin. The basis of virulence of the bacillus appears to be due to the cord factor and sulfatides. Sulfatides potentiate action of cord factor. Sulfatides are peripherally present glycolipids seen in virulent strains of mycobacteria. The cord factor causes damage to mitochondrial membranes and functional damage to respiration and oxidative phosphorylation. In the human cells, the cell wall, tuberculoprotein, bacterial polysaccharide and lipids contribute in their own way to pathogenicity of tuberculosis including delayed hypersensitivity and formation of tubercles.

The fate of the tubercle bacilli entering the body is dependent on the dose, virulence and the way the bacteria entered the body. Mostly the bacteria enter by inhalation. They enter the alveolar macrophages where they are phagocytosed. Here they multiply and these

Table 26.2: Differences between *M. tuberculosis* and *M. bovis*

	M. tuberculosis	*M. bovis*
Morphology	Slender, thinner with a tendency to curve	Straight, stouter and shorter
Staining	Beaded/Barred appearance	Uniform staining
Growth on egg containing medium	Eugonic	Dysgonic
Growth in semisolid medium	Aerobic	Microaerophilic
Glycerol	Stimulates the growth	Does not stimulate growth
Pyruvate	Usually does not stimulate growth	Stimulates the growth
Pigment production	Yellowish	White or no color
Niacin test	+	—
Nitrate reduction	+	—
Pyrazinamide	S	R
Pathogenicity in rabbits	Not pathogenic	Pathogenic

phagocytes act as vehicles transporting the infection to different parts of the body. Intracellular multiplication of the bacteria is stopped only when cellular immunity sets in about 6 to 8 weeks after infection.

In children, primary infection leads to the formation of a primary complex. This is called Ghon's focus. This consists of a subpleural focus of tuberculous pneumonia in the lung parenchyma usually found in the lower lobe or the lower part of upper lobe together with enlarged lymph nodes. The primary complex undergoes spontaneous healing. Rarely the primary infection leads to hematogenous spread and the development of miliary tuberculosis, meningitis and lesions in different organs such as spleen, liver and kidneys.

The adult type of tuberculosis is due to reactivation of the primary infection (post-primary progression). The adult type of pulmonary lesion may heal by resorption, fibrosis and occasionally calcification or go on to chronic fibrocaseous tuberculosis with tubercle formation. Caseation cavitation and shedding of tubercle bacilli in sputum (open tuberculosis) develop in this case.

Clinical Types

Pulmonary

- Childhood type
- Adult type

Extrapulmonary

- Miliary
- CNS
- Pleural
- TB pericarditis
- TB liver
- TB cecum
- TB skin
- TB adrenal
- TB larynx
- TB kidney
- TB salpingo-oophoritis
- TB peritonitis
- TB endometritis
- TB lymphadenitis
- TB bones/joints
- TB oral cavity

In fact in all parts of the body can be affected except thyroid, heart muscle and pancreas.

Epidemiology

World

The World Health Organization (WHO) estimates that the largest number of new TB cases in 2005 occurred in the South-East Asia Region, which accounted for 34% of incident cases globally. However, the estimated incidence rate in sub-Saharan Africa is nearly twice that of the South-East Asia Region, at nearly 350 cases per 1,00,000 population.

There were an estimated 8.8 million new tuberculosis (TB) cases in 2005, including 7.4 million in Asia and sub-Saharan Africa. A total of 1.6 million people died of TB, including 195, 000 patients infected with HIV. Both the highest number of deaths and the highest mortality per capita are in the Africa Region. The TB epidemic in Africa grew rapidly during the 1990s, but this growth has been slowing each year, and incidence rates now appear to have stabilized or begun to fall.

It is estimated that 1.8 million people died of tuberculosis in 2008. There were an estimated 9.4 million new cases of tuberculosis in 2008 of which the majority were in Asia and Africa. It is thought that the rates of new tuberculosis infections and deaths per capita have probably been falling globally for several years now. In total, 12,904 TB cases (a rate of 4.2 cases per 100,000 persons) were reported in the United States in 2008. Both the number of TB cases reported and the case rate decreased; this represents a 2.9% and 3.8% decline, respectively, compared to 2007. However, the total number of new tuberculosis cases is still slowly rising due to population growth.

India

India is home to over 3.4 million tuberculosis patients—about one-fifth of the global figure—making it the most TB prevalent country, reported by the World Health Organization.

It revealed that 325,172 people in India had died of the disease in 2005 alone. In 2006, India recorded 1.9 million new cases. Of all fresh cases in the country, 1.2 percent were infected with HIV and 2.8 percent of all new cases have been diagnosed with multi-drug resistant TB (MDR-TB).

Of the 1.9 million TB cases reported in 2006, 89,905 were those who had a relapse and had to take the treatment again. It is reported that the Southeast Asia region, with 4.97 million TB cases, carries over one-third of the global burden of TB.

Source of Infection

- Human smear positive patient
- Bovine—through infected milk. This has reduced after boiling and pasteurization of milk.

Mode of Infection

It is transmitted from person to person via the aerial route. The droplets are expelled during coughing, sneezing and talking. If the host is susceptible, then infection can result. Fomites are not important in transmission of tuberculosis.

Laboratory Diagnosis

Laboratory diagnosis of tuberculosis includes diagnosis of pulmonary tuberculosis and extra-pulmonary tuberculosis.

Pulmonary Tuberculosis

- *Clinical features*
  - Chronic cough is the major respiratory symptom
  - Sputum is scanty or nonpurulent
  - Hemoptysis is frequent
  - Crepitations in chest can be heard.

Laboratory investigations: These can be specific or nonspecific.

Nonspecific
- ↑ ESR (Raised ESR)
- Anemia
- Lymphocytosis.

Specific Investigations
Samples to be collected:
- Sputum
- Bronchial washings
- Laryngeal swab
- Gastric lavage
- Tissue biopsies.

Collection and Transport: The most common clinical specimens received for isolation of acid fast bacilli are pulmonary secretions. Spontaneously coughed or induced sputum, bronchial aspirations and lavages and gastric contents (expected to contain swallowed sputum) are all acceptable. Patients who are able to produce sputum should be given clear instructions as to the collection of such a specimen.

Purulent material from the 1st productive deep cough of the morning should be expelled into a sterile container without contaminating saliva or nasal secretions. Collected secretions which accumulate during the night yields more.
- Patient should rinse his or her mouth out vigorously with water and not any mouthwash before producing sputum.
- Sputum should be collected after deep inspiration.
- Approximately 5 to 10 mL of sputum should be collected in a sterile container such as a screw top plasticine cup or a universal container.
- Patients who are unable to produce sputum may be induced to cough up deep respiratory secretions by allowing them to breathe nebulized warm 10 percent NaCl, or 10 percent glycerine or 15 percent sodium chloride solutions for up to 10 minutes. Such specimens should be labeled induced sputum so that they are not mistaken for saliva because they appear watery. Specimen should be transported immediately. If the specimen must be kept it should be refrigerated where mycobacteria can survive. Do not use pooled sputum samples collected over several hours. For optimal recovery of mycobacteria, 3 to 5 separate specimens

collected over a period of several days are recommended.

Gastric aspirates should be used for:

- Patients unable to produce sputum
- Uncooperative patients
- Small children
- Patients too ill to expectorate usually swallow sputum during night that pools in the stomach. Because of the relative acid resistance of mycobacteria and the slow rate of host metabolism during sleep such swallowed sputum retains acid fast bacilli. Therefore, gastric contents can be collected for culture specimens first thing in the morning or after the patient has fasted for 8 hours.

A disposable plastic gastric tube is inserted through the nose or mouth and gently threaded down the esophagus into the stomach. Patient is instructed to sip small amounts of water to help to move the tube down. When the tube reaches the stomach, the gastric contents are aspirated into a 50 mL syringe and immediately placed in a sterile container. Then 20 to 30 mL of sterile distilled water is injected into the stomach through the tube or swallowed by the patient. This fluid which is the gastric lavage is aspirated into a syringe and added to the original specimen. This is taken to the lab where it is neutralized with pellets of NaOH until pH 7.0 is reached. Can be done on three successive mornings.

Processing: Either the sputum is used as such, or it is digested and shaken with an equal amount of 1 percent sodium acetylcysteine or 1 percent buffered pancreatin which liquefies the sputum. It can then be subjected to concentration methods to increase the yield of *M. tuberculosis*.

Concentration Methods: Sometimes we have to concentrate the samples to be able to detect *Mycobacterium tuberculosis* easily. These concentration methods can be:

a. Used for microscopy alone.
b. Used for culture and animal inoculation.

a. *Used for microscopy alone:*
   1. Treatment with antiformin.
   2. Treatment with sodium hypochlorite.
   3. Treatment with detergents like tergitol.
   4. Flotation method using hydrocarbons.
   5. Autoclave method.

These concentration methods kill the bacteria without altering their morphology and staining properties. The concentration method decontaminates, concentrates the sample and homogenises it.

b. *For culture and animal inoculation*: Certain methods which concentrate the bacteria without inactivating them can be used for culture and animal inoculation.

1. *Petroff's method*
   i. Sputum is mixed with an equal volume of 4 percent NaOH.
      a. This is an emulsifier.
      b. It works as a decontaminant.
      c. It shortens the decontamination time.
      d. It preserves viable mycobacteria.
   ii. It is incubated with frequent shaking till it becomes clear on an average for 20 minutes.
   iii. It is then centrifuged at 3000 rpm for 30 minutes.
   iv. The sediment is neutralized with N/10 HCl. This can then be used for culture and animal inoculation.
2. *Hanks flocculation technique.*
3. *Treatment with trisodium phosphate.*

Direct Microscopy: The material is picked up directly or after concentration from the specimen and put on to the surface of the slide in a thin layer. Slides should be heat fixed and stained with Ziehl-Neelsen stain or Kinyoun's cold acid fast stain (Chapter 3).

It has been estimated that at least 1 lakh acid fast bacteria should be present per mL of the sputum for them to be readily seen in direct smears. A negative report should not be given till at least 100 fields have been examined taking about 10 minutes. A positive report can be given only if 2 to 3 typical bacteria are seen.

The positive smear is graded as below:

1 + if → 3 to 9 bacilli are seen in the entire smear

2 + if → 10 or more bacilli are seen in the smear

3 + if → 10 or more bacilli are seen in most oil-immersion fields

Fluorescent staining can also be done in those labs which have a fluorescent microscope. Fluorescent stains are much more sensitive than the conventional carbol fuchsin stains. The fluorescent bacilli stand out brightly against a dark background. The stain used is auramine rhodamine or auramine phenol. It is much quicker to examine.

Precautions

1. It is important to wipe the oil-immersion lens from the objective lens after examining a positive smear since stained bacilli can float off the slide into the oil and may give rise to a false positive test.
2. Demonstration of acid fast bacilli microscopically provides only presumptive evidence as saprophytic mycobacteria may present a similar appearance. Most saprophytic species stain uniformly without any barred or beaded appearance and are usually only acid fast without being alcohol fast.
3. As saprophytic mycobacteria are present in tap water, rubber tubes, cork and bark, they can get into clinical specimens. Saprophytic bacilli are not present in respiratory secretions but they are a problem with gastric as pirates, feces and specimens from urogenital tract.

The advantage of microscopy is simplicity and speed. We can also find out if the patient is an open case.

Culture: It is a very sensitive method for detection of low number of organisms. We can also differentiate between the various species. Culture can be positive with as few as 10 to 100 bacilli/mL of sputum. The concentrated material is inoculated into at least 2 bottles of LJ medium. The cultures are examined for growth after incubation at 37° for 4 days (for rapidly growing mycobacteria, fungi and contaminant bacteria) and at least 2 weekly thereafter. A negative report is given if no growth appears after 6 to 8 weeks.

The generation time of bacilli is 14 to 15 hours. Optimum temperature is 37°C (Temperature range is 25 to 40°C).

Both solid and liquid media are used, the details of which are discussed in the section on culture.

Biochemical Tests: Relevant biochemical tests are done as explained in the section earlier.

For the identification of tubercle bacilli, see the flow chart.

Animal Inoculation: Concentrated material is inoculated I/M and not S/C into the thigh of 2 healthy guinea pigs who are 12 weeks old.

Subcutaneous inoculation may cause a local ulcer that may be infectious. Animals are weighed before and after inoculation. Progressive loss of weight is an indication of tuberculosis. One animal is killed at 4 weeks and the other at 8 weeks if the first does not show any signs.

Autopsy Findings

1. A caseous lesion at the site of inoculation. Pus may spurt on incision.
2. Enlarged caseous draining lymph nodes-femoral, inguinal, lumbar, portal, mediastinal, cervical. Severity of lesion diminishes as the distance from the site of inoculation increases.
3. Enlarged spleen showing irregular necrotic areas.
4. Tubercles in the peritoneum.
5. A few tubercles in the lungs.
6. Kidneys are unaffected.

Differential diagnosis:

- *Y. pseudotuberculosis*
- *Salmonella*
- *Brucella*
- Pyogenic cocci
- Some fungi

Confirm by demonstration of acid fast bacilli in lesions.

Rabbit is used to distinguish between human and bovine types. Bovine is more virulent for rabbits:

- Catalase negative and INH resistant strains do not produce progressive disease in guinea pigs.
- Animals inoculated with strains of low virulence may have to be observed for 12 weeks or longer for evidence of infection.
- Strains from South India are of low virulence to guinea pigs.

Drug Sensitivity

As drug resistance is an important problem in tuberculosis, it is desirable that sensitivity tests should be performed with the isolates as an aid to treatment.

There are three types of tests:
1. Absolute concentration method
2. Resistance ratio method
3. Proportion method

Absolute concentration method: A number of media containing the serial concentration of the drug are inoculated and the MIC calculated from the medium with the least drug concentration that inhibits growth.

Resistance ratio method: Two sets of media containing graded concentration of drugs are inoculated—one with the test strain and one with the standard strain of known sensitivity.

Proportion method: This test indicates the average sensitivity of a strain taking into account that any population of tubercle bacilli will contain cells with varying degree of sensitivity to drug.

Polymerase Chain Reaction

PCR detection of *Mycobacterium tuberculosis* by a polymerase chain reaction from a clinical sample can be done if the lab is equipped to do so. It can amplify and identify the DNA of a single *Mycobacterium tuberculosis* too. This method is very helpful in case of a difficult diagnosis. False positive reactions may occur.

Extrapulmonary Tuberculosis

Specimens which are to be collected are:

1. CSF
2. Urine
3. Pleural fluid
4. Joint aspirate
5. Ascitic fluid
6. Feces
7. Lung biopsy FNAC
8. Endometrial biopsy
9. Skin biopsy
10. Bronchial washings

Processing is the same as for pulmonary tuberculosis with a few differences.

1. *In tubercular meningitis*: The CSF is examined by smear, culture and animal inoculation. On standing, a spider web clot is formed in CSF which contains enmeshed tubercle bacilli.
2. *Pleural fluid and other exudates* are collected with citrate to prevent coagulation. They are then centrifuged and the sediment cultured.
3. *In renal tuberculosis* bacillary shedding may be intermittent. It is advisable to test 3 to 6 consecutive morning samples of urine. Each specimen is sent to the lab on the day of collection. 100 mL of the daily sample is centrifuged at 3000 rpm for 30 minutes. Deposit is neutralized if necessary and stored in the refrigerator. Each day's specimen is treated in this manner and pooled. Pooled material is concentrated and used for culture and animal inoculation.

Tuberculin Testing

Introduction

Tuberculin may be defined as a substance or a mixture of substances derived from *M. tuberculosis* capable of giving rise to a delayed type of hypersensitivity in a sensitized person.

This reaction is induced by sensitized T cells which on contact with specific antigen release lymphokines that in turn affect leukocytes, macrophages and tissue cells.

When a small dose of tuberculin is injected intradermally in an individual sensitized to tuberculoprotein by prior infection or immunization, an indurated inflammatory reaction occurs at the site within 48 to 72 hours. In unsensitized individuals, tuberculin infection gives no response.

Tuberculin–Old and New

Tuberculin was initially used by Koch who prepared a protein extract of tubercle bacillus by concentrating ten fold by evaporation, a 6 to 8 week culture filtrate of the bacillus grown in 5 percent glycerol broth. This was called old tuberculin. Now, we use a standardized tuberculin protein purified derivative/RT 23 with Tween 80 as a stabilizer which is now available through the WHO. This is called new tuberculin.

Techniques of Doing the Test

- Cutaneous reaction of Von Pirquet (rubbing tuberculin into scarified skin)
- Percutaneous reaction of Moro (rubbing into skin as an ointment)
- Patch test of Vollmer and Goldberger
- Graded I/D test of Mantoux
- Multiple puncture by Heaf injector.

Mantoux Test

Graded doses of tuberculin are injected intradermally on the forearm using a tuberculin syringe with 27 gauge needle. 0.1 mL is injected in adults and 0.05 mL in children.

On examination after 48 to 72 hours, a positive reaction is indicated by edema and induration at the site measuring 10 mm in diameter. Erythema alone is not taken as a positive reaction. The transverse diameter is the one which is measured.

Interpretation of Mantoux Test

- All persons with prior infection with the tubercle bacillus whether clinical or subclinical give a positive test.
- *Specific reaction*: This is characterized by a large reaction (an induration of > 10 mm or more to 1 TU of PPD RT-23). This is considered as positive infection with *Mycobacterium tuberculosis*.
- *Nonspecific reaction*: This is characterized by a small reaction (6 to 9 mm induration) to ITU of tuberculin. This represents in most cases infection with one or more atypical bacteria.
- Negative reaction < 5 mm.
- If a child less than 2 years is tuberculin positive it is an indirect evidence of an active tuberculous lesion in the body.
- Size of tuberculin reaction is related to the risk of developing tuberculosis at a later date. Those who react with 20 mm or more of induration have more chances of developing tuberculosis than those with an induration of 10 mm. Negative reactors with < 5 mm induration have more risk of developing tuberculosis than those with 6 to 9 mm induration. Those with 6 to 9 mm induration have the least chance of developing tuberculosis.
- Where skin tests are preformed in contacts of infectious cases of tuberculosis, subjects with initial skin test reaction of < 10 mm should be retested at 6 weeks.
- If a positive test is seen in nonvaccinated individuals it indicates disease.
- Tuberculin sensitivity decreases gradually. It gradually disappears in 4 to 5 years in absence of subsequent contact with the bacteria. In endemic area this sensitivity is maintained by repeated exposure to the bacillus.
- A false negative reaction is called anergy. It can occur in many conditions:
  - Miliary tuberculosis
  - Measles
  - Immunosuppressed states
  - Sarcoidosis
  - Malnutrition
  - Convalescence from viral infection
  - Defective CMI
  - Malignancy
- False positive reaction may be seen in infections with related mycobacteria.

Uses of Mantoux Test

1. To see the prevalence of infection as such in school children.
2. To see contact tracing of infectious cases of tuberculosis in families and close relatives of young children who give a positive reaction.
3. As an aid to clinical diagnosis of suspected infection in very young children.
4. As an indication of early infection in older children who give strongly positive reaction. These require follow-up with X-ray.

5. Post-vaccination check on efficacy of the BCG vaccination.
6. To measure the prevalence of infection in a community.

Serology

- No serological test is useful in the diagnosis of tuberculosis.
- The tests available are:
  - ELISA, radioimmunoassay, IHA, CIEP, CFT
  - The results are erratic and negative in early cases.

BCG

It stands for Bacille Calmette-Guérin. In 1921 two French workers, Calmette and, Guérin introduced a live vaccine prepared from a bovine strain that had been cultured for 239 subcultures on a bile potato medium for a period of 13 years.

This has been used for immunoprophylaxis of tuberculosis since early times with variable results.

Intradermal injection of BCG in animals led to initial tubercle formation and multiplication of the bacteria but later the lesions disappeared and led to immunity. BCG vaccination in a tuberculin negative human led to tuberculin positivity.

The immunity produced by BCG vaccination is similar to the immunity following natural infection but the disease does not progress.

Many field trials have been conducted to assess the efficacy of the BCG vaccine. The results have varied widely from 80 percent efficacy to a total absence of protection. The reasons given for this disparity are probably due to differences in the prevalence and virulence of tubercle bacilli in various communities, the age, nutritional status, type and potency of vaccines and presence of other mycobacteria.

The complications of BCG vaccination are rare and respond to treatment. They are:

1. *Local*—An abscess, ulcer, keloid or small satellite BCG tubercles may develop in the neighborhood of the vaccination site.
2. *Regional*—There may be enlargement of the draining lymph nodes and abscess formation.
3. *General*—There may be fever or ear infection.

Status of BCG

1. Routine immunization with BCG should continue. It is given to infants at birth intradermally over the deltoid.
2. It has also now been concluded that BCG does protect against tuberculosis especially in infants and children. Even if they do get the disease, it runs a milder course. It is also believed to prevent skeletal, meningeal and miliary forms of tuberculosis.
3. It is also believed that immunization with BCG leads to stimulation of the reticulo-endothelial system and gives some protection against leprosy and leukemia.

Some studies have tried *M. microti* as a live vaccine against tuberculosis but it causes unacceptable severe local reactions.

MYCOBACTERIUM LEPRAE

INTRODUCTION

Leprosy is caused by *Mycobacterium leprae*. The lepra bacillus was first observed by Hansen in 1868. It has not been possible to grow the bacillus in culture.

MORPHOLOGY

M. leprae is a straight or slightly curved rod 1 to 8 μ × 0.2 to 0.5 μ in size. It is Gram-positive and stains more readily than the tubercle bacillus. It is acid fast but 5 percent H_2SO_4 is used for decolorization after staining with carbol fuchsin. The bacilli are seen singly and in groups, intracellularly or lying free outside the cells. In groups, the bacilli are bound together by a lipid like substance called glia. These masses are known as globi. The parallel rows of bacilli in the globi present a cigar bundle appearance.

CULTIVATION

It has not been possible to culture lepra bacilli either in bacteriological media or in tissue culture. In 1962, Indian Cancer Research Center, Bombay, isolated an acid fast bacteria growing on human fetal spinal ganglion cell culture. It has been adapted for growth on LJ medium but its relation to the lepra bacillus is uncertain.

There have been many attempts to transmit leprosy to animals. In 1960, Shepard showed that lepra bacilli could multiply in the foot pads of mice kept at a low temperature (20°C). Now, this is a standard procedure for work with leprosy bacteria. Following intradermal inoculation into foot pads of mice a granuloma develops at the site in 1 to 6 months. Another animal which is used is the nine banded armadillo. The generation time of the lepra bacteria is about 12 to 13 days.

RESISTANCE

Lepra bacteria can remain viable in warm humid environment for about 2 weeks. They can survive exposure to ultraviolet light for 30 minutes and direct sunlight for 2 hours.

EPIDEMIOLOGY

- Leprosy occurs in humans only
- The only source of infection is the patient
- The mode of infection may be either through the respiratory tract or through the skin
- Asymptomatic infection appears to be quite common in endemic areas
- Leprosy is not highly communicable. Only 5 percent of spouses show leprosy disease. Intimate and prolonged contact is necessary for infection to take place.

Worldwide—15 to 20 million people suffer from leprosy of which 3 million are in India.

Andhra Pradesh and Tamil Nadu, have the maximum number of cases. Orissa, West Bengal and Nagaland are next followed by Gujarat, Jammu & Kashmir, Uttar Pradesh and Himachal.

LEPROSY—THE DISEASE

Leprosy is a chronic granulomatous disease of man involving primarily the skin, peripheral nerves and nasal mucosa but can affect any tissue or organ. The disease can be of 4 types:

- Lepromatous
- Tuberculoid
- Dimorphous
- Indeterminate.

The type of disease is a reflection of the immune status of the host. Therefore, it is not the same and changes with chemotherapy and change in host resistance.

Lephromatous

- The host resistance is low
- The bacilli are seen in large numbers as globi inside the lepra cells or extracellularly
- Superficial nodular lesions called lepromata develop which consist of granulation tissue. The nodules ulcerate and become infected and cause distortion and disfigurement
- The bacilli invade the mucosa of the nose, mouth and upper respiratory tract and are shed in large numbers in nasal and oral secretions
- Bacillema is present
- Prognosis is poor
- Lepromatous type is more infective than other types
- Most of the reticuloendothelial system, eyes, testis, kidneys and bones are involved
- Cell mediated immunity is deficient
- Lepromin test is negative
- Humoral immunity is high.

Tuberculoid

- This is seen in patients with high degree of resistance
- Skin lesions are few and sharply demarcated consisting of macular anesthetic patches
- Neural involvement occurs early and may lead to deformities in hands and feet
- Bacilli are less in lesions and infectivity is minimal
- Cell mediated immunity is adequate
- Lepromin test is positive
- Antibodies are rare
- Prognosis is good.

Borderline or Dimorphous

The term borderline or dimorphous means lesions having characteristics of both tuberculoid and lepromatous. It may shift to the lepromatous side or tuberculoid side.

Indeterminate

This type is an early unstable tissue reaction which is not characteristic of either lepromatous or tuberculoid. In some healing may occur and in others, the lesions may progress to tuberculoid or lepromatous type.

Ridley and Jopling have introduced a scale for classifying the spectrum of leprosy into 5 groups:

1. Tuberculoid (TT)
2. Borderline tuberculoid (BT)
3. Borderline borderline (BB)
4. Borderline lepromatous (BL)
5. Lepromatous (LL).

LABORATORY DIAGNOSIS

- Bacteriological diagnosis is easy in the lepromatous but may be difficult in the tuberculoid cases.

  Diagnosis means the demonstration of acid fast bacilli in the lesions.
- The specimens are collected from:
  - Nasal mucosa
  - Skin
  - Ear lobules

A blunt narrow scalpel is introduced into the nose and the internal septum scraped to remove a piece of mucous membrane which is then transferred to a slide and made into a smear. Samples from the skin should be obtained from the center. The skin is pinched up tight to minimize bleeding and a cut about 5 mm long is made with a scalpel, deep enough to get into the layers. After wiping off blood or lymph that may have exuded the scalpel blade is turned transversely to scrape the sides and bottom of the cut so as to obtain a little tissue pulp which is taken on a slide.

About 5 to 6 different areas of the skin are sampled including the skin over the buttocks, forehead, chin, cheek and ears. The smears are stained by Ziehl-Neelsen technique using 5 percent instead of 20 percent H_2SO_4 for decolorization.

Biopsy of the nodular lesions and thickened nerves and lymph node puncture may be required.

LEPROMIN TEST

The lepromin test is a skin test described by Mitsuda in 1919. The lepromin test is not used to diagnose leprosy nor does it indicate prior contact with the lepra bacillus. It is used to:

1. Classify the lesions of leprosy patients. The lepromin test is positive in tuberculoid, negative in lepromatous and variable in dimorphous and indeterminate types of disease.
2. To assess the prognosis and response to treatment. A positive reaction indicates good prognosis and a negative one bad. If its gets converted to positive during treatment, its a good sign.
3. It is advisable to employ only lepromin positive persons for work in leprosaria as lepromin negative persons are more prone to develop the disease.

The earlier lepromin which was used was the crude Mitsuda's-antigen. The original antigen (lepromin) was boiled, emulsified lepromatous tissue rich in lepra bacilli. It showed a typical bi phasic response. The first was called early reaction of Fernandez that consisted of erythema and induration developing in 24 to 48 hours and remaining for 3 to 5 days. The second was the late reaction of Mitsuda appearing in 3 weeks reaching a peak in 4 weeks and then subsiding in the next few weeks. Most people use the late reaction as evidence of lepromin positivity.

Now Mitsuda's crude antigen is modified in many ways to provide a pure and more standardised antigen with less of tissue and more of bacillary components. Such partially purified preparations are called lepromins. Those which contain bacillary protein components only are called leprolins and give only the early reaction. Armadillo derived lepromin is now widely used.

Attempts are now being made to develop a specific vaccine using lepra bacilli grown in armadillos.

ATYPICAL MYCOBACTERIA

INTRODUCTION

Mycobacteria other than human or bovine tuberculosis that may occasionally cause human disease resembling tuberculosis have been called atypical, anonymous or unclassified mycobacteria.

FEATURES OF ATYPICAL MYCOBACTERIA

- They normally live in soil or water and cause opportunistic infections in man
- They are also called paratubercle, tuberculoid and mycobacteria other than tubercle bacteria (MOTT)
- They are not directly transmitted from man to man
- Atypical mycobacteria are different from saprophytic bacteria such as *M. smegmatis* and *M. phlei* which cannot infect man or animals
- Atypical mycobacteria are of low virulence. Human infection with them is common but disease is rare. They are unable to cause progressive disease when injected into guinea pigs
- Atypical mycobacteria are becoming much more important these days because tuberculosis has been brought under control
- Some of them cause pulmonary disease similar to tuberculosis. Others cause lymphadenitis, urinary infections and cutaneous and subcutaneous lesions
- Atypical mycobacteria are found more often in developed countries, e.g. in South East USA where a large proportion of the population is infected. These areas have low grade tuberculin reactions
- Atypical mycobacteria are resistant to antituberculous drugs particularly streptomycin and INH. Treatment is difficult and a combination of drugs or surgery may become necessary.

CLASSIFICATION

Based on pigment production and rate of growth atypical mycobacteria have been divided into 4 groups by a scientist called Runyon in 1959.

Group I—Photochromogens

- These strains produce no pigment in the dark but when the young culture is exposed to light for 1 hour in the presence of air, and reincubated for 48 hours a yellow orange pigment develops.
- Slow growing.
- For example: *M. kansasii* which causes chronic pulmonary disease resembling tuberculosis particularly in old persons with pre-existing lung diseases.
- These bacilli are isolated from soil and milk and there is no man to man transmission.
- They are urease positive and reduce nitrate.

Group II—Scotochromogens

- These strains form pigmented colonies (yellow-orange-red) even in the dark.
- They are present in the environment and can contaminate cultures of tubercle bacilli.
- They do not usually cause human disease except for *M. scrofulaceum* which may cause scrofula (cervical adenitis in children).
- They are urease positive.

Group III—Nonphotochromogens

- These strains do not form pigment even on exposure to light.
- Colonies are similar to tubercle bacilli.
- The medically important species are *M. intracellulare*, *M. avium* and *M. xenopi*.

M. Intracellulare

This causes chronic pulmonary disease similar to tuberculosis:

- It is called Battey bacillus because of the name of the hospital from where they were first identified
- Soil is the reservoir of infection
- It also causes renal infection and lymphadenopathy
- Rifampicin and streptomycin are recommended for treatment.

M. Avium

This is very similar to Battey bacillus and therefore, it is considered by some to belong to the same species. It causes tuberculosis in fowls and may also infect pigs. Human infection is rare and may cause cervical adenitis in children or lung disease in elderly.

- It is easier to treat than Battey bacillus. *M. avium* is put into a complex along with *M. intracellulare* and also *M. scrofulaceum* called MAIS complex. *M. avium-intracellulare-scrofulaceum* complex.
- *M. xenopi*: It was isolated from toads.
- Occasionally causes chronic lung disease or renal disease in man.

M. avium and *M. xenopi* are thermophiles capable of growing at 45°C. They are isolated from water taps mostly hot water taps in hospitals.

Group IV—Rapid Growers

- This is a heterogenous group of mycobacteria.
- They are capable of rapid growth.
- Colonies appear within 7 days of incubation at 37°C or 25°C.
- Within this group photochromogenic, scotochromogenic, and nonchromogenic species occur.

Table 26.3: Differences between *M. ulcerans* and *M. marinum*

	M. ulcerans	*M. marinum*
Distribution	Usually found in tropics	Found in temperate countries.
Clinical course	Following infection through minor injuries, the area becomes indurated and becomes a chronic progressive ulcer	Human infection originates from contaminated swimming pools or fish tanks. The lesion begins as a papule and breaks down to form an indolent ulcer which follows abrasions and occurs on the prominences (elbow, knees, ankles, nose, finger or toes). It is self-limited and undergoes healing. It was called swimming pool granuloma
Bacilli in ulcer	Abundant. Smears from the edge of the ulcer show large clumps of bacilli which are acid fast and alcohol fast	Bacilli are scanty in smears from ulcers
Growth	The bacilli grow on Löwenstein-Jensen medium slowly in 4–8 weeks. Temperature of incubation is between 30–33°C but not at 25° or 37°C	Growth occurs in about 2 weeks at 30°C (range 25°–35°C Colonies are nonpigmented in the dark but become intense orange yellow to red on exposure to light
Mouse foot pad	Inoculation into foot pad of mice leads to edema of the limb, and ulceration	Foot pad inoculation in mice leads to a severe lesion
Toxin production	A toxin produced by *M. ulcerans* causes inflammation and necrosis when injected into the skin of guinea pigs. Only known toxin produced by mycobacterium species No tuberculin reaction	It is not pathogenic for guinea pigs but intradermal inoculation in rabbits leads to a superficial granulomatous lesion Low grade tuberculin reaction

- Medically important species are:
  - *M. fortuitum*
  - *M. chelonae*
  - Both of them cause chronic abscesses in man.

The abscesses are mostly after injection of vaccines. The pulmonary lesions are similar to typical tuberculosis. No standard chemotherapy is available.

SKIN PATHOGENS

Two mycobacteria are exclusively skin pathogens: *M. ulcerans and M. marinum*

- They multiply optimally at skin temperature
- Systemic invasion does not occur
- Regional lymph nodes are not involved
- Cause chronic ulcers and granulomatous lesions on the skin.

Differences between *M. ulcerans* and *M. marinum* are shown in the Table 26.3.

CHAPTER

27

Gram-positive Rods: Anaerobic—*Clostridium Tetani*

LESSON PLAN

- Classification of Anaerobic Bacteria
- *Clostridium*
- General Properties of Genus Clostridia
- Classification of Clostridia
- *Clostridium Tetani*
  - Morphology
  - Culture
  - Biochemical Reactions
  - Resistance
  - Toxins
  - Pathogenicity
  - Tetanus
  - Laboratory Diagnosis
  - Prevention of Tetanus
- Gas Gangrene and *Clostridium Welchii*
- *Clostridium Botulinum*

Genus—Clostridium
Species—Clostridium tetani

CLASSIFICATION OF ANAEROBIC BACTERIA

Anaerobic bacteria are those that do not grow in the presence of oxygen and require an anaerobic environment for growth. They outnumber aerobic bacteria, especially in the human intestine where they are present as commensals. They also cause many dreaded diseases like tetanus, gas gangrene botulism or syphilis. A very simple classification of anaerobic bacteria is as follows:

I. Cocci
   A. Gram-positive
      1. Peptococcus
      2. *Peptostreptococcus*
      3. Sarcina
   B. Gram-negative
      1. Veillonella

II. Bacilli—Endospore forming—Clostridia
   Nonsporing

Gram-positive	Gram-negative
Lactobacillus	*Bacteroides*
Bifidobacterium	*Fusobacterium*
Actinomyces	
Propionibacterium	

III. Spirochaetes
   1. *Treponema*
   2. *Borrelia*

CLOSTRIDIUM

Introduction

The genus *Clostridium* consists of gram-positive, anaerobic, spore forming bacilli. The spores are wider than the bodies of bacteria giving the bacteria a swollen appearance resembling a spindle. Hence, the name *Clostridium* (kloster meaning spindle). This genus consists of bacteria that are responsible for three major diseases of man-gas gangrene, food poisoning and tetanus. Many species are pathogenic but most are saprophytes found in soil, water and decomposing plant and animal matter.

GENERAL PROPERTIES OF GENUS CLOSTRIDIA

- Clostridia vary greatly in their shape, size and appearance on stain (pleomorphism).
- They are rod shaped, 3 to 8 μ × 0.4 to 1.2 μ in size.
- Sporulation occurs with different frequency in different species.
  Spores may be
  - **Central or equatorial**—bacteria appear spindle shaped-*Cl. bifermentans.*
  - **Subterminal**—the bacteria appear club shaped-*Cl. welchii.*
  - **Oval and terminal**—appearing like a tennis racket-*Cl. tertium.*
  - **Spherical and terminal**—drumstick appearance-*Cl. tetani.*
- Clostridia are motile with peritrichate flagella except-*Cl. welchii* and some *Cl. tetani.*
- Clostridia are gram-positive organisms but in older cultures are gram variable.
- Clostridia are anaerobic. Some are more exacting anaerobes than others.
- Growth is slow on solid media. Blood agar and Robertson's cooked meat broth are used for growth. Robertson's cooked meat broth contains unsaturated fatty acids which take up oxygen, the reaction being catalyzed by hematin in the meat.
- Clostridia can produce disease only when conditions are appropriate. Pathogenic clostridia have powerful exotoxins. *Clostridium botulinum* is totally noninvasive and botulism is due to the ingestion of preformed toxin in the blood. *Clostridium tetani* has invasive properties and is confined to the primary site of lodgment. Tetanus results from the action of the potent exotoxin it produces. The gas gangrene clostridia besides being toxigenic are also invasive and can spread along tissues and cause septicemia.

CLASSIFICATION OF CLOSTRIDIA

A. **Gas Gangrene Group**
   1. ***Confirmed pathogens***
      - *Cl. welchii*
      - *Cl. septicum*
      - *Cl. oedematiens*
   2. ***Less pathogenic***
      - *Cl. histolyticum*
   3. ***Doubtful pathogens***
      - *Cl. bifermentans*
      - *Cl. sporogenes*

B. **Tetanus**—*Cl. tetani*

C. **Food poisoning**
   1. Gastroenteritis—*Cl. welchii (Type A)*
   2. Botulism—*Cl. botulinum*

CLOSTRIDIUM TETANI

Introduction

Clostridium tetani is the causative organism of tetanus. It is widely distributed in soil and in the intestines of man and animals. It is present all over and is a common contaminant in wounds (Fig. 27.1) shows the morphology of *Cl. tetani.*

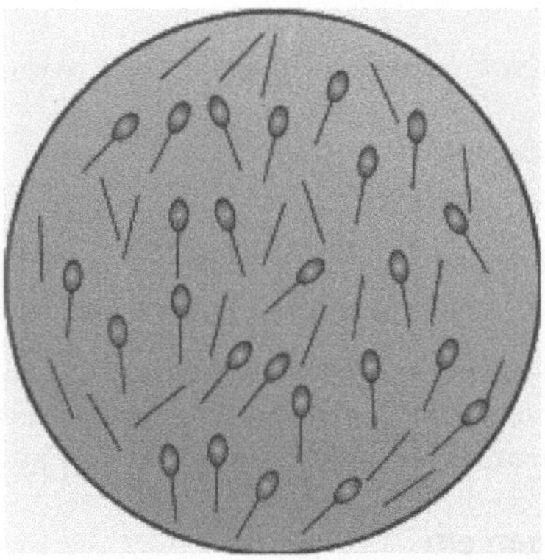

Fig. 27.1: *Cl. tetani*—both with and without spores

Morphology

It is a gram-positive, slender bacteria. The spores are round, present at the ends and are bulging giving the bacteria a drumstick appearance. It is noncapsulated and motile by flagella present all around the body (peritrichous).

Culture

- It is an obligatory anaerobe that grows only in the absence of oxygen.
- Optimum temperature for growth is 37°C. pH is 7.4.
- It grows on ordinary media.
  - Blood agar.
  - Robertson's cooked meat medium.
  - Nutrient agar slopes.
  - MacConkey's medium.

Surface growth is very translucent and fine and has a tendency to swarm.

Biochemical Reactions

Indole positive
MR, VP negative

It does not ferment any sugar.

Resistance

Autoclaving is the best to kill spores. The spores are resistant to most antiseptics.

Toxins

Clostridium tetani produces at least two distinct toxins.

- Tetanolysin
- Tetanospasmin

Tetanolysin—Its pathogenic role is not very clear, probably it acts as a leukotoxin.

Tetanospasmin—This is the toxin responsible for the clinical manifestations of tetanus. It is a good antigen and specifically neutralized by antitoxin.

Pathogenicity

Clostridium tetani has little invasive power. The toxin produced locally is absorbed by the motor nerve endings and transported to the central nervous system along the nerve axis. The tetanus toxin blocks synaptic inhibition. This causes uncontrolled spread of impulses and simultaneous contraction of the muscle groups resulting in muscle rigidity and spasm.

Tetanus

Tetanus results from the infection of a wound or raw surface with the tetanus bacteria or the I/V injection of contaminated substances. It is characterized by tonic muscle spasms that start at the site of infection but then become general and involve the whole of the somatic muscular system.

Usually the disease follows injury that may be small, or results after surgical operations due to contamination.

Simple contamination of a wound does not lead to tetanus. Until anaerobic conditions are available, the spores are dormant. Destruction and necrosis of tissue, lack of drainage in the areas, presence of contaminated matter of the soil, infection with other bacteria, all favor an anaerobic environment and development of tetanus. The incubation period is variable but is commonly 6 to 12 days.

Tetanus is more common in the rural areas that are crowded and unhygienic. In rural India, tetanus is the fourth commonest cause of death.

Laboratory Diagnosis

The diagnosis of tetanus should always be made on clinical grounds and treatment started. The lab reports should confirm the findings.

Laboratory diagnosis may be made by:

1. Demonstration of *Clostridium tetani* by microscopy, culture or animal inoculation.

Microscopy is not completely reliable. Diagnosis by culture is more dependable. Culture isolation is more likely from tissue obtained from the necrotic depths of wounds than from wound swabs. The culture media on which they can be inoculated are:

1. Blood agar
2. Robertson's cooked meat broth.

Blood agar: On blood agar, *Clostridium tetani* produces swarming growth that may be detected on the opposite half of the plate after one to two days incubation anaerobically.

Robertson's cooked meat broth: *Cl. tetani* grows well in Robertson's cooked meat broth with turbidity and some gas formation. The meat is not digested but is turned black on prolonged incubation.

Toxigenicity Testing

Two methods have been used to test for toxins.

1. The first method involves the testing of toxigenic *Cl. tetani* strains (tetanolysin toxin) by incorporating antitoxin to *Cl. tetani* in one-half of the horse blood agar plates. Tetanolysin produces hemolysis on blood agar. Therefore, toxigenic *Cl. tetani* strains show haemolysis around the colonies, only on the half without the antitoxin. But this method tests for tetanolysin and not for tetanospasmin which is the pathogenic toxin.
2. The second method involves testing for toxigenicity in the tail of a mouse. Toxigenic strains cause the development of symptoms and death of the animal.

Prevention of Tetanus

Tetanus is a preventable disease. The disease is due to the action of toxin; hence the most dependable method of prevention is to build-up antitoxic immunity by active immunization. Prevention can be done by:

1. Surgical method
2. Antibiotics
3. Immunization—passive, active or combined.

Surgical Prevention

This aims at the removal of foreign bodies, necrotic tissue and blood clots so that an anaerobic environment favorable for the tetanus bacillus is not provided.

Antibiotics

Antibiotics have no action on toxin. Hence, antibiotic prophylaxis does not replace immunization. It kills tetanus bacilli and pyogenic bacteria so that production of toxin is prevented.

Immunization

Immunization is of two types—passive and active.

Passive immunization: This involves administration of tetanus antitoxin. It is given immediately after the wounding. The recommended dose is 1500 international units administered subcutaneously or intramuscularly.

Passive immunization is an emergency procedure to be used only once.

Active immunization: It is the most effective method of prophylaxis.

It can prevent tetanus following unnoticed injuries. It is given in the form of a toxoid. Tetanus toxoid is given either alone or along with diphtheria toxoid.

A course of immunization consists of 3 doses of tetanus toxoid given I/M with an interval of 4 to 6 weeks between the first two doses and 6 to 12 months between the 2nd and 3rd doses.

A booster dose is given after 10 years and then every 3 years.

GAS GANGRENE AND *CLOSTRIDIUM WELCHII*

Clostridium welchii (*Clostridium perfringens*) is a normal inhabitant of the large intestines of man and animals. It is found in the feces and contaminates the skin of the perineum, buttocks and thighs. The spores are commonly found in soil, dust and air. This is most important of the clostridia causing gas gangrene. It also produces food poisoning and necrotic enteritis in man and many serious diseases in animals.

Gas Gangrene

Gas gangrene is a rapidly spreading edematous myonecrosis occurring with severe wounds of many muscle masses that have been contaminated with pathogenic clostridia particularly with *Clostridium welchii*. It occurs as a disease of the war in which extensive wounds with heavy contamination are very common. The disease follows road accidents or other types of injury involving crushing of large muscle masses.

The diagnosis of gas gangrene is made on clinical grounds and the function of the lab is only to provide confirmation. The specimens are collected from the muscles at the edge of the affected area from the tissue in the necrotic areas, and from the exudates in the deeper part of the wound. Gram's stained films and cultures are done to diagnose the infection.

CLOSTRIDIUM BOTULINUM

Clostridium botulinum, causes botulism a severe form of food poisoning. Botulism can be of two types—wound and infant botulism. Diagnosis may be confirmed by the demonstration of the bacillus or the toxin in food or feces.

Botulism is a severe form of food poisoning caused by the ingestion of the food containing toxin (Botulin) produced by *Clostridium botulinum*. Botulism is associated with inadequately processed, home-canned foods, but occasionally commercially produced foods are implicated as the source of outbreaks. Sausages, meat products, canned vegetables, and seafood products have been the most frequent vehicles for food borne botulism.

Resistance

Botulinum toxin is heat-labile, or unstable if heated to a certain temperature, and can be destroyed if heated and held at 80 degrees Centigrade (176 degrees Fahrenheit) for ten minutes or longer.

Pathogenicity

Human botulism is primarily caused by *Clostridium botulinum* that produces toxin type A, B and E. Botulin toxin is one of the most powerful known toxins: about one microgram is lethal to humans. The toxin enters the body in one of four ways: by colonization of the digestive tract by the bacterium in children (infant botulism) or adults (adult intestinal toxemia), by ingestion of toxin from foodstuffs (food borne botulism) or by contamination of a wound by the bacterium (wound botulism). All forms lead to paralysis that typically starts with the muscles of the face and then spreads towards the limbs. In severe forms, it leads to paralysis of the breathing muscles and causes respiratory failure.

Symptoms

Classic symptoms of botulism include double vision, blurred vision, drooping eyelids, slurred speech, difficulty in swallowing, dry mouth, and muscle weakness. Infants with botulism appear lethargic, feed poorly, are constipated, and have a weak cry and poor muscle tone. In food borne botulism, symptoms generally begin 18 to 36 hours after consuming contaminated food, but they can occur as early as 6 hours or as late as 10 days after consumption. Botulinum toxin causes flaccid paralysis by blocking motor nerve terminals at the myoneural junction.

Laboratory Diagnosis

The most direct and effective way to confirm the clinical diagnosis of botulism in the laboratory is to demonstrate the presence of toxin in the serum or feces of the patient or in the food the patient consumed. Currently, the most sensitive and widely used method for detecting toxin is the mouse neutralization test, that involves injecting serum or stool into mice and looking for signs of botulism. This test typically takes 48 hours. Culturing of specimens takes 5–7 days. Some cases of botulism may go undiagnosed because symptoms are transient or mild, or are misdiagnosed as Guillain-Barre syndrome.

Prevention

Metal cans containing food in which bacteria, possibly Cl. botulinum, are growing may bulge outwards due to gas production from bacterial growth, such cans should be discarded. Consumption of uncooked or under-processed foods such as meat products and seafood should be avoided.

CHAPTER

28

Gram-negative Rods: Enterobacteriaceae—*Escherichia*, *Citrobacter*, *Klebsiella* and *Proteus*

LESSON PLAN

- Enterobacteriaceae
  - Classification
- *Escherichia Coli*
  - Morphology
  - Culture
  - Biochemical Reactions
  - Toxin Production
  - Antigenic Structure
  - Pathogenicity
  - Laboratory Diagnosis
- *Citrobacter*
  - Some Facts
- *Klebsiella*
  - Species of *Klebsiella*
- *Proteus*
  - Morphology
  - Culture
  - Biochemical Reactions
  - Antigenic Structure
  - Pathogenicity
  - Laboratory Diagnosis

The clinically significant gram-negative rods that we will be studying in this text are the following:

1. *Enterobacteriaceae*
2. *Vibrio*
3. *Pseudomonas*
4. *Haemophilus*

ENTEROBACTERIACEAE

Introduction

It is a large and complex family composed of gram-negative rods that are found in the human or animal intestine (Entero). They have the following features:

1. Members may or may not be capsulated.
2. They may be motile by peritrichate flagella or non-motile.
3. They are aerobic and facultatively anaerobic.
4. They grow readily on ordinary media.
5. They are catalase positive, ferment glucose producing acid and gas or acid only.

Differences exist between family members.

Classification

There are many ways in which *Enterobacteriaceae* can be classified. The earlier classification was based on lactose fermentation. The bacteria were divided into three groups.

1. Those that fermented lactose were called lactose fermenters and included genus *Escherichia* and *Klebsiella*.
2. Those that fermented lactose late included *Shigella sonnei and Citrobacter*.
3. Those that did not ferment lactose were called lactose non-fermenters and included *genus Salmonella, Shigella* and *Proteus*.

The lactose fermenters are usually non-pathogenic in the intestinal tract and non-lactose fermeters are intestinal pathogens.

The other classification groups bacteria that have a number of common morphological and biochemical properties.

Family Enterobacteriaceae

Tribe 1 Escherichieae

Genus:

1. *Escherichia* 2. *Edwardsiella*
3. *Citrobacter* 4. *Salmonella*
5. *Shigella*

Tribe 2 Klebsielleae

Genus:

1. *Klebsiella* 2. *Enterobacter*
3. *Hafnia* 4. *Serratia*

Tribe 3 Proteeae

Genus:

1. *Proteus*

Tribe 4 Erwinieae

Genus:

1. *Erwinia*

ESCHERICHIA COLI

Introduction

This genus was named after Escherich who was the first to describe the colon bacillus *E. coli* that lives in the human or animal intestine. When it is voided in feces it remains in the environment for some days. Detection of *E. coli* in drinking water is taken as evidence of recent pollution with human or animal feces.

Morphology

E. coli is a gram-negative, straight rod measuring 1–3 μ × 0.4–0.7 μ arranged singly or in pairs. It is motile by peritrichate flagella though some strains may be non-motile. Capsules and fimbriae are found in some strains. Spores are not formed.

Many strains have a combination of characters. This is because of conjugation and transduction between bacterial strains.

Culture

- It is an aerobe and facultative anaerobe.
- Temperature range required for growth is 10 to 46°C (optimum 37°C).
- Good growth occurs on ordinary media.
- Media used are nutrient agar, blood agar, MacConkey's agar and nutrient broth. On nutrient agar or blood agar, the colonies are large, greyish white, moist, smooth, opaque or partially translucent discs. Many strains especially the pathogenic ones are beta hemolytic on blood agar. On MacConkey's medium the colonies are bright pink due to lactose fermentation. Their morphology is the same as that on nutrient agar or blood agar In nutrient broth, the growth occurs as general turbidity and a heavy deposit.

Biochemical Reactions

Lactose, mannitol, sucrose, maltose and many other sugars are fermented with the production of acid and gas. The four biochemical tests that are used very widely are *IMViC*. This stand for indole, methyl red, Voges Proskauer and citrate tests. *E. coli* is indole and MR positive and VP and citrate negative (IMViC) (+ + – –). Gelatin is not liquefied. H_2S is not formed, urea is not split and growth does not occur in KCN medium.

Toxin Production

As in the case of gram-negative bacteria, *E. coli* possesses endotoxic activity associated with O antigen. Some strains of *Escherichia coli* produce two types of exotoxins:

- Enterotoxins
- Hemolysins

Enterotoxins: Some strains of *E. coli* that produce diarrhea form enterotoxins. Two types of *E. coli* enterotoxins have been identified—heat labile and heat stable. A strain of *Escherichia coli* may produce either one or both types of enterotoxins.

Hemolysins: Three types of hemolysins are found to be produced by *Escherichia coli*.

Antigenic Structure

Serotyping of *Escherichia coli* is based on three antigens:

- Somatic antigen O
- Capsular antigen K
- Flagellar antigen H.

So far, 164 types of O antigens,
103 types of K antigens,
75 types of H antigens—have been recognized.

Three types of K antigen (envelope) antigen located in the capsule or microcapsule have been discovered so far — L, A and B. Only one of them is present on any one strain. Several different serotypes of *Escherichia coli* are found in normal intestine. Most of them do not have K antigens. Of the strains that possess K antigens most are of L type. The K antigen encloses the O antigen and makes the strain inagglutinable by the O antiserum. It may contribute to virulence by inhibiting phagocytosis. The L and B types are heat labile but A is heat stable.

The normal colon strains belong to the early O groups (1, 2, 3, 4), where as the entero-pathogenic strains belong to the later O groups (26, 55, 86, 111, etc.).

Pathogenicity

Escherichia coli is associated with four diseases:

1. Urinary tract infections
2. Diarrhea/Gastroenteritis
3. Pyogenic infections
4. Septicemia.

Urinary Tract Infection

- *E. coli* is the single major causative organism of urinary tract infection.
- The *E. coli serotypes* commonly responsible for urinary tract infections are those of the gps 1, 2, 4, 6, 7.
- The infections of the lower urinary tract are caused by fecal coliforms. The infections of the upper urinary tract are hematogenous.

Diarrhea

E. coli is the major member of the aerobic bacterial flora of the human intestine and is usually non-pathogenic in this location. There are four groups of *E. coli* which can cause diarrheal disease particularly in infants and also in older children and adults.

These four groups are:

1. Enteropathogenic *Escherichia coli*
2. Enterotoxigenic *Escherichia coli*
3. Enteroinvasive *Escherichia coli*
4. Enterohemorrhagic *Escherichia coli*.

Enteropathogenic Escherichia coli: This was first isolated from infantile diarrhea and later when serotyping schemes developed it was possible to establish a relationship between these *Escherichia coli* and diarrhea. These include 25 serotypes. Some examples are $O_{26}B_6$, $O_{55}B_5$, $O_{86}B_7$, $O_{111}B_4$, etc. EPEC (enteropatho-genic *E. coli)* cause diarrhea in developed countries. The pathogenic mechanism is believed to be a shigella-like toxin and also that these bacteria adhere tightly to the intestinal cells leading to structural damage.

Enterotoxigenic E. coli: This is the most common causative organism of traveller's diarrhea. (This means diarrhea seen in persons from developed countries within a few days of their visit to one of the developing countries). There are special methods to detect the toxins done in reference laboratories. Most strains of ETEC belong to the serotypes 6, 8, 15, 25, 27, 63, 78, 148, 159. These are different from EPEC types.

Enteroinvasive E. coli: These strains invade the intestinal epithelial cells just like dysentery bacilli and so they are called enteroinvasive. They belong to the stools of older children and adults with dysentery like disease. When we inject (EIEC) into the eyes of guinea pigs it causes keratoconjunctivitis (Serenys test). The invasion of Hela cells in tissue culture also provides another diagnostic method.

EIEC strains are atypical biochemically. Many strains ferment lactose late or not at all and may be anaerogenic. There is a marked antigenic relationship between EIEC strains and shigellae.

Enterohemorrhagic E. coli: This was identified only in 1983 following food borne outbreaks of hemorrhagic colitis caused by *E. coli* 0157H7. EHEC produces a cytotoxin that appears to be identical to shigella shiga toxin. This toxin has been called verotoxin because of its effect on vero cells in culture.

Pyogenic Infections

E. coli may cause superficial infections such as wound infections and abscesses or deep infections such as peritonitis, cholecystitis and meningitis. *E. coli* is a common cause of meningitis in the newborn.

Septicemia

E. coli and *Pseudomonas aeruginosa* have rep-laced staphylococci as the commonest cause of septicemia in many hospitals. This syndrome of gram-negative septicemia consists of fever, hypotension and endotoxic shock. Mortality is high.

Laboratory Diagnosis

Diarrhea

Normally a stool sample is plated on blood agar and MacConkey's agar. There is no single test that can identify all strains of *Escherichia coli* responsible for diarrhea. Various specialized tests are employed for the detection of types of *Escherichia coli*.

Urinary Tract Infection

Normal urine is sterile but during voiding it becomes contaminated with the genital commensals and gives bacterial growth. So we try and obtain midstream samples.

What are Midstream Samples?

It indicates the middle part of the urine flow that is collected and supposed to have minimum contamination with the surrounding genital area. In males as well as females the genital area should be cleaned before giving a sample. The first portion of the urine that flushes out commensal bacteria from the anterior urethra is discarded. The next portion of urine is collected directly into a sterile wide mouthed container and transported to the lab. If there is a delay of more than 1 to 2 hours the specimen should be refrigerated.

What is Significant Bacteriuria in Urine Culture?

Kass was a scientist who introduced the term significant bacteriuria. He fixed the count at 100000 bacteria/mL. Kass and his team established that if there is urinary tract infection, the urine contains 100,000 bacteria or more/mL. Counts of 10,000 bacteria or less/mL are due to contamination during voiding and are of no significance. Counts between these two need to be carefully evaluated considering the clinical condition of the patient.

We use a standard loop that delivers 0.001 mL of urine (fixed volume) onto the plate and then see if the plate has 100 colonies for the count to be significant. An antibiotic sensitivity test is done to see which antibiotics are most suitable for treatment.

Certain quick tests are available for the diagnosis of significant bacteriuria. They are:

a. *Griess nitrate test*: This test is based on the absence of nitrite in the normal urine. The presence of nitrite detectable by a simple test indicates the presence of nitrate reducing bacteria in the urine.
b. *Catalase test*: The presence of catalase is seen by frothing on addition of hydrogen peroxide which indicates bacteriemia.
c. *Triphenyltetrazolium chloride* (TTC) test is based on the production of a pink red precipitate in the reagent caused by the respiratory activity of growing bacteria.
d. *Microscopic demonstration*: Bacteria are seen in Gram's stained films of urine.

e. *Dipslide culture methods*: Agar coated slides are immersed in urine or even exposed to the stream of urine during voiding, incubated and the growth estimated by colony counting or by color change of indicators. None of the screening methods are as sensitive as culture.

Pyogenic Infections

Blood agar and Mac-Conkey's medium is used. The isolate is identified by biochemical methods and an antibiotic sensitivity test is done.

Septicemia

Isolation of bacteria is done by blood culture. This is explained in detail in the chapter on *Salmonella*.

CITROBACTER

Some Facts

- Motile bacteria
- Utilize citrate
- Grow in KCN medium (Medium containing potassium cyanide)
- Produce H_2S and ferment lactose late or not at all
- Normal intestinal inhabitant
- It may cause infections of the urinary tract, gallbladder, middle ear and meninges
- Earlier called paracolons
- Some strains (Ballerup-Bethesda group) exhibit antigenic sharing with salmonellae and cause confusion in the diagnostic laboratory.

KLEBSIELLA

Introduction

The genus *Klebsiella* consists of non-motile, capsulated rods that grow very well on ordinary media forming large dome-shaped, lactose fermenting mucoid colonies that are sticky. Klebsiella are widely distributed in nature occurring both as commensals in intestine and as saprophytes in soil and water. They are classified into three species.

- *Klebsiella pneumoniae*
- *Klebsiella ozaenae*
- *Klebsiella rhinoscleromatis.*

Species of *Klebsiella*

Klebsiella Pneumoniae

- This bacteria was first isolated by Freidlander in 1883 from fatal cases of pneumonia and is called Freidlander's bacillus.
- It ferments sugars (glucose, lactose, sucrose and mannitol) with the production of acid and abundant gas.
- It is IMViC (– – + +), indole and MR are negative, VP and citrate are positive.
- It forms urease.
- It is the second most common member of our aerobic bacterial flora.

Diseases Produced

Pneumonia: Pneumonia due to *Klebsiella* is an uncommon disease and occurs with some predisposing factors such as:
- Old age
- Diabetes
- Alcoholism
- Chronic bronchopulmonary disease.

The outcome is poor, case fatality is 80 percent. There is involvement of one or more lobes of the lung and massive mucoid inflammatory exudate. Necrosis and abscess formation is more common than pneumococcal pneumonia.

Serotypes 1, 2, 3 are usually responsible for pneumonia. Positive blood cultures are only seen in 25 percent of cases.

Urinary tract infection: *Klebsiella* is a common cause of UTI and they are resistant to most antibiotics.

Others: It also causes *pyogenic infections* such as abscesses, meningitis and septicemia. Rarely it can cause *diarrhea*.

Klebsiella Ozaenae

It causes a disease which is characterized by foul smelling nasal discharge. Identification is difficult due to variation in the biochemical reactions of strains. *K. ozaenae* belongs to capsular types 3 to 6.

Klebsiella Rhinoscleromatis

It causes rhinoscleroma that is a chronic granulomatous hypertrophy of the nose. It is found in Southeastern Europe, India and Central America. The bacilli are seen intracellularly in lesions. It can be identified by biochemical reactions and belongs to capsular type 3.

PROTEUS

Introduction

Proteus are gram-negative lactose non-fermenting bacilli. They are called proteus after the Greek God Proteus who could assume any shape. Proteus is characterized by swarming (spreading) growth on agar.

Morphology

They are gram-negative rods 0.5 μ × 1 to 3 μ in size.

- Pleomorphism exists with long filaments and granular forms.
- They have peritrichate flagella and exhibit swimming motility, best seen at 20°C.
- They are non-capsulated and non-sporing.
- Many strains are fimbriate.

Culture

They are aerobic and facultatively anaerobic.

- Good growth occurs on ordinary media.
- Cultures give out an odor described as fishy.
- Discrete colonies can be seen in only very young cultures. After that the actively motile cells spread over the surface of the plate in waves. This is called swarming.

Swarming on the one hand helps in diagnosis but on the other proteus gets mixed-up with other bacteria and it is difficult to identify other bacteria. To inhibit swarming several methods are used:

1. Increasing the concentration of agar to 6 percent
2. Incorporation of chloral hydrate (1:500)
   Sodium azide (1:5000)
   Alcohol (5 to 6%)
   Sulphonamide
   Surface active agents
   Boric acid (1:1000).

Swarming does not occur on MacConkey's medium on which smooth colorless colonies are formed. Non-motile strains do not swarm.

Swarming is a feature of *Proteus vulgaris* and *Proteus mirabilis* but does not occur with other species at 37°C though it may be induced by growing on soft agar at 20 to 28°C.

In broth, proteus produces uniform turbidity and a slight powdery deposit.

Biochemical Reactions

A very distinctive feature of proteus is the deamination of phenylalanine to phenyl pyruvic acid (PPA) that is positive in proteus and negative in all other bacteria.

- All members are urea positive except *Pr. inconstans*
- MR positive
- VP negative
- All ferment glucose producing acid and gas except *Pr. rettgeri* and *Pr. inconstans*—These are anaerogenic
- Lactose is not fermented.

Genus *Proteus* is divided into five species that are differentiated on the basis of biochemical reactions. They are *Proteus vulgaris, Proteus mirabilis, Proteus morganii, Proteus rettgeri, Proteus inconstans.*

The other differences are given in the Table 28.1.

Antigenic Structure

The bacteria have thermostable somatic (O) antigen and thermolabile flagellar (H) antigens.

The H and the O antigens of proteus are of interest. Weil and Felix in 1916 observed that flagellated strains growing on agar formed a thin surface film resembling the mist produced by

Table 28.1: Biochemical reactions of the various species of *Proteus*

	Proteus vulgaris	*Pr. mirabilis*	*Pr. morganii*	*Pr. rettgeri*	*Pr. inconstans*
Gas from glucose	+	+	+	d	d
Acid from sucrose	+	d	–	d	d
Acid from maltose	+	–	–	–	–
Acid from mannitol	–	–	–	+	–
Indole	+	–	+	+	+
H_2S	+	+	–	–	–
Citrate	d	d	–	+	+
Urease	+	+	+	+	–

d—variable

breathing on glass and named this form **Hauch** meaning film of breath. Non-flagellated variants grew as isolated colonies without the surface film and were called Ohne Hauch form (meaning without film of breath). These names were shortened to be called 'H' and the 'O' forms and later on, the H type was called flagellar forms and O, the somatic forms. We now refer to the loose fluffy masses as H type agglutination and fine granular appearance as somatic agglutination or O type agglutination.

Weil and Felix also observed that certain non-motile strains of *Proteus vulgaris* called the X strains were agglutinated by sera from typhus fever patients. This heterophile agglutination due to the sharing of an alkali stable carbohydrate hapten by certain strains of proteus and rickettsia form the basis of Weil Felix reaction for the diagnosis of some rickettsial infection.

Three non-motile strains are employed as the antigens for this agglutination test—*Proteus vulgaris* strains OX2, OX19 and *Pr. mirabilis* OXK that contain O antigen types 1, 2, 3 respectively.

Pathogenicity

- Proteus species are saprophytes and are found everywhere.
- They occur as commensals in the intestine and sometimes on the skin over the moist parts of the body.
- They are opportunist pathogens and may cause many types of infection. They are known to cause hospital acquired infection especially in burns.
- Urinary tract infection is the commonest disease caused by proteus.
- It also produces pyogenic lesions of various types such as abscesses and infections of wounds, ear or respiratory tract.

Laboratory Diagnosis

- Proteus can be isolated easily from clinical samples.
- Culture is done on MacConkey's agar and blood agar. Steps are taken to inhibit swarming so that other bacteria can be identified too.
- The species identification is done by biochemical tests.
- ***Pr. mirabilis*** is the most commonly isolated species in clinical samples.
- Antibiotic sensitivity testing is done to identify drug resistance.

CHAPTER

29 Gram-negative Rods: Enterobacteriaceae—*Salmonella*—*Salmonella Typhi*

LESSON PLAN

- Introduction
- Morphology
- Culture
  - Basal Media
  - Enriched Medium
  - Differential and Selective Solid Media
  - Enrichment Media
- Biochemical Reactions
- Resistance
- Antigenic Structure
  - H Antigen
  - O Antigen
  - Vi Antigen
- Classification of *Salmonella*
- Pathogenicity
  - Enteric Fever
  - *Salmonella* Gastroenteritis
  - *Salmonella* Septicemia

Genus—Salmonella
Species—Salmonella typhi

INTRODUCTION

The genus *Salmonella* consists of gram-negative rods belonging to family *Enterobacteriaceae* that can cause enteric fever, gastroenteritis, septicemia and a carrier state in man. These bacteria are found in the intestine of many vertebrate animals.

Salmonellae are oxidase negative, generally motile, non-lactose fermenting, urease negative and citrate positive rods.

The most important member of the genus is *Salmonella typhi*, the causative agent of typhoid fever. The typhoid bacillus was first observed by Eberth in 1880 and was isolated by Gaffky in 1884. It came to be known as the Eberth Gaffky bacillus or *Eberthella typhi*. *Salmonella* genus has about 2000 serotypes or species all of which can cause disease. They are divided into two groups.

1. The enteric fever group, consisting of typhoid and paratyphoid bacilli that are only found in humans.
2. The food poisoning group that are mainly found in animals but can also infect man producing gastroenteritis, septicemia or localized infection.

MORPHOLOGY

Salmonella are gram-negative rods 2 to 4 μ × 0.6 μ in size, non-sporing and non-capsulate. Most serotypes are motile with peritrichous flagella but *S. gallinarum* and *S. pullorum* are non-motile. Most strains form fimbriae.

CULTURE

- Salmonellae are aerobic and facultatively anaerobic.
- They grow on simple lab media in the temperature range of 15 to 45°C (optimally at 37°C) pH (6 to 8).

- Many culture media can be used to culture salmonellae. They may be divided into:

Basal Media

i. *Nutrient agar*: After 24 hours at 37°C, the colonies of most strains are large (2 to 3 mm in diameter), grey white, moist circular discs with a smooth convex surface and entire edge.
ii. *Peptone water and nutrient broth*: In liquid media, most strains give abundant growth with uniform turbidity. A thin surface pellicle usually forms.

Enriched Medium

Blood Agar

The colonies on blood agar are similar to nutrient agar.

Differential and Selective Solid Media

These media are valuable for the isolation of salmonellae from faeces and other materials contaminated with bacteria of other kinds.

i. *MacConkey's agar*: After 18 to 24 hours at 37°C, the colonies are pale yellow or colorless, 1 to 3 mm in diameter, different from the pink red colonies of lactose fermenting commensal coliform bacteria, e.g. *Escherichia coli*.
ii. *Brilliant green MacConkey's agar*: The addition to MacConkey's agar of brilliant green 0.004 g/liter is inhibitory to *E. coli*, *Proteus* species and other commensal enterobacteria. *Salmonella* appear as low, convex, pale green, translucent colonies 1 to 3 mm in diameter. Lactose fermenting, bacteria produce blue-purple colonies.
iii. *Leifson's deoxycholate citrate agar (DCA)*
   - The colonies of *Salmonellae* on DCA are almost the same or slightly smaller in size than those on MacConkey's agar.
   - They are pale, nearly colorless, smooth, shiny and translucent. Sometimes they have a black center and are surrounded by a zone of cleared medium. These are easily distinguished from the opaque pink colonies of lactose fermenting coliform bacilli that are inhibited on this selective differential medium. DCA is also selective for *Shigellae* that gives colonies similar to that of *Salmonella* and it is therefore the most widely used plating medium for the isolation of intestinal pathogens from feces.

   DCA (Deoxycholate Citrate Agar)

   DCA is Neutral red lactose agar + 2 solutions (A and B)

   Neutral Red Lactose Agar

Meat extract	– 20 g
Peptone	– 20 g
Agar	– 90 g
Neutral red 2 percent in 50 percent ethanol	– 5 mL
Lactose	– 40 g
Water	– 4 liters

   Solution A

   - Sodium citrate
   - Sodium thiosulphate
   - Ferric ammonium citrate
   - Sterile water

   Solution B

   - Sodium deoxycholate
   - Sterile water

   Complete Medium

• Neutral red lactose agar	100 mL
• Solution A	5 mL
• Solution B	5 mL

   The finished medium is pale pink in color.
iv. *Wilson and Blair's Brilliant Green Bismuth Sulphite Agar (BBSA)*: This medium is very good for the isolation of *S. typhi*. Cultures should be seen after 24 hours and then again after 48 hours. Colonies are 1 mm in diameter and appear green or pale brown. All salmonellae that produce hydrogen sulphide have a black center or a metallic sheen.

Salmonella typhi and S. paratyphi B reduce sulphite to sulphide and form black colonies. *E. coli* is inhibited by brilliant green and by bismuth sulphite. After 18 hours, *Salmonella* colonies may be clear green, black centerd or black but after 48 hours, are uniformly black and surrounded by a dark zone and metallic sheen. Other organisms like coliforms are usually inhibited but may form green or brown colonies without a dark halo or metallic sheen. This medium is highly selective for salmonellae being inhibitory to coliforms, proteus and shigellae.

v. *Taylor's Xylose Lysine Deoxycholate Agar (XLD)*: XLD was developed by a scientist Taylor in 1965 as a selective medium for shigellae because he found that *Shigella dysenteriae* and *Shigella flexneri* are inhibited by concentrations of deoxycholate, brilliant green, selenite and tetrathionate in the selective media mostly used for salmonellae. Sodium deoxycholate is incorporated in XLD to restrain the growth of *E. coli* and prevent spreading by proteus but at a concentration of only 0.1 percent or 0.25 percent instead of 0.5 percent as in DCA. The ingredients of the XLD agar are:
   - Yeast extract
   - Xylose
   - Lactose
   - Sucrose
   - Lysine
   - Sodium chloride
   - Sodium deoxycholate
   - Sodium thiosulphate
   - Ferric ammonium citrate
   - Phenol red
   - Agar
   - Water.

Interpretation of XLD

1. Shigellae do not form acid from xylose, lactose and sucrose in the medium within 24 hours, and hence give red colored colonies in the presence of phenol red in alkaline medium (phenol red in alkaline medium is red). Some strains of proteus (*Pr. morganii*) *Pr. rettgeri*, and providenciae also form red colonies.
   H_2S negative salmonellae, e.g. *S. paratyphi* do not form a black center and their colonies are red.
2. Salmonellae neutralize the acid they form from the limited amount of xylose by decarboxylating the lysine. Hence, the color of the colonies is red in alkaline medium.
   Most salmonella produce H_2S that reacts with ferric ammonium citrate in the medium to produce black centers in their red colonies.
3. Yellow (acid) colonies are formed by most other enterobacteria. (Phenol red gives yellow color in the presence of acid).
   a. *E. coli* forms so much acid from lactose and sucrose that is not neutralized by decarboxylation of lysine.
   b. *Citrobacter* and *Proteus* do not ferment lactose but xylose. They also do not decarboxylate lysine and hence do not neutralize the acid as salmonellae do.

To summarize:

- Red colonies without black centers
  - *Shigella*
  - H_2S negative salmonellae
  - Some strains of Proteus < *Pr. morgani* / *Pr. rettgeri*
  - *Pseudomonas*
- Red colonies with black centers
  Most strains of *Salmonella*.
- Yellow colonies
  Most strains of *E. coli*, *Klebsiella*, *Enterobacter*, *Citrobacter*, *Proteus* and *Serratia*.

Enrichment Media

These are liquid media used to assist the isolation of salmonellae from feces, sewage, food stuffs and other materials containing a mixed bacterial flora. The number of salmonella colonies increase that can then be put onto a differential agar medium, e.g. MacConkey's or DCA after 18 to 24 hours.

Enrichment mediums can be the following:

1. *Tetrathionate broth*: It enriches salmonellae including *S. typhi* and sometimes shigellae but permits the growth of proteus species. The complete tetrathionate medium is as follows:
   - Calcium carbonate
   - Nutrient broth
   - Thiosulphate solution
   - Iodine solution
   - Phenol red.

   The solutions of Iodine and Thiosulphate should be prepared separately and then added to broth along with $CaCO_3$. The medium should be used within a few hours of adding the iodine solution to other reagents.
2. *Kauffmann Muller tetrathionate broth with brilliant green*: The addition of brilliant green inhibits the growth of proteus and so improves the selectivity of tetrathionate broth but makes it too inhibitory to *S. typhi* and shigellae. As an alternative to brilliant green the addition of 40 mg novobiocin per liter of medium serves to overcome interference by proteus.
3. *Rappaport's malachite green magnesium chloride broth*: This has been reported to be more efficient than other enrichment media for the isolation of salmonellae from feces, water and food stuffs.
4. *Selenite F Broth*: This is the most commonly used enrichment medium for specimens that may contain salmonellae or shigella. It is excellent for *S. typhi* and *S. dublin* but some salmonellae, e.g. *S. paratyphi A* and *S. cholerasuis* and some shigellae fail to multiply. The F in selenite F broth stands for feces. The selenite in the enrichment medium inhibits coliform bacilli while permitting salmonellae and many shigellae to grow. The constituents are:
   - Sodium hydrogen selenite.
   - Peptone
   - Lactose
   - Sodium hydrogen phosphate
   - Sodium dihydrogen phosphate
   - Sterile water.

   3 g stool specimen is first inoculated in 15 mL saline. After the debris has settled down the supernatant is inoculated into the selenite F broth. The selenium salts are toxic and care should be taken while handling.
5. *Strontium chloride broth*: This was found to be superior to selenite F broth for the isolation of a wide range of salmonellae from feces and sewage.

BIOCHEMICAL REACTIONS

Salmonellae ferment glucose, mannitol and maltose forming acid and gas. *S. typhi* and *S. gallinarum* do not form gas. Lactose and sucrose are not fermented. The other biochemical reactions are as follows:

- Indole is negative
- MR positive
- VP negative
- Citrate + (*S. typhi* and *S. paratyphi A* are citrate negative)
- Urea negative

  H_2S is produced except by *S. paratyphi A*, *S. cholera suis* and *S. sendai*.

Decarboxylase tests: Salmonellae decarboxylate the amino acids, lysine, ornithine and arginine. *S. typhi* is ornithine negative and *S. paratyphi* A is lysine negative.

RESISTANCE

The bacilli are destroyed at 55° in 1 hour. Boiling or chlorination of water and pasteurization of milk destroy the bacilli. In polluted water and soil they survive for weeks and in ice for months. They are killed within 5 minutes with 5 percent phenol.

ANTIGENIC STRUCTURE

Salmonellae have the following antigens based on which they are classified:

1. Flagellar H antigen
2. Somatic O antigen
3. Surface antigen Vi found in some species.

Several strains have fimbriae. Fimbrial antigens are not important in identification but cause confusion due to their nonspecific nature and widespread sharing among enterobacteria.

H Antigen

This antigen present on the flagella is a heat labile protein. It is destroyed by boiling or by treatment with alcohol but not by formaldehyde. When mixed with antisera, H suspensions agglutinate rapidly and produce large loose fluffy clumps. The H antigen is strongly immunogenic and induces antibody formation rapidly and in high titer following infection or immunization. The flagellar antigen is in two phases—1 or 2.

O Antigen

The somatic O antigen is a phospholipid protein polysaccharide complex that is a part of the cell wall. It is the same as endotoxin. The O antigen is unaffected by boiling, alcohol or weak acids. When mixed with antisera, O antigen suspensions form compact, chalky, granular clumps.

The O agglutination takes place slowly and at a higher temperature 50°–55°C than H agglutination (37°C). The O antigen is less immunogenic than the H antigen and the titer of O antibody induced after infection or immunization is lower than that of H antibody.

Vi Antigen

Many strains of *S. typhi* do not agglutinate with O antiserum when freshly isolated. This is due to the presence of a surface antigen enveloping the O antigen. Felix and Pitt who first described this antigen believed that it was related to virulence and named it the Vi antigen (Vi = virulence). It is heat labile. Bacilli inagglutinable with O antiserum become agglutinable after boiling or heating at 60° for one hour. The Vi antigen tends to be lost on serial subculture. It may act by coating the bacterial surface and preventing the antibacterial and opsonic effect of the O antibody. In experiments strains possessing Vi antigen were found to cause clinical disease more consistently than those lacking the antigen.

The Vi antigen is poorly immunogenic and only low titres of antibody are produced following infection. Detection of Vi antibody is not helpful in diagnosis of cases and hence the Vi antigen is not employed in the Widal test. The Vi antibody disappears early in convalescence. It's persistence indicates the development of the carrier state. The Vi antigen affords a method of epidemiological typing of *S. typhi* strains based on Vi bacteriophages.

CLASSIFICATION OF *SALMONELLA*

Kauffmann-White scheme: This scheme first developed in 1934 classifies salmonellae into different O groups or O serogroups each of which contains a number of serotypes having a common O antigen not found in other O groups. They are A, B, C_1 C_2 C_3 C_4, D_1 D_2 D_3, E_1 E_2 E_3 E_4, F G H I and others. Groups A-E contain all salmonellae that are important pathogens in man and animals. Each O group is characterized by a particular antigen, e.g. group A is characterized by O antigen 2, group B by O antigen 4 and group D by O antigen 9. See Table 29.1 for some classification of the common salmonella species.

Some groups are divided into subgroups whose members are distinguished by a second O antigen. Within each O group, the different serotypes are distinguished by a particular H antigen. See appendix 1 for the detailed Kauffmann-White classification.

Table 29.1: Classification of some common *Salmonella* species

O Group	*Serotype (species)*	*O antigens*	*H Ag*
A	*S. paratyphi A*	1, 2, 12	a
B	*S. paratyphi B*	1, 45, 12	b
	S. typhimurium	1, 4, 5, 12	i, 1, 2
C_1	*S. paratyphi C*	6, 7 (Vi)	c, 1, 5
D	*S. typhi*	9, 12 (Vi)	d–

The serotypes that share same antigenic formula are differentiated from one another by biochemical tests. The detailed classification is shown in the appendix 1.

PATHOGENICITY

Salmonellae are strict parasites of animals or man. *S. typhi, S. paratyphi A* and *S. paratyphi B* are confined to man. Other salmonellae are parasitic in various animals.

Salmonellae cause the following clinical syndromes in man:
1. Enteric fever
2. Septicaemia with or without local suppurative lesions
3. Gastroenteritis or food poisoning.

Enteric Fever

Clinical Spectrum

The term enteric fever includes typhoid fever caused by *S. typhi* and paratyphoid fever caused by *S. paratyphi A, B* and *C*.

The infection is acquired by ingestion. On reaching the gut, the bacilli attach themselves to the intestinal villi and penetrate in to the lamina propria and submucosa. They are phagocytosed there by polymorphs and macrophages. They then enter the mesenteric lymph nodes where they multiply and via the thoracic duct enter the blood stream. They stay in the blood for a short time from the blood, bacilli are seeded in the liver, gallbladder, spleen, bone marrow, lymph nodes, lungs and kidneys where further multiplication takes place. Towards the end of the incubation period, there occurs a massive bacteremia from these sites of multiplication which indicates the onset of clinical disease. Bile is a good culture medium for the bacillus, it multiplies in the gallbladder and is discharged continuously into the intestine. It involves peyers patches and lymphoid follicles of the ileum that become inflamed, undergo necrosis and slough off leaving behind ulcers.

Incubation period is 14 days. The clinical course may vary from mild fever to a fatal disease. The clinical features are:
1. Step ladder pyrexia
2. Soft palpable spleen
3. Hepatomegaly.

The onset is usually gradual with headache, malaise, anorexia, a coated tongue and abdominal discomfort with either constipation or diarrhea.

Rose spots that fade on pressure appear on the skin during the second or third week.

The most important complications are intestinal perforation, hemorrhage and circulatory collapse. Convalescence is slow. In about 5–10 percent of cases, relapse occurs during convalescence. *S. paratyphi A* and *B* cause paratyphoid fever that resembles typhoid fever but is generally mild. *S. paratyphi C* may cause paratyphoid fever but it leads to frank septicemia with suppurative complications.

Epidemiology

S. paratyphi A is found in India and other Asian countries, Eastern Europe and South America, *S. paratyphi B* in Western Europe, Britain and North America and *S. paratyphi C* in Eastern Europe and Guyana.

Enteric fever is endemic in all parts of India. It has been estimated to affect 150 to 300 per 100,000 population. The proportion of typhoid to paratyphoid A is 10:1. Paratyphoid B is rare and C, very rare. The disease occurs in all ages but it is commonest in the 5–20 year age group.

Source of infection is a carrier. Patients who continue to shed typhoid bacilli in feces for 3 weeks to 3 months after clinical cure are called convalescent carriers. Those who shed the bacilli for >3 months but <1 year are called temporary carriers and those who shed the bacilli for over one year are called chronic carriers. About 2–4 percent of patients become chronic carriers. The bacilli persist in the gallbladder or the kidney and are eliminated in the feces (fecal carrier) or urine (urinary carrier). Food handlers or cooks who become carriers are very dangerous.

Typhoid epidemics are water, milk or food borne. Water borne epidemics have become rare due to better control of drinking water. Milk borne epidemics have also become rare.

Food borne epidemics may be due to contamination of tinned foodstuffs, vegetables or shellfish that are eaten raw or undercooked.

Laboratory Diagnosis

Bacteriological diagnosis of enteric fever consists of isolation of bacilli from the patient and the demonstration of antibodies in his serum.

A positive blood culture is diagnostic while isolation from feces/urine is not that significant. Demonstration of antibodies is not conclusive evidence of current infection.

Blood culture: Bacteremia occurs early in the disease and blood cultures are positive in 90 percent of cases in the first week of fever, 75 percent of cases in the second week, 60 percent in the third week and 25 percent thereafter till the fever subsides. Blood cultures become negative on treatment with chloramphenicol.

About 5 to 10 mL of blood is collected by venepuncture and inoculated into a culture bottle containing 50 to 100 mL of 0.5 percent bile broth. Blood contain substances that inhibit the growth of the bacilli and hence it is essential that broth is taken in sufficient quantity to provide four-fold dilution of blood. Sometimes sodium polyanethol sulphonate (liquoid) is added to counteract the bactericidal action of blood.

Processing: After overnight incubation at 37°C, the bile broth is subcultured on MacConkey's agar. Pale, non-lactose fermenting colonies appear on this medium and are picked out for biochemical tests and motility. Final identification of the isolate is by slide agglutination. A loopful of the growth from an agar slope is emulsified in 2 drops of saline on a slide. One emulsion acts as a control, to show that the strain is not autoagglutinable. If *S. typhi* is suspected (i.e. when no gas is formed from glucose), a loopful of typhoid O antiserum, factor 9 is added to one drop of bacterial emulsion on the slide and agglutination looked for after rocking the slide gently. Quick agglutination indicates that the isolate belongs to salmonella group D. Then we check with the flagellar anti D.

When the isolate is a non-typhoid salmonella, it is tested for agglutination with O and H antisera for groups A, B, C. For identification of unusual serotypes the help of the National Salmonella Reference center should be taken which is located in Kasauli.

If salmonellae are not obtained from the first subculture from bile broth, subcultures should be repeated every other day till growth is obtained. Cultures should be declared negative only after incubation for 10 days. To decrease the risk of contamination, Castanedas' method of culture may be used. In this a double medium is used. The bottle of bile broth has an agar slant on one side. After inoculation of blood, the bottle is incubated in the upright position. For subculture, the bottle is tilted so that broth runs over the surface of agar. It is reincubated in the upright position. If salmonellae are present, colonies will appear on the slant.

Clot culture: An alternative to blood culture is clot culture. Here 5 mL of blood is withdrawn from the patient into a sterile test tube and allowed to clot. The serum is pipetted off and used for the Widal test. The clot is broken up with a sterile glass rod and added to a bottle of bile broth. The incorporation of streptokinase (100 units/mL) in broth facilitates lysis of the clot. Clot cultures give a higher rate of isolation than blood cultures as the bactericidal action of the serum is canceled.

Stool culture: Salmonellae are shed in the stool throughout the course of the disease and even in convalescence. A positive stool culture is almost as significant as a blood culture. Isolation from stool is successful when enrichment and selective mediums are used. Repeated sampling increases the rate of isolation. Samples are put into selenite and tetrathionate broth and then replated on to MacConkey's and DCA medium.

Urine culture: Salmonella are shed in the urine irregularly and infrequently. Hence urine culture is less useful than the culture of blood or feces. Cultures are generally positive only in the 2nd or the 3rd week and in only 25 percent of cases. Repeated sampling improves the rate of isolation. Clean voided urine samples are centrifuged and the deposit inoculated into enrichment and selective media as for fecal culture.

Other materials for culture:

- Bone marrow cultures
- Culture of bile obtained by duodenal aspiration
- Cerebrospinal fluid.

Widal test: As we know, this is a serological test to test for the antibodies against H and O antigens for typhoid and paratyphoid bacteria. Two different types of tubes are used for the test. A narrow tube with a conical bottom—Dreyer's agglutination tube for the H agglutination and a short round bottomed tube (Felix) tube for the O agglutination.

Serial dilutions of the serum samples are made and H and O antigen suspensions of *S. typhi* and *S. paratyphi* A and B are added to them. These are incubated in a water bath at 37°C overnight. The agglutination titers of the serum are read. H agglutination leads to the formation of loose cotton woolly clumps while O agglutination is a disc-like pattern at the bottom of the tube.

Interpretation of Widal Test

1. The antibody titer will depend on the stage of the disease. The antibodies usually appear by the end of the 1st week so that blood taken earlier may give a negative result. The titer steadily increases till the 3rd or 4th week after which it comes down.
2. We must test two or more serum samples because a rising titer is more meaningful than a single high reading.
3. Titers of > 1:100 for O antibodies and > 1:200 for H antibodies are significant. But it must be interpreted keeping in mind the antibody levels of the normal sera in the area.
4. Antibodies may be present on account of previous disease, in apparent infection or immunization. This must be taken into consideration.
5. H antibodies last for longer time than O antibodies.
6. Individuals immunized with TAB vaccine has antibodies to *S. typhi, S. paratyphi* A and B whereas in case of infection, antibodies will be seen only against the infecting species.
7. Persons who have had prior infection or immunization may develop an anamnestic response during an unrelated fever. But this rise is only temporary whereas in enteric fever the rise is sustained. Cases treated with chloramphenicol may show poor antibody response.

Demonstration of circulating antigen: Typhoid antigen is present in the blood in the early phase of the disease and also in the urine of patients. This can be detected by using laboratory tests.

Other lab tests:

1. Leukopenia with relative lymphocytosis is seen.
2. Eosinophils are low.

Diagnosis of carriers: The detection of carriers is important for epidemiological and public health purposes.

The identification of fecal carriers is by isolation of the bacillus from feces or from bile.

It is important to test repeated samples for the detection of urinary carriers.

The Widal test has no role.

The demonstration of Vi antibody indicates the carrier state. Confirm by culture.

Bacteriophage typing: As we know bacteriophages are viruses that kill bacteria. Different bacterial species are divided into phage types depending on the specific bacteriophages they are attacked by. A bacteriophage has been discovered that acts on the Vi antigen of the typhoid bacillus (Vi phage II). This is called phage A. Phage types A and E1 are the most common phages types and are present throughout India.

Prophylaxis: Typhoid fever can be effectively controlled by improvement in sanitation and proper water supply.

Three vaccines are available for typhoid these days (approximately equal efficacy 50 to 75%).

1. *Heat-phenol inactivated vaccine* for parenteral use. TAB vaccine S/C infection of two doses 0.5 mL at an interval of 4–6 weeks. This is not much used.
2. *An oral live attenuated Ty 21a* supplied as enteric coated capsules. Four doses are taken, one every other day. The capsules must be refrigerated and taken with cool liquids (37°C or less) at least 1 hour before meals. All four doses must be taken. Side-effects are minimum.
3. *A Vi capsular polysaccharide [Vi (CPS)]* vaccine for parenteral use. The Vi CPS vaccine is given as a single intramuscular injection. Adverse effects consist of local irritation at the site of infection, fever and headache. A booster dose of the heat inactivated vaccine is recommended every 3 years. Booster doses of *Vi CPS* is given every 2 years. The optimal booster dose of the Ty 21a is not known but it is recommended repeating the 4-dose series every 5 years. The live attenuated vaccine should not be given in immunosuppressed patients.

Treatment and drug resistance: Earlier ampicillin, chloramphenicol and septran were given for the treatment of enteric fever. Now resistance has set in and therefore fluoroquinolones (Ciprofloxacin) and Ceftriaxone can be used. Chloramphenicol was sensitive till 1972 when resistant strains emerged in Mexico and Kerela.

Multiple drug resistance is being seen in salmonella now.

Salmonella Gastroenteritis

Salmonella gastroenteritis or food poisoning is generally a zoonotic disease. The source of infections is animals or animal products.

The most common salmonella species that causes infection is *S. typhimurium*. The others are *S. enteritidis, S. newport, S. anatum*, etc.

Human infection results from the ingestion of contaminated food. The most frequent sources of salmonella food poisoning are poultry, meat, milk, cream and eggs. Food contamination also results from droppings by rats, lizards or small animals.

The disease develops after a short incubation period of 24 hours or less with diarrhea, vomiting, abdominal pain and fever. It usually subsides in 2 to 4 days but in some, prolonged enteritis develops with passage of mucus and pus in feces resembling dysentery. In a few, typhoidal or septicemic type of fever may develop.

Laboratory diagnosis is made by isolating the *Salmonella* from the stool. By taking a proper history the causative agent of the food poisoning can be detected. Isolation of salmonellae from the article of food confirms the diagnosis.

Control of *Salmonella* food poisoning requires the prevention of food contamination. Treatment is symptomatic. Antibiotics should not be used in uncomplicated cases.

Salmonella Septicemia

Certain Salmonellae, (*S. cholerasuis*) may cause septicemic disease with focal suppurative lesions such as osteomyelitis, deep abscesses, endocarditis, pneumonia and meningitis. Gastroenteritis may or may not be present. The case fatality is as high as 25 percent. *Salmonella* may be isolated from blood or pus. Stool culture may be positive. Septicemic salmonellosis should be treated with appropriate antibiotics.

APPENDIX 1

Antigens of some representatives of the genus *Salmonella* (Kauffmann-White classification)

O group	*Serotype ('species')*	*O antigens[a] (and Vi)[b]*	*H antigens*	
			Phase 1	*Phase 2*
A	*S. paratyphi A*	1, 2, 12	a	–
	A. paratyphi A var. durazzo	2, 12	a	–
B	*S. paratyphi B*	1, 4, 5, 12	b	1, 2
	S. paratyphi B var. odense	1, 4, 12	b	1, 2
	S. java	1, 4, 5, 12	b	(1, 2)
	S. limete	1, 4, 12, 27	b	1, 5
	S. typhimurium	1, 4, 5, 12	i	1, 2
	S. typhimurium var. copenhagen	1, 4, 12	i	1, 2
	S. agama	4, 12	i	1, 6
	S. abortus-equi	4, 12	–	e, n, x
	S. abortus-ovis	4, 12	c	1, 6
	S. agona	4, 12	f, g, s	–
	S. brandenburg	4, 12	l, v	e, n, z_{15}
	S. bredeney	1, 4, 12, 27	l, v	1, 7
	S. derby	1, 4, 5, 12	f, g	–
	S. heidelberg	1, 4, 5, 12	r	1, 2
	S. saint-paul	1, 4, 5, 12	e, h	1, 2
	S. salinatis	4, 12	d, e, h	d, e, n, z_{15}
	S. stanley	4, 5, 12	d	1, 2
	S. indiana	1, 4, 12	z	1, 7
C_1	*S. paratyphi C*	6, 7 (Vi)	c	1, 5
	S. cholerae-suis	6, 7	c	1, 5
	S. cholerae-suis var. kunzendorf	6, 7	(c)	1, 5
	S. decatur	6, 7	c	1, 5
	S. typhi-suis	6, 7	c	1, 5
	S. bureilly	6, 7	y	1, 5
	S. infantis	6, 7	r	1, 5
	S. menston	6, 7	g, s, t	–
	S. montevideo	6, 7	g, m, s	–
	S. oranienburg	6, 7	m, t	–
	S. thompson	6, 7	k	1, 5
C_2	*S. bovis-morbificans*	6, 8	r	1, 5
	S. newbport	6, 8	e, h	1, 2
D	*S. typhi*	9, 12, (Vi)	d	–
	S. ndolo	9, 12	d	1, 5
	S. dublin	1, 9, 12, (Vi)	g, p	–
	S. enteritidis	1, 9, 12	g, m	–
	S. gallinarum	1, 9, 12	–	–
	S. pullorum	(1), 9, 12	–	–
	S. panama	1, 9, 12	l, v	1, 5
	S. miami	1, 9, 12	a	1, 5
	S. sendat	1, 9, 12	a	1, 5
E_1	*S. anatum*	3, 10	e, h	1, 6
	S. give	3, 10	l, v	1, 7
	S. london	3, 10	l, v	1, 6
	S. meleagridis	3, 10	e, h	l, w
	S. weftevrden	3, 10	r	26
E_2	*S. cambridge*	3, 15	e, h	l, w
	S. newington	3, 15	e, h	1, 6
E_3	*S. minneapolis*	(3), (15), 34	e, h	1, 6

Contd...

Contd...

O group	*Serotype ('species')*	*O antigens[a] (and Vi)[a]*	*H antigens*	
E_4	*S. senftenberg*	1, **3**, **19**	g, s, t	–
	S. simsbury	1, **3**, **19**	–	z_{27}
F	*S. aberdeen*	**11**	i	1, 2
G	*S. cubana*	1, **13**, 23	z_{29}	–
	S. poona	**13**, 22	z	1, 6
H	*S. heves*	**6**, **14**, 24	d	1, 5
	S. onderstepoort	1, **6**, **14**, 25	e, h	1, 5
I	*S. brazil*	**16**	a	1, 5
	S. hvittingfoss	**16**	b	e, n, x
Others	*S. kirkee*	**17**	b	1, 2
	S. adelaide	**35**	f, g	–
	S. locarno	**57**	z_{29}	z_{42}

[a] Numbers in bold type indicate the antigens characterizing the O group.
Numbers in brackets are antigens that are not always present.

CHAPTER 30

Gram-negative Rods: Enterobacteriaceae—*Shigella*

LESSON PLAN

- Introduction
- Morphology
- Culture
- Resistance
- Biochemical Reactions
- Classification
  - Subgroup A–*Shigella Dysenteriae*
  - Subgroup B–*Shigella Flexneri*
  - Subgroup C–*Shigella Boydii*
  - Subgroup D–*Shigella Sonnei*
- Pathogenicity
  - Dysentery
- Epidemiology
- Laboratory Diagnosis
  - Samples
  - Macroscopic Examination
  - Microscopic Examination
  - Culture
  - Biochemical Tests
  - Slide Agglutination Tests
  - Colicin Typing
  - DNA Hybridization
  - Serology
- Treatment

Genus—Shigella

Species—S. dysenteriae, S. boydii, S. flexneri, S. sonnei

INTRODUCTION

Genus *Shigella*, a part of the family *Enterobacteriaceae* are gram-negative rods causing bacillary dysentery. Dysentery as we know is a clinical condition characterized by the passage of loose stools mixed with blood and mucus. The two common types of dysentery are:

(i) amoebic, and (ii) bacillary. We will be studying amoebic dysentery in the section on Parasitology. Shiga was the first scientist who isolated the causative agent of bacillary dysentery from an epidemic of dysentery in Japan and hence the name of the genus *Shigella*.

MORPHOLOGY

Shigellae are short gram-negative rods, 2 to 4 µ × 0.6 µ in size. They are non-motile, non-sporing and non-capsulated. Fimbriae may be present in some strains.

CULTURE

- They are aerobes and facultative anaerobes.
- Temperature range for growth is 10°C to 40°C. Optimum temperature is 37°C.
- Optimum pH for growth is 7.4.
- They grow readily on ordinary media but not as easily as *E. coli* and *Klebsiella species*.
- The various culture media that can be used for the growth of shigellae are:
  - *Solid*
  - Nutrient agar

- Blood agar
- MacConkey's agar
- DCA (Deoxycholate citrate agar)
- XLD (Xylose lysine deoxycholate) agar.
- *Liquid*
- Peptone water
- Nutrient broth
- Selenite F broth

After overnight incubation, on solid media the colonies are small, 2 to 3 mm in diameter, round convex, translucent discs. There are differences in the color of the colonies on different media.

Nutrient agar: The colonies are colorless or greyish.

Blood agar: The colonies are greyish. MacConkey's agar—The colonies are colorless due to the absence of lactose fermentation. An exception is *Shigella sonnei* that ferments lactose late and forms pale pink colonies. Since MacConkey's medium is not a selective medium for shigella, growth of other intestinal bacteria occurs as well, that causes difficulty in isolation of shigellae.

Deoxycholate citrate agar: This is an excellent selective medium for isolation of shigellae from feces. The colonies are the same as that which appear on MacConkey's medium. They are also similar to the colonies of salmonella on this medium except that they are smaller and more translucent and do not form a black center. On prolonged incubation *S. sonnei* forms pink papillae.

XLD agar (Xylose lysine deoxycholate): This is the best selective medium for shigellae, probably a little better than DCA too, because it is not inhibitory to some strains. Colonies are red without black center.

Peptone water and nutrient broth: On overnight incubation, good growth of shigellae occurs with uniform turbidity.

Selenite F broth: This is an enrichment medium for shigella especially *S. flexneri serotype 6*.

The growth of shigellae is inhibited on Wilson and Blair's bismuth sulphite medium.

RESISTANCE

- Boiling or chlorination of water and pasteurization of milk destroy the bacilli.
- They are killed by 1 percent phenol in 15 minutes. Shigellae are killed at 56°C in 1 hour by moist heat.
- In water and ice they remain viable for 1 to 6 months.
- In stool samples they die within a few hours due to acidity produced by commensal bacteria. They can survive for some days in feces if preserved at 4°C or in buffered glycerol saline.
- Can survive for 1 to 3 weeks in cool, damp and dark conditions, when feces dry on cloth or on lavatory seats.
- *S. sonnei* is more resistant and survives better in the environment.

BIOCHEMICAL REACTIONS

- Shigellae are MR positive.
- Reduce nitrates to nitrites.
- Catalase is produced except by *Shigella dysenteriae* type 1, and *Sh. flexneri* serotype 4a.
- Glucose is fermented with the production of acid without gas except for the Newcastle and Manchester biotypes of *Sh. flexneri* type 6, and *Sh. boydii* serotype 14 that form gas.
- Fermentation of mannitol is important because *Sh. flexneri*, *Sh. boydii* and *Sh. sonnei* ferment mannitol, whereas *Sh. dysenteriae* do not.
- Indole is positive in all *Shigellae* except in *Shigella dysenteriae* serotype 1, *Sh. flexneri* serotypes 6 and *Sh. sonnei* that are indole negative.
- Lactose and Sucrose is not fermented except by *Sh. sonnei* which ferments them late.
- H_2S, urease and citrate are negative (Flow chart 30.1 and Table 30.1).

CLASSIFICATION

Shigella are divided into four species or sub-groups (group A, B, C, D) based on a combination of biochemical and serological characteristics. Shigellae possess one or more

Flow chart 30.1: Identification of *Shigella spp* based on biochemical reactions

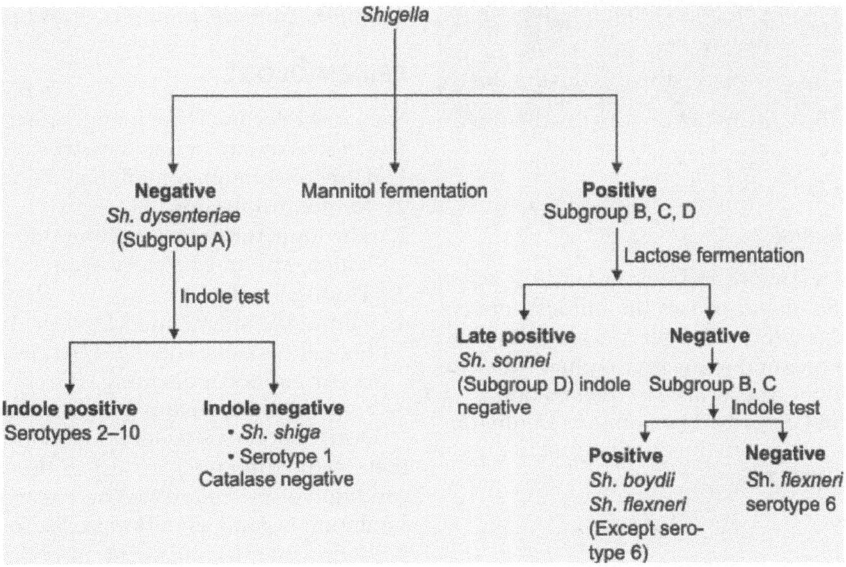

major antigens and a large number of minor somatic O antigens. Serotypes are within a species. Fimbrial antigens and K antigens are also present in some species.

Subgroup A

Shigella Dysenteriae

This species of mannitol non-fermenting bacilli consist of 10 serotypes. Type 1 is called shiga bacillus. This was originally described by *Shiga*. It is indole negative and it is the only member of the family that does not form catalase. It is also different in that it forms exotoxins. These include:

1. *Neurotoxin*: This causes paralysis and death when injected into mice or rabbits.
2. *Enterotoxin*: This causes fluid accumulation in ligated rabbit ileal loop.
3. *Cytotoxin*: This damages cell cultures of monkey kidney and Hela.

Sh. neurotoxin is the earliest exotoxin to be detected in gram-negative bacilli. *Sh. dysenteriae* causes the most severe type of dysentery.

Subgroup B

Shigella Flexneri

This group is named after Flexner who described the first of mannitol fermenting shigellae from Philippines. This group is biochemically heterogenous and antigenically the most complex. Based on type specific and group specific antigens they have been classified into 6 serotypes. In addition, two antigenic variants called X and Y are recognized that lack the type specific antigens. Serotype 6 is always indole negative and occurs in 3 biotypes some of which form gas from sugars (Table 30.1).

Subgroup C

Shigella Boydii

This group consists of dysentery bacilli that resemble *Sh. flexneri* biochemically but not antigenically. This group is named after Boyd who first described these strains from India. Fifteen serotypes have been identified. They are less common.

Table 30.1: Biotypes of *Sh. flexneri type 6*

Biotype	*Fermentation* *Glucose*	*Mannitol*
Boyd 88	Acid	Acid
Manchester	Acid + Gas	Acid + Gas
Newcastle	A or AG	—

Subgroup D

Shigella Sonnei

This ferments lactose and sucrose late. It is indole negative. *Sh. sonnei* causes the mildest form of bacillary dysentery. *Sh. sonnei* is classified into 17 colicin types and exists in two phases that are different in the appearance of their colonies.

It was first described by Sonne in Denmark.

PATHOGENICITY

Dysentery

Shigellae cause bacillary dysentery. Infection occurs by ingestion. The minimum infective dose is low. The bacteria invade the mucosal epithelial cells, that then spread and involve surrounding cells. Inflammatory reaction develops with capillary thrombosis leading to necrosis of patches of epithelium which slough off causing superficial ulcers. Though some shigellae have an exotoxin such as *Sh. dysenteriae* type 1, invasive property is much more important in causing dysentery.

Bacillary dysentery has a short incubation period (1 to 7 days), usually 48 hours. The onset and clinical course are variable depending upon the virulence of the infecting strain. The main clinical features are frequent passage of loose, scanty stool with blood and mucus along with griping pain and tenesmus. Fever and vomiting may or may not be present.

Complications can be present especially with *Sh. dysenteriae* type 1 such as arthritis, toxic neuritis, conjunctivitis, parotitis, etc. The severity of the disease varies from acute severe dysentery to mild diarrhea. Man is the only natural host. Experimentally the disease can be produced only in monkeys. Animals that can be used to establish diagnosis are mice, guinea pigs and rabbits.

EPIDEMIOLOGY

Source of infection is the man (cases or carriers). The modes of transmission may be:

1. Direct—through contaminated fingers (hand to mouth infection).
2. Through **fomites**—such as door handles, water taps and lavatory seats.
3. Through water.
4. Through contaminated food or drink. Shigellosis especially *Sh. sonnei* infection can occur as food poisoning. Rarely flies may transmit the infection as mechanical vectors.

Distribution of shigellosis is worldwide but the strain differs according to the economic condition of the country. Where environmental sanitation is good as in Britain, *Sh. sonnei* is the predominant infecting agent. In USA, *Sh. sonnei* and *Sh. flexneri* are common. In India, *Sh. flexneri* is the most common species (50 to 85%) followed by *Sh. dysenteriae* (8 to 25%), *Sh. sonnei* (2 to 24%) and *Sh. boydii* (0 to 8%).

In India many localized outbreaks have been observed from Kerala in 1981 and West Bengal in 1983. The epidemic strains show drug resistance.

LABORATORY DIAGNOSIS

1. *Sample*
   - *Fresh feces*: The feces should be inoculated without delay or transported in a suitable medium such as Sach's buffered glycerol saline, pH 7 to 7.4.
   - *Direct swab of an ulcer*: This is taken by sigmoidoscopic examination. It is best to use for inoculation, mucus flakes, if they are present in the sample.
2. *Macroscopic examination*: Macroscopically, the stool sample is very little, more of it is blood and mucus. It is bright red in color and odorless.

3. *Microscopic examination*: A saline preparation shows abundant cellular exudate containing pus cells and macrophages with phagocytosed red blood cells. It should be distinguished from amoebic dysentery. The red blood cells may appear in Rouleaux form.
4. *Culture*:
   - The solid media which can be used are:
     Nutrient agar
     Blood agar
     MacConkey's agar
     DCA
     XLD agar.
     We can use blood agar and MacConkey's agar or DCA for routine stool culture to detect shigellae.
   - The liquid media that can be used are Selenite F broth.

   After overnight incubation at 37°C, the plates are inspected for non-lactose fermenting colonies that are then tested for motility and biochemical reactions.
5. *Biochemical tests*: Any non-motile bacteria, that is urease, citrate and H_2S negative, should be subjected to detailed biochemical tests for *Shigella*.
6. The subgroups and serotypes are identified by slide agglutination tests.
7. The other methods of diagnosis include colicin typing, DNA hybridization and serology.

TREATMENT

Bacillary dysentery is a self-limited condition and recovers spontaneously. Antibiotics should be given after sensitivity testing in severe cases.

CHAPTER

31

Gram-negative Rods: *Vibrio—Vibrio Cholerae*

LESSON PLAN

- Introduction
- *Vibrio Cholerae*
  - Morphology
  - Cultural Characteristics
  - Biochemical Reactions
  - Classification
  - Pathogenicity
  - Epidemiology
  - Laboratory Diagnosis
  - Cholera Vaccination
- Halophilic Vibrios
  - *Vibrio Parahaemolyticus*

Genus—Vibrio
Species—Vibrio cholerae

INTRODUCTION

Vibrios are gram-negative, non-acid fast, rigid, curved rods that are comma-shaped. They are actively motile by means of a polar flagellum. The term vibrio is derived from the vibratory motility (vibrare—meaning to vibrate). They are non-sporing and non-capsulated. Vibrios have been included in the chapter under gram-negative rods for convenience.

The representative member of this genus is Vibrio cholerae, the causative agent of cholera. It was first isolated by Koch in 1883 from cholera patients in Egypt.

VIBRIO CHOLERAE

Morphology

Vibrio cholerae is a short, curved, cylindrical rod 1.5 μ × 0.2 to 0.4 μ in size with slightly pointed ends. The cell is typically comma-shaped but pleomorphism is frequent in old cultures (Fig. 31.1). In stained films of mucus flakes from acute cholera cases, the vibrios are arranged in parallel rows described by Koch as fish in stream appearance. It is actively motile with a single polar flagellum. The motility is of darting type and when acute cholera stool or a young culture is examined under the microscope, the actively motile vibrios suggest a swarm of gnats.

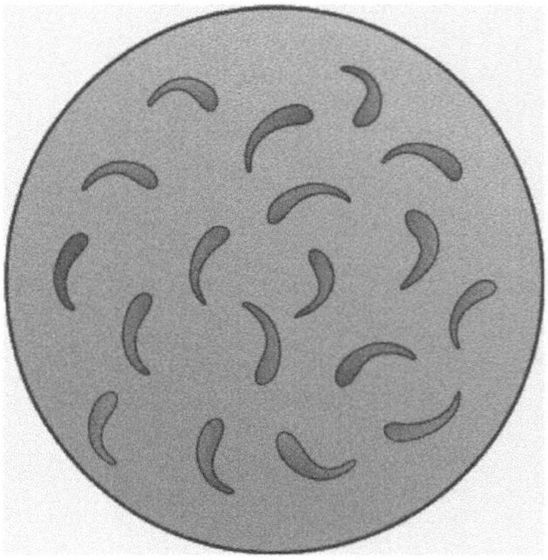

Fig. 31.1: Morphology of cholera vibrios

Cultural Characteristics

Vibrio cholerae is strongly aerobic, and growth is slow anaerobically. It grows within a temperature range of 16 to 40° (optimum 37°C).

- Growth is better in an alkaline medium, the range of pH = 6.4–9.6 (optimum 8.2).
- The culture media used for its culture are:

Basic Media

- Nutrient agar
- MacConkey's agar
- Blood agar
- Peptone water.

Nutrient agar: After overnight growth, the colonies are moist, translucent, round discs about 1 to 2 mm in diameter, with a bluish tinge in transmitted light. They have a distinct odor.

MacConkey's agar: The colonies are colorless at first but become reddish on prolonged incubation due to late fermentation of lactose.

Blood agar: The colonies are initially surrounded by a zone of greening that later becomes clear due to hemodigestion.

Peptone water: Growth occurs in 6 hours as a fine surface pellicle that breaks up on shaking into membranous pieces.

Special Media

a. *Transport medium*
   1. *Venkatraman-Ramakrishnan (VR medium)*: This medium is prepared by dissolving 20 g crude seasalt and 5 g peptone in one liter distilled water and adjusting the pH to 8.6 to 8.8. It is dispersed in screw-capped bottles in 10 to 15 mL amounts. About 1 to 3 mL of stool is added to each bottle. In this medium, vibrios remain viable for weeks.
   2. *Cary-Blair medium*: This is a buffered solution of sodium chloride, sodium thioglycollate, disodium phosphate and calcium chloride at pH 8.4. It is a suitable transport medium for salmonella, shigella and vibrios.

b. *Enrichment Media*
   1. *Alkaline peptone water at pH 8.6*: It is an excellent medium for enriching *V. cholerae* from a fecal specimen before plating it on a selective agar medium. It has:
      - Peptone 10 g
      - Sodium chloride (NaCl) 10 g
      - Distilled water 1 liter
   2. Monsur's taurocholate tellurite peptone water pH 9.2.

      Both of these are good transport as well as enrichment media. Alkaline peptone water is commonly used for the isolation of vibrios.

c. *Plating media*
   1. *Alkaline bile salt agar* (BSA) pH (8.2).
   2. *Monsur's gelatin taurocholate trypticase tellurite agar (G TTA)* medium. Cholera vibrios produce small translucent colonies with a greyish black center and a turbid halo. The colonies become 3 to 4 mm in size in 48 hours.
   3. *TCBS (medium)*: This medium contains thiosulphate, citrate, bromothymol blue and sucrose. Cholera vibrios produce large yellow convex colonies that may become green on continued incubation.

Vibrio colonies may be identified by the string test. A loopful of growth from culture is mixed with a drop of 0.5 percent, sodium deoxycholate in saline on a slide. If the test is positive, the suspension loses its turbidity, becomes mucoid and forms a string when the loop is drawn slowly away from the suspension.

Biochemical Reactions

- Carbohydrate metabolism is fermentative producing acid but no gas. Cholera vibrios ferment glucose, mannitol, maltose, mannose and sucrose but not inositol, arabinose or lactose.
- Indole is formed and nitrates are reduced to nitrites. These two properties contribute to the cholera red reaction that is tested by adding a few drops of H_2SO_4 to a 24-hour peptone water culture.

- Cholera vibrios produce a reddish pink color due to the formation of nitrosoindole.
- Catalase and oxidase test are positive.
- MR and urease test are negative.
- Vibrios decarboxylate lysine and ornithine but do not utilize arginine. Gelatin is liquefied. We will later see how the VP reaction and hemolytic reaction is used to classify vibrios.

Classification

Gardner and Venkatraman Classification

They divided the vibrios into two large groups

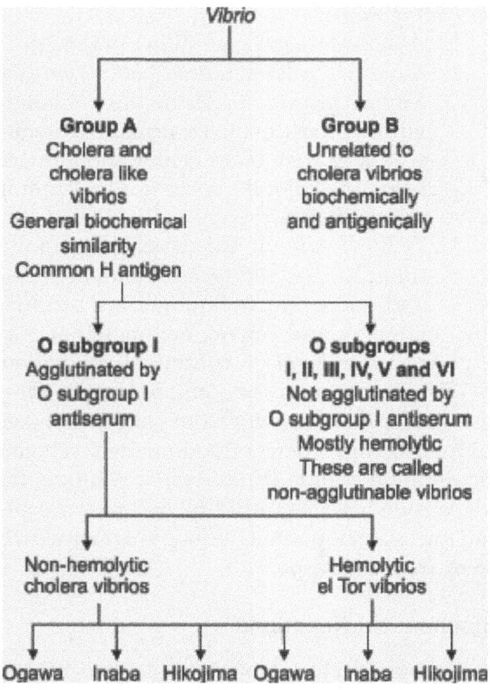

Group A consists of cholera vibrios and biochemically similar vibrios possessing a common H antigen and group B, a heterogenous collection of vibrios distinct from group A.

Group A vibrios are divided into six subgroups: I-VI based on the O antigens. Vibrios belong to O subgroup I. Vibrios resembling (*V. cholerae and el Tor vibrios*) but not agglutinated by O subgroup I antiserum are called non-agglutinating or NAG vibrios. They are also known as non-cholera vibrios or NCV. They are from time to time associated with outbreaks of diarrheal disease.

Vibrios belonging to O subgroup I are divided by the Greig test into non-hemolytic cholera vibrios and the hemolytic el Tor vibrios both of which are antigenically indistinguishable.

Based on differences in minor O antigens both hemolytic and non-hemolytic O subgroup I vibrios are divided into three serotypes—Ogawa, Inaba and Hikojima.

The el Tor vibrios: Gotschlich in 1905 isolated a vibrio from six Haj pilgrims who had died of dysentery or gangrene of the colon at the Tor quarantine station on the Sinai Peninsula. These were called the el Tor vibrios. They were identical to cholera vibrios in all respects except that they were VP positive and hemolytic. As they were isolated from human intestines and water samples they were considered non-pathogenic. Slowly the el Tor vibrios spread to Southeast Asia and started the 7th pandemic of cholera that is yet to subside. Earlier the strains isolated were hemolytic but later the majority of isolates were non-hemolytic.

The differences between the two are shown in Table 31.1.

Table 31.1: Differences between classical and el Tor vibrios

Test	*Classical cholera*	*el Tor vibrios*
Hemolysis	–	+
Voges-Proskauer	–	+
Chick erythrocyte agglutination	–	+
Polymyxin B sensitivity	+	–
Group IV phage susceptibility	+	–

VP test: As already studied in biochemical tests.

Hemolysis test: The modified test involves taking equal volumes (0.5 mL) of a 24-hour heart infusion broth culture and 1 percent sheep erythrocyte suspension, mixed, incubated at 37°C for 2 hours and examined for hemolysis after holding at 4°C overnight.

Chick red cell agglutination test: A loopful from an agar culture is taken and emulsified in a drop of saline on a slide and one drop of 2.5 percent chick erythrocyte suspension added. Clumping of erythrocytes within a minute denotes a positive test. All el Tor strains are positive and classical cholera vibrios negative.

Sensitivity to polymyxin B: This is tested by the disc diffusion method using discs containing 50 units of the antibiotic. All strains of classical cholera vibrio are sensitive to polymyxin at this concentration and all strains of el Tor vibrio are resistant.

Sensitivity to cholera phage group IV: All strains of classical cholera vibrio are lysed by Mukerjee's group IV phage at routine test dilution while all el Tor strains are insusceptible. This is considered to be the most dependable test available for differentiating between el Tor and classical strains.

Heiberg Classification

Heiberg classified vibrios into 8 groups based on the fermentation of mannose, sucrose and arabinose. Cholera vibrios belong to group I (Table 31.2).

Table 31.2: Heiberg grouping of vibrios

Group	*Mannose*	*Sucrose*	*Arabinose*
I	A	A	–
II	–	A	–
III	A	A	A
IV	–	A	A
V	A		–
VI	–	–	–
VII	A	–	A
VIII	–	–	A

Pathogenicity

Cholera

Cholera is an acute diarrhoeal disease caused by *V. cholerae*. In serious cases, there is profuse watery diarrhea and vomiting that may lead to shock and death is less than 24 hours. In treated cases, the disease may last 4 to 6 days. Since there is a lot of loss of extracellular fluid volume, the common complications are muscular cramps, renal failure and pulmonary edema.

Cholera like symptoms can be produced by either classical vibrio in which case the disease is severe or el Tor vibrios in which the disease is less severe. NAG vibrios may produce a disease clinically similar to cholera. The same clinical picture can be caused by enterotoxigenic E. coli. The incubation period varies from less than 24 hours to about 5 days. The clinical illness may begin slowly with mild diarrhea, or suddenly with sudden massive diarrhea. The initial diarrheal stools contain fecal material but the later stools assume the rice water appearance with flecks of mucus in a colorless fluid. The stool has a fishy odor. Purging is painless and effortless. Vomiting that starts along with diarrhea consists of a clear watery fluid secreted by the upper part of the small intestine.

In human infection, the vibrios enter orally through contaminated food or drink. If they survive the barrier of gastric acidity, they multiply in the alkaline contents of the intestine. Vibrios do not penetrate the gut wall and do not invade the blood stream but secrete an enterotoxin that acts on the intestinal epithelium to cause outpouring of fluid. The cholera exotoxin is a protein with a molecular weight of 84,000. It has two fractions A (active) and B (binding). Neither fraction alone has any significant toxicity. Fraction B is the part responsible for binding to the ganglioside receptor on the host cell membrane. Fraction A can be broken down into 2 polypeptide chains termed A1 and A2. The A1 subunit is the part responsible for activation of adenyl cyclase and subsequent watery diarrhea.

Epidemiology

There have been seven pandemics. The six pandemics have been caused by classical cholera vibrios and the seventh has been caused by el Tor vibrios. Infection with el Tor vibrios leads to a higher proportion of mild cases, higher incidence of carriers and greater chances for endemicity as compared to classical cholera.

In India, most of the isolates are of the el Tor type. Transmission is maintained by a cycle involving the vibrio excretor and the environment particularly a water source. Person to person transmission is relatively unimportant. The only natural source of infection is man. Both convalescent and chronic carriers exist. In the chronic carrier the vibrio survives in the gall-bladder and is shed intermittently particularly when the carrier suffers from diarrhea.

Cholera is mainly a disease of poverty and insanitation.

Laboratory Diagnosis

The laboratory diagnosis is not so much for the treatment of individual cases but for control of the outbreak.

- Stool collected in the acute stage of disease is the most valuable specimen for laboratory diagnosis.
- The best specimen, however, is collected by introducing into the rectum a No. 26 or 28 rubber catheter lubricated with paraffin and letting the liquid stool flow directly into a screw-capped container. Rectal swabs may be used, that absorb the fluid stool. They are useful in collection of specimens from convalescent carriers who no longer have watery diarrhea. They are moistened with transport medium.
- After collection of the stool it is necessary to preserve the sample in VR fluid or Cary-Blair medium because cholera vibrios die within a few hours. If the sample can reach the lab in a few hours, it may be transported in enrichment media such as alkaline peptone water or Monsur's medium. If transport medium is not available strips of blotting paper may be soaked in watery stool and sent to the lab packed in plastic envelopes. Whenever possible, the plates should be inoculated and sent to the laboratory. When they reach the lab:
  - The specimens sent in enrichment media should be incubated for 6 to 8 hours.
  - The specimens sent in holding media should be inoculated into enrichment media to be incubated for 6 to 8 hours before being streaked on a selective or non-selective media.
  - We should also do direct plating before enrichment wherever possible.

Selective Media

- Monsur's GTTA
- TCBS.

Non-selective Media

- Bile salt agar.
- Meat extract agar.
- Gelatin agar.
- Generally the plates are examined after overnight incubation at 37°C. Colonies suggestive of vibrios should be picked up with a straight wire and tested by slide agglutination with cholera O subgroup I serum. If positive, agglutination should be repeated using monospecific Ogawa and Inaba sera for serotyping. If agglutination is negative with one colony, it is essential to repeat the test with at least 5 more colonies. If slide agglutination is positive, the isolate is tested for chick red cell agglutination. Isolates that are not agglutinated by the O subgroup I serum should not be ignored, as NAG vibrios are also known to produce cholera-like disease. Any vibrio which is agglutinated by H antiserum but not by cholera O subgroup I antiserum is considered to be a NAG vibrio.
- The isolate is subjected to detailed biochemical testing. The strain may be sent

to the International Reference Center for Vibrio phage typing at the NICED Calcutta.
- Serological examination is of little use in diagnosis of cases.
- For examination of water samples for vibrios, enrichment or filtration methods may be used. In the enrichment method, 900 mL of water is added to 100 mL (ten-fold concentrated) peptone water, incubated at 37°C for 6 to 8 hours and a second enrichment done before plating on selective media. For the filtration technique, the water to be tested should be filtered through the Millipore membrane filter that is then placed directly on the surface of a selective medium and incubated.

Colonies appear after overnight incubation. Sewage should be diluted in saline, filtered through gauze and treated as for water.

Cholera Vaccination

The incidence of cholera among travelers is very low, and the vaccine is also only marginally effective. So the WHO does not routinely require immunization even for persons travelling to and from endemic areas.

Cholera vaccine contains a suspension of killed vibrios. Two injections are given intramuscularly 2 to 6 weeks apart followed by booster injections every 6 months during periods of possible exposure. Protection depends largely on booster doses. An inactivated oral vaccine appears to be more effective than the parenteral vaccine. A live attenuated vaccine is being investigated. This is a stable mutant of the cholera vibrio that produces only fraction B of the toxin without fraction A. This strain is totally avirulent but is expected to provide local antibacterial as well as antitoxic immunity.

HALOPHILIC VIBRIOS

Vibrios that have a high requirement of sodium chloride are called halophilic vibrios. Their natural habitat is sea water and marine life. Some halophilic vibrios have been shown to cause human disease:
- *V. parahaemolyticus,*
- *V. alginolyticus*—Its status as a human pathogen is uncertain. It is associated with marine wound infections.
- *Vibrio vulnificus*—Lactose fermenting, isolated from wound patients in the USA.

Vibrio Parahaemolyticus

V. parahaemolyticus was originally isolated in 1951 in Japan as the causative agent of an outbreak of food poisoning due to sea fish. It is now considered an important cause of food poisoning throughout the world. It is found in sea animals and also pond fishes.
- In morphology it resembles cholera vibrios except that it is capsulated, shows bipolar staining and is pleomorphic.
- It produces peritrichous flagella when grown on solid media. Polar flagella are formed on liquid media.
- It grows in media containing NaCl (upto 8%). Optimum salt concentration is 2 to 4 percent.
- On TCBS agar, the colonies are green with an opaque, raised center and flat translucent periphery.
- Oxidase, calalase, nitrate, indole and citrate are positive.
- Pathogenic *V. parahaemolyticus* when grown in high salt blood agar (Wagatsuma agar) are hemolytic. This is called the Kanagawa phenomenon and is due to a heat stable hemolysin.

CHAPTER

32

Gram-negative Rods: *Pseudomonas—Pseudomonas Aeruginosa*

LESSON PLAN

- Introduction
- *Pseudomonas Aeruginosa*
  - Morphology
  - Culture
  - Biochemical Reactions
  - Classification
  - Resistance
  - Pathogenicity
  - Laboratory Diagnosis
- *Pseudomonas Mallei*
- *Pseudomonas Pseudomallei*

Genus—Pseudomonas
Species—Pseudomonas aeruginosa

INTRODUCTION

The genus *Pseudomonas* includes aerobic, non-sporing, gram-negative bacilli motile by polar flagella.

Most of the members of the genus are saprophytes, being found in water, soil or wherever decomposing organic matter is found. They can be opportunistic pathogens too, e.g. *Pseudomonas aeruginosa* associated with hospital acquired infection and infection of burns and two other species *P. pseudomallei* and *P. mallei* that cause fatal infections in healthy persons or animals.

PSEUDOMONAS AERUGINOSA

Morphology

It is a thin gram-negative bacillus 1.5 to 3 μm × 0.5 μm in size, actively motile by a polar flagellum. It is non-capsulated. Sometimes when grown in the absence of sucrose, an extracellular polysaccharide slime layer may be formed.

Strains isolated from clinical specimens have pili.

Culture

- It is strongly aerobic.
- No growth anaerobically.
- Growth occurs at a wide range of temperature (5 to 42°C), optimum is 37°C.
- It grows well on ordinary media producing large, opaque, irregular colonies with a musty smell.
- The culture media used are nutrient agar, blood agar, MacConkey's agar and DCA.
- On nutrient agar they produce large opaque irregular colonies with a greenish pigment.
- On blood agar they produce similar colonies, that are hemolytic.
- On MacConkey's agar and DCA, they form non-lactose fermenting colonies.
- In broth, they produce dense turbidity with a surface pellicle.

Pigment Production

Pseudomonas aeruginosa produces many pigments—pyocyanin and fluorescein being important among them. Pyocyanin is a bluish-green phenazine pigment soluble in water and chloroform and produced only by *Pseudomonas aeruginosa*. Fluorescein is a greenish-yellow pigment soluble in water but not in chloroform. Fluorescein is produced by other species also. Other pigments produced are pyoverdin (green), pyorubin (red) and pyomelanin (black). Some strains are non-pigmented. Pyocyanin inhibits the growth of other bacteria so that pseudomonas can be isolated from a mixed bacterial flora.

Biochemical Reactions

- The metabolism is oxidative and non-fermentative
- Glucose is utilized oxidatively forming acid only.
- Indole, MR, VP and H_2S tests are negative
- Catalase and oxidase are positive.

Classification

The typing methods used for classification are:

1. Serotyping
2. Pyocin (Bacterocin typing)
3. Bacteriophage typing.

Based on O antigen, it has been divided into 27 serotypes using slide agglutination. Pyocin typing is more popular.

Resistance

- The bacteria is killed at 55° in one hour.
- It is resistant to chemical agents and even grows in bottles of disinfectants. Selective media have been made using these chemical agents. This is the reason why it thrives in hospital conditions.
- It is naturally resistant to many antibiotics but sensitive to:
  - Gentamicin
  - Tobramycin
  - Carbenicillin
  - Pipercillin
  - Ceftazidime.

Pathogenicity

The bacteria produces **blue pus** and it is named after this (aeruginosa means verdigris that is bluish-green in color). It can cause infections in the community or the hospital. The commonest infection in the community caused by *Pseudomonas aeruginosa* is suppurative otitis media which is chronic. In the hospital it causes localized or generalized infections. Localized infections are infections of the wounds and bedsores, eye infections and urinary tract infections following catheterization. Generalized infections include infections in burns, post-tracheostomy pulmonary infection and iatrogenic meningitis following lumbar puncture. *Pseudomonas aeruginosa* is one of the agents responsible for infantile diarrhea.

Pseudomonas aeruginosa is an important cause of hospital acquired infection due to its resistance to common antibiotics and antiseptics that help it to establish itself widely in the hospitals. Equipments such as respirators, bed pans and medicines such as lotions, ointments and eyedrops may be contaminated.

The virulence factors of *Pseudomonas aeruginosa* are Exotoxin A, proteases, elastases hemolysins and a slime layer.

Laboratory Diagnosis

As *Pseudomonas aeruginosa* is a frequent contaminant, isolation of the bacillus from a specimen should not mean that it is the causative agent. Repeated isolations confirm the diagnosis.

The culture medium used for *Ps. aeruginosa* should be one that has a selective agent and special constituents to enhance pigment production. Some of the media used are:

1. *Pseudomonas* isolation agar (PIA) with selective agent irgasan.
2. Cetrimide containing Pseudosel agar.
3. Enrichment broth containing acetamide.

Pyocin Typing

The bacteriocins of *Pseudomonas aeruginosa* are called pyocins. Four different types of pyocins are recognized. Strains are immune to their own pyocin but act on other strains. The standard procedure (Govan 1978) used a cross-streaking technique in which pyocin production by the test strain was detected by inhibitory activity against a standard set of 13 indicator strains of *Pseudomonas aeruginosa*. Pyocin typing is used for epidemiological purposes.

Two other species of Pseudomonas that cause human disease are:

- *Pseudomonas mallei*
- *Pseudomonas pseudomallei.*

PSEUDOMONAS MALLEI

This bacteria causes a disease in equine animals (glanders) but can be transmitted to other animals and man as well. In humans it causes fever, mucopurulent discharge and extreme weakness. The disease in humans is mainly an occupational infection. It can also result from infection by lab cultures. It is a very dangerous bacteria to work with.

PSEUDOMONAS PSEUDOMALLEI

It is the causative agent of melioidosis, a glanders like disease usually in rodents. The human disease is like an acute septicemia with respiratory involvement and multiple abscess formation. The human disease is believed to be transmitted from rats, either through fleas or through food contaminated with rat excreta.

CHAPTER 33

Gram-negative Rods: *Haemophilus*—*Haemophilus Influenzae*

LESSON PLAN

- Introduction
- *Haemophilus Influenzae*
  - Morphology
  - Culture—X and V Factors
  - Biochemical Reactions
  - Resistance
  - Antigenic Properties
  - Pathogenicity
  - Epidemiology
  - Laboratory Diagnosis
- *Haemophilus Aegyptius*
- *Haemophilus Ducreyi*

Genus—Haemophilus
Species—Haemophilus influenzae

INTRODUCTION

The genus *Haemophilus* contains small, non-motile, non-sporing, gram-negative bacilli that are parasitic in man or animals. They are characterized by their requirement of one or both of two accessory growth factors (X and V) present in blood (*Haemophilus* means blood loving). Since it was observed by Pfeiffer from sputum of patients of influenza it was called influenza bacillus.

Three species are pathogenic in man:
1. *Haemophilus influenzae* which is common in respiratory tract infections and sometimes causes meningitis, conjunctivitis or otitis media.
2. *Haemophilus aegyptius* (the Koch-Weeks bacillus) the cause of acute contagious conjunctivitis.
3. *Haemophilus ducreyi* which is the cause of venereal infection (chancroid or soft sore).

Other species are commonly commensal in the human mouth and throat and rarely cause opportunistic infections.

HAEMOPHILUS INFLUENZAE

Morphology

H. influenzae is a small (1.5 μ × 0.3 μ) gram-negative, non-motile, non-sporing bacillus showing a lot of pleomorphism (Fig. 33.1). In sputum, smears it is seen as clusters of cocco-bacillary forms whereas in CSF from meningitis cases, long bacillary and filamentous forms predominate. Strains from acute infections are capsulated.

Culture

The bacteria has fastidious growth requirements.
- The accessory growth factors (bacterial vitamins) named X and V present in blood are both essential for growth. The other species requiring both X and V factors are *H. aegyptius* and *H. haemolyticus*.

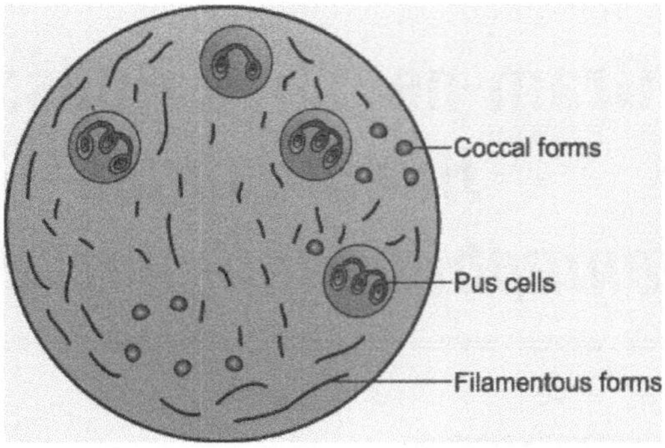

Fig. 33.1: *H. influenzae* showing pleomorphism in a CSF smear

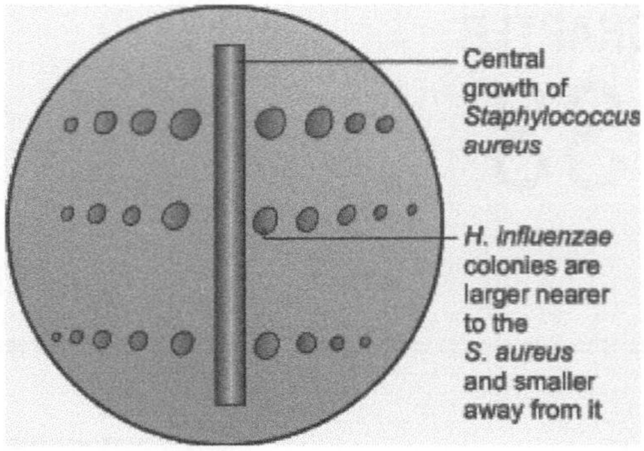

Fig. 33.2: Satellitism showing requirement of V factor by *Haemophilus influenzae*

- *What is X factor?* X factor is a heat stable iron porphyrin haematin. It is necessary for the synthesis of catalase, oxidase, peroxidase and other enzymes in aerobic respiration.
- *What is V factor?* V factor is heat labile factor present in red blood cells and in many animal and plant cells. It is made by some fungi and bacteria (e.g. *Staph. aureus*) in excess of their requirements and released into the surrounding medium. The V factor can be supplied as coenzyme I or II or nicotinamide adenine dinucleotide (NAD). It acts as a hydrogen acceptor in the metabolism of the cell.
- It is aerobic but grows anaerobically also, the optimum temperature is 37°C. Some strains require 10 percent CO_2.
- It grows on blood agar but growth is scanty as the V factor is not freely available being locked inside the red blood cells. Therefore, the V factor has to be supplied from outside. When *Staph. aureus* is streaked across a plate of blood agar on which a specimen containing *H. influenzae* is inoculated, after overnight incubation, the colonies of *H. influenzae* will be large and well-developed alongside the streak of *Staph. aureus* and smaller further away. This is called satellitism and demonstrates the dependence of *H. influenzae* on the factor that is available in higher concentration near the staphylococcal growth and only in smaller quantities away from it (V factor) (Fig. 33.2).
- Another way to obtain V factor is to prepare chocolate agar because the V factor is released from within the red blood cells and hence this media is superior to plain blood agar for growing *H. influenzae*.
- Clear transparent media may be prepared by boiling and filtering a mixture of blood and nutrient broth (Levinthal's medium) or by adding a peptic digest of blood to nutrient agar (Fildes agar).
- After 24 hours at 37°C, the colonies are usually 0.5 mm to 1 mm in diameter, circular, low convex smooth, pale grey and transparent. On Fildes agar they are transparent and have a slightly blue iridescence. In growth on most media they have a fishy, seminal smell.
- *H. influenzae* has often to be isolated from specimens such as throat swabs and sputum that yield a mixture of throat commensal bacteria liable to over grow and mask the haemophili. Growth of viridan's streptococci, neisseriae, diphtheroid bacilli, and albus staphylococci are suppressed on blood agar or heated blood agar containing 0.2 to 0.5 units/mL of penicillin or 5 to 19 units/mL of bacitrain. Filde's agar is also moderately selective.

Biochemical Reactions

Fermentation reactions are irregular. Indole, urease and ornithine are positive. Catalase and oxidase are positive.

Resistance

H. influenzae is a delicate bacterium readily destroyed by heating, refrigeration, drying or any disinfectant. In cultures, the cells die within two or three days due to autolysis. For preservation, chocolate agar slopes are used.

Antigenic Properties

Capsulated strains are classified by **Pittman** into 6 types (a–f) based on capsular antigens that are polysaccharide in nature and resemble pneumococcal capsular antigens. Type b strains account for most infections. Typing is done by agglutination, the Quellung test or by precipitation of the extracted polysaccharide with specific antisera.

Species of *Haemophilus*

1. *H. influenzae*	2. *H. aegyptius*
3. *H. suis*	4. *H. haemolyticus*
5. *H. ducreyi*	6. *H. aphrophilus*
7. *H. parainfluenzae*	8. *H. gallinarum*
9. *H. paragallinarum*	10. *H. parasuis*

Pathogenicity

H. influenzae stays in the human throat or nosopharynx. Sixty to eighty percent of healthy children carry the bacillus in the upper respiratory tract.

Diseases due to *H. influenzae* can be considered under two groups.

In one group—the bacillus acts as a primary pathogen causing suppurative infections, e.g. *Haemophilus* meningitis, laryngoepiglottitis, otitis media, pneumonia, arthritis, endocarditis and pericarditis. These infections are usually seen in children and are caused by capsulated strains, type b being responsible for most cases. In the second group, the bacillus causes secondary or superadded infections usually of the respiratory tract. These include chronic bronchitis, bronchiectasis and sinusitis. These are usually seen in adults and are caused by non-capsulated strains.

Epidemiology

Infection is transmitted by the respiratory route. Carriage in the upper respiratory tract is common but such strains are usually non-capsulated and not responsible for acute infections.

Immunity is type specific. As a large majority of infections are produced by type b strains, the possibility of active immunization by the specific capsular polysaccharide is being tried. A type b polysaccharide vaccine has been tried but due to poor immune reactions, the protection was incomplete. Cross-reactions have also been demonstrated.

Laboratory Diagnosis

1. In meningitis, the presence in the CSF of pleomorphic gram-negative bacilli that do not stain well should give suspicion of *H. influenza* infection. The finding of very large numbers of small gram-negative bacilli in a sputum Gram's stained smear should alert us for suspected haemophilus infection.
2. If type b antiserum is available, the Quellung phenomenon can be seen.
3. Capsular polysaccharide antigen may be present in CSF in meningitis and in urine in systemic infections. Its demonstration by precipitation or counterimmunoelectrophoresis with specific antiserum is useful in diagnosis.
4. For isolation, CSF should be plated on a suitable medium such as blood agar or chocolate agar and incubated in an environment containing 5 to 10 percent CO_2 and high humidity. A strain of staphylococcus should be streaked across the plate. After overnight incubation at 37°C, small opaque colonies appear that show satellitism.
5. Blood cultures are often positive in cases of laryngoepiglottitis and pneumonia.
6. Isolation from the sputum requires culturing several samples from the patient and also different parts of the sputum specimen.

HAEMOPHILUS AEGYPTIUS

Koch in 1883 observed a small bacillus in conjunctivitis cases in Egypt. It is worldwide in distribution and causes a highly contagious form of conjunctivitis (pink eye). It is especially common in the tropics and subtropics and may occur in epidemic forms.

HAEMOPHILUS DUCREYI

Ducrey in 1890 demonstrated this bacterium in chancroid lesions. Chancroid or soft sore is a venereal disease characterized by tender, non-indurated, irregular ulcers on the genitalia.

H. ducreyi is a short ovoid bacillus with a tendency to occur in end to end pairs or short chains. It is gram-negative and shows bipolar staining.

CHAPTER 34

Gram-negative Rods: Moraxellaceae—*Acinetobacter*

LESSON PLAN

- Introduction
- Morphology
- Culture
- Resistance
- Antibiotic Resistance
- Antigenic Properties
- Risk Groups
- Epidemiology
- Pathogenicity
- Laboratory Diagnosis
  - Sample
  - Microscopic Examination
  - Culture
  - Molecular Methods
- Transmission
- Treatment
- Prevention

Genus—Acinetobacter
Species—Acinetobacter baumanii

INTRODUCTION

The genus *Acinetobacter* is a group of gram-negative, non-motile and non-fermentative bacteria belonging to the family Moraxellaceae. 'Acineto' arrived from a Greek word 'Akineto' meaning 'non-motile'. Its natural habitats are water and soil, and it has been isolated from foods, arthropods, and the environment. In humans, *Acinetobacter* can colonize skin, wounds, and the respiratory and gastrointestinal tracts. Acinetobacter colonization is particularly common in patients who are intubated and in those who have multiple intravenous lines or monitoring devices, surgical drains, or indwelling urinary catheters.

There are at least 25 different types of Acinetobacter species. Based upon routine laboratory identification methods they are divided into three main complexes:

- *Acinetobacter calcoaceticus-baumanii complex*: Non-hemolytic
- *Acinetobacter lwoffii*: Non-hemolytic
- *Acinetobacter haemolyticus*: Non-hemolytic.

Acinetobacter calcoaceticus: *Acinetobacter baumannii* complex consists of the species *Acinetobacter calcoaceticus*, *A. baumannii*, genomic species 3, and genomic species 13TU which are genetically highly related and difficult to distinguish phenotypically. Except for *A. calcoaceticus*, all the other three are important nosocomial species. *Acinetobacter* species play a significant role in the colonization and infection of inpatients. Out of the two important species of Acinetobacter namely, *A. baumannii* and *A. lwoffii*, *Acinetobacter baumannii* accounts for more than 80% of isolates causing human disease and is often associated with hospital acquired infections.

MORPHOLOGY

The genus Acinetobacter consists of gram-negative bacilli or coccobacilli (1.5-2.5 um × 1.0–1.5 um), non-motile and non-sporing organisms. Acinetobacter infections have been clinically prominent in tropical countries. They have been a recurrent problem during wars and natural disasters, and have recently caused multihospital outbreaks in temperate climates.

CULTURE

- *Acinetobacter* grows easily on an ordinary media. They are aerobes and facultative anaerobes. They produce smooth, opaque, pale yellow to white-greyish colonies of 2-3 mm diameter on the solid medium.
- On MacConkey agar they produce colorless (non-lactose fermenting) colonies. They are often partially lactose fermenting.
- They are oxidase negative, catalase positive, nitrate negative and indole negative.
- *A. baumannii* strains oxidize and produce acid from glucose, xylose, galactose, manose, rhamnose and lactose.
- *A. lwoffii* produces smaller colonies on ordinary, non-pigmented mediums and does not oxidize glucose.

RESISTANCE

Some strains of *Acinetobacter* can survive environmental desiccation for weeks, a characteristic that promotes transmission through fomite contamination in hospitals. *A. baumannii* can survive on the human skin or dry surfaces for weeks. *Acinetobacter* is killed at 15 minutes of boiling or spraying with 70 percent ethanol.

Antibiotic Resistance

Members of the genus *Acinetobacter* have the ability to develop resistance to new antibiotics extremely rapidly. One such example is carbapenem resistant *Acinetobacter*. Multidrug resistance typically results from the accumulation of multiple mutations and/or the acquisition of resistance genes from other bacterial genera. This may occur by a variety of mechanisms, including the transfer of plasmids, transposons and integrons carrying clusters of genes encoding resistance to several unrelated families of antibiotics simultaneously. Multidrug resistant Acinetobacter are only sensitive these days to Colistin or Polymyxin. There is a danger of spread of antibiotic resistant *Acinetobacter* in Hospital settings.

ANTIGENIC PROPERTIES

Acinetobacter LPS (Lipo-polysaccharide) contains an O-polysaccharide chain (O-antigen). Elucidation of the chemical structure of several O-polysaccharides has revealed that they generally are branched and contain amino sugars. Thus, O-polysaccharide-specific monoclonal antibodies may serve as tools to discriminate *Acinetobacter* strains based on their O-antigens and to track clinically important groups.

RISK GROUPS

Acinetobacter poses very little risk to healthy people. However, people who have weakened immune systems, chronic lung disease, cancer, AIDS or diabetes may be more susceptible to infections with *Acinetobacter*. Hospitalized patients, especially very ill patients on a ventilator, patients with open wounds, burns, receiving broad-spectrum antibiotic treatment and prolonged hospital stay are also at greater risk for *Acinetobacter* infection.

EPIDEMIOLOGY

- Outbreaks of *Acinetobacter* infections, often caused by multiresistant strains, have been widely reported, commonly in intensive care units (ICUs) in North America and Europe.
- The *Acinetobacter* outbreaks that occurred between August 1999 and November 2001 in The Netherlands were caused by *A. baumannii* in seven hospitals and by *Acinetobacter* genomic species 13TU in one hospital. The overall impact of Acinetobacter on morbidity and mortality is not known, and crude mortalities have been found to fluctuate between 17 and 52 percent.

- A study was conducted in Jawaharlal Institute of Postgraduate Medical Education and Research (JIPMER) Hospital, Pondicherry, India for 24 months period (October 1998 to September 2000) on the admitted patients with *Acinetobacter* infections. It revealed that most of the infections were nosocomial, and majority of these were acquired in intensive care units (ICUs). *A. baumannii* accounted for 41.8 per cent of all pneumonia acquired in the ICU. It is also found that MDR *A. baumannii* is the species responsible for majority of the *Acinetobacter* outbreaks in the hospital and is also associated with high mortality. Other species such as A. lwoffii, A. junnii and *A. haemolyticus* are encountered as opportunistic pathogens among immunosuppressed patients.

PATHOGENICITY

Acinetobacter causes a variety of diseases, ranging from pneumonia to serious blood or wound infections and the symptoms vary depending on the disease.

Acinetobacter is a causative agent of nosocomial pneumonia, particularly ventilator-associated cases. Predisposing factors for nosocomial *Acinetobacter pneumonia* include endotracheal intubation, tracheostomy, previous antibiotic therapy, ICU residence, recent surgery and underlying pulmonary disease. Typical symptoms of pneumonia could include fever, chills, or cough. Acinetobacter may also "colonize" or live in a patient without causing infection or symptoms, especially in tracheostomy sites or open wounds. It can cause suppurative infections in virtually every organ system—meningitis, peritonitis, endocarditis and soft tissue infections.

LABORATORY DIAGNOSIS

Samples are obtained as per the infection suspected.

- In case of pneumonia, respiratory specimens should be obtained which includes endotracheal secretions, sputum, throat swabs, etc.
- Blood can be the collected for bloodstream infections.
- Midstream urine is the appropriate specimen in case of urinary tract infections.

Culture

Samples are processed for culture. Acinetobacter grows on routine laboratory media, including sheep blood agar: colony appears smooth, mucoid, and nonpigmented (yellowish to gray).

MacConkey's medium: Colonies are colorless (non-lactose fermenting) colonies or partially lactose fermenting.

Molecular Methods

Identification at the species level can be done by adapting molecular methods like PCR and DNA sequencing.

TRANSMISSION

Acinetobacter can be spread to high risk group persons by person-to-person contact or contact with contaminated surfaces.

TREATMENT

Acinetobacter is found to develop resistance against aminoglycosides, penicillin and chloramphenicol. Increasing resistance against floroquinolones and carbapenems in patients with prolonged treatment with broad-spectrum antibiotics is also reported. The drugs of choice may be ceftazidime, trimethoprim-sulfamethoxazole, colistin and polymyxin B that are still effective against nosocomial *Acinetobacter*.

In vitro susceptibility of multidrug resistant *Acinetobacter* to various synergistic combinations of antimicrobials including carbapenems, colistin, rifampin and ampicillin-sulbactam is also reported.

PREVENTION

Acinetobacter lives on the skin and may survive in the environment for several days. Hence, careful attention to infection control procedures such as hand hygiene, use of personal protective equipments (gloves, gown, mask, etc.) while handling patients and samples and environmental cleaning can reduce the risk of transmission.

CHAPTER

35

Spirochaetes—*Treponema Pallidum*

LESSON PLAN

- Introduction
- *Treponema Pallidum*
  - Morphology
  - Culture
  - Resistance
  - Antigenic Structure
  - Pathogenesis and Clinical Findings
  - Laboratory Diagnosis
  - Immunity
  - Treatment
  - Prevention
- Diseases Related to Syphilis
  - Bejel
  - Yaws
  - Pinta
- Other Spirochaetal Organisms
  - *Borrelia Recurrentis*
  - *Borrelia Burgdorferi*
  - *Leptospira*
- Fusospirochaetal Disease

INTRODUCTION

Spirochaetes are a large group of motile spiral organisms. They have an axial filament lying between the cell membrane and cell wall. This is formed from endoflagella and is responsible for movement. Three genera are pathogenic for humans:

Treponema—that causes syphilis, bejel, yaws and pinta.

Borrelia—that causes relapsing fever and Lyme's disease.

Leptospira—that causes leptospirosis (systemic infection with fever, jaundice and meningitis).

TREPONEMA PALLIDUM

Morphology

- Slender spirals measuring 0.2 μm in width and 5 to 15 μm in length. The spiral coils are regularly spaced at a distance of 1 μm from one another (Fig. 35.1).
- Organisms are actively motile, rotating steadily around their central axial filaments even when they are attached to cells.
- The organism so thin that it is not visible with an ordinary microscope.
- Immunofluorescence and dark field illumination microscopes are used to see it
- *Treponema pallidum* does not stain well with aniline dyes but it reduces silver nitrate to mettalic silver that is deposited on the surface so that treponemes can be seen in tissues (Levaditi's silver impregnation).
- Treponemes reproduce by transverse fission.

Culture

Treponema pallidum has never been cultured with certainity on artificial media, in fertile eggs or in tissue culture. Non-pathogenic treponemes (e.g. Reiter Strain) can be cultured anaerobically

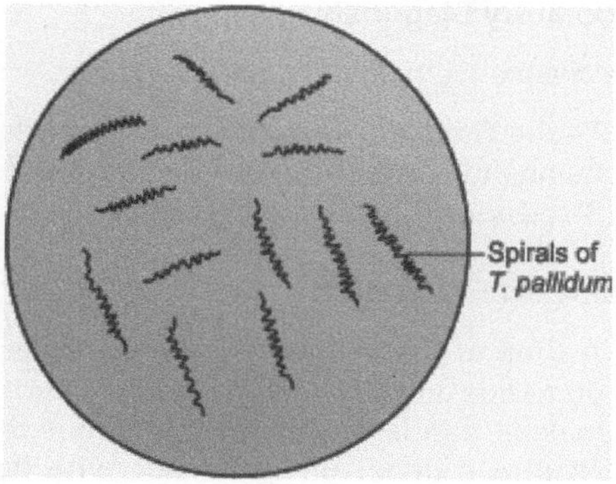

Fig. 35.1: Typical organisms of *T. pallidum* from tissue fluid in dark field microscopy

in vitro. They are saprophytes antigenically related to *T. pallidum*. They grow in a defined medium of 11 amino acids, vitamins, salts, minerals and serum albumin. In proper suspending fluids and in the presence of reducing substances, *T. pallidum* may remain motile for 3 to 6 days at 25°C. In whole blood or plasma stored at 4°C, organisms remains viable for at least 24 hours.

Resistance

- *T. pallidum* is very delicate and is killed by drying and raising the temperature to 41°C or 42°C.
- *T. pallidum* is inactivated by contact with oxygen, distilled water, soap, bismuth and common antiseptic agents and antibiotics.

Antigenic Structure

The antigens of *T. pallidum* have not been well-defined. Two main types of antibodies develop in the serum against *T. pallidum*:

1. Development of an antibody like substance reagin that gives positive complement fixation and flocculation tests with aqueous suspensions of lipids extracted from normal mammalian tissues. This antibody reacts in standard or non-specific serological tests for syphilis, such as Wassermann, Kahn and VDRL.
2. Anti-treponemal antibodies that can participate in indirect immunofluorescence and immobilize and kill live motile *T. pallidum*.

Pathogenesis and Clinical Findings

Acquired Syphilis

- Natural infection with *T. pallidum* is limited to the human host.
- Human infection is usually transmitted by sexual contact and the infectious lesion is on the skin or mucous membrane of genitalia. In 10 to 20 percent of cases, the primary lesion is intrarectal perianal or oral. It can be anywhere on the body.
- *T. pallidum* can probably penetrate intact mucous membranes or it may enter through a break in the epidermis.
- Spirochaetes multiply locally at the site of entry and some spread to nearby lymph nodes and then reach the bloodstream.
- In 2 to 10 weeks after infection, a papule develops at the site of infection and breaks down to form an ulcer with a clear hard base (hard chancre). The inflammation is characterized by a predominance of lymphocytes and plasma cells. This is called the primary lesion.
- Two to ten weeks later the secondary lesions appear. This consists of a red maculopapular rash anywhere on the body and moist pale papules (condylomas) in the anogenital region, axilla and mouth. Syphilitic meningitis, choreoretinitis, hepatitis, nephritis or periostitis may develop.
- The secondary lesions subside spontaneously. Both primary and secondary lesions are rich in spirochaetes and highly infectious. In some cases syphilitic infection may remain subclinical and the patient may pass through the primary or secondary stage without symptoms and signs and yet develop tertiary lesions.

- In about 30 percent of cases early syphilitic infection progresses spontaneously to complete cure without treatment.
- In another 30 percent, the untreated infection remains latent (serological tests are positive).
- In the remainder (40%) the disease progresses to the tertiary stage characterized by the development of granulomatous lesion (gum-mas) in skin, bones and liver, degenerative changes in the central nervous system (meningovascular syphilis) or cardiovascular lesions (aortitis, aortic aneurysm, aortic valve insufficiency). In all tertiary lesions, treponemes are very rare and hypersensitivity contributes to the tissue response. Occasionally treponemes may be found in the eye or CNS in tertiary syphilis.

Congenital Syphilis

A pregnant syphilitic woman can transmit *T. pallidum* to the fetus through the placenta in the 10th or 15th week of gestation. Some of the infected fetuses die and miscarriages result, others are stillborn at term. Some others are born live but develop signs of congenital syphilis in childhood.

These are:
- Interstitial keratitis
- Hutchinson's teeth
- Saddle nose
- Periostitis
- Central nervous system anomalies.

Adequate treatment of the mother during pregnancy prevents congenital syphilis. In congenital infection the child makes IgM anti-treponemal antibody.

Experimental disease: Rabbits can be experimentally infected in skin, testis and eye with human *T. pallidum*. The animal develops a chancre rich in spirochaetes and organisms persist in lymph nodes, spleen and bone marrow of the animal for the entire life.

Laboratory Diagnosis

Specimens

- Tissue fluid expressed from early surface lesions for demonstration of spirochaetes.
- Blood serum for serological reactions.

Dark Field Examination

- A drop of tissue fluid or exudate is placed on a slide and a coverslip pressed over it to make a thin layer. The preparation is then examined under oil-immersion with dark field illumination for typical motile spirochaetes. Treponemes disappear from lesions within a few hours after the beginning of antibiotic treatment.

Immunofluorescence

Tissue fluid or exudate is spread on a glass slide, air dried, and fixed. It is stained with a fluorescein labelled antitreponeme serum and examined by means of immunofluorescence microscopy for typical fluorescent spirochaetes.

Serological Tests for Syphilis (STS)

These use either treponemal or non-treponemal antigens.

Non-treponemal tests: The antigens employed are lipids extracted from normal mammalian tissue. The purified cardiolipin from beef heart is a diphosphatidylglycerol. To this are added sensitizers lecithin and cholesterol. This combined antigen can react with syphilitic reagin. Reagin is a mixture of IgM and IgA antibodies directed against some antigens widely distributed in normal tissues. It is found in patient's serum samples after 2 to 3 weeks of untreated syphilitic infection and in spinal fluid after 4 to 8 weeks of infection. Two types of tests are used to test for the reagin antibody.

- *Flocculation test* (VDRL–Venereal Disease Research Laboratories), RPR (Rapid Plasma Reagin). These tests are based on the principle that particles of the lipid antigen (beef heart cardiolipin) remain dispersed with normal serum but forms visible clumps when they combine with reagin more so if the suspension is agitated. Positive VDRL reverts to negative in 6 to 18 months after effective treatment of syphilis.

- *Complement fixation (CF) Wassermann, Test.*

Complement fixation tests are based on the principle that reagin containing sera fix complement in the presence of cardiolipin antigen.

Both the tests above can give quantitative results. We can perform dilution of the serum and express the titre as the highest dilution that gives a positive result.

Non-treponemal tests are subjected to false positive results. They can either be due to technical difficulties or biological false positives because of the presence of reagins in a variety of human disorders such as malaria, leprosy, measles, infectious mononucleosis, vaccinations, collagen vascular disease (SLE, polyarteritis nodosa, rheumatic disorders) and other conditions.

Non-treponemal antibody tests may become negative spontaneously in progressive tertiary syphilis. Thus, a negative VDRL does not rule-out disease activity.

Treponemal antibody tests: FTA (Fluorescent treponemal antibody).

A test employing indirect immunofluorescence (killed *T. pallidum* + patient's serum + labelled antihuman gammaglobulin) shows excellent specificity and sensitivity for syphilis. The presence of IgM-FTA in the blood of newborn is good evidence of *in utero* infection (congenital syphilis). This test is the most sensitive test for the diagnosis of syphilis.

TPI test: This test demonstrates *T. pallidum* immobilization (TPI) by specific antibodies in the patient's serum after the second week of infection. Dilutions of serum are mixed with the complement and with live actively motile *T. pallidum* extracted from the testicular chancre of a rabbit and the mixture is observed microscopically.

If specific antibodies are present, spirochaetes are immobilized. In normal serum active motion continues. The test requires live treponemes from infected animals. This is the most specific test for the diagnosis of syphilis.

Treponema pallidum haemagglutination assay (TPHA): Red blood cells are treated to adsorb treponemes on their surface. When mixed with serum containing antitreponemal antibodies, the cells become clumped. The test is similar to the FTA test in specificity and sensitivity but it becomes positive somewhat later in the course of infection.

VDRL and FTA can also be performed on spinal fluid. Antibodies do not reach the cerebrospinal fluid from the bloodstream. They are formed in the central nervous system in response to syphilitic infection.

Immunity

A person with active or latent syphilis or yaws appears to be resistant to superinfection with *T. pallidum*. However, if early syphilis or yaws is treated adequately and the infection is eradicated the individual again becomes fully susceptible. The various immune responses usually fail to eradicate the infection or arrest its progression.

Treatment

Penicillin is the drug of choice for treponemes.

Prevention

1. Prompt and adequate treatment of all discovered cases.
2. Follow-up on sources of infection and contacts.
3. Sex hygiene.
4. Prophylaxis—Mechanical prophylaxis (condoms) and chemoprophylaxis (penicillin after exposure).

DISEASES RELATED TO SYPHILIS

- These diseases are all caused by treponemes indistinguishable from *T. pallidum.*
- All give positive treponemal and non-treponemal serological tests for syphilis.
- None are sexually transmitted.
- All are commonly transmitted by direct contact.
- None of the causative organisms have been cultured on artificial media.

Bejel

Endemic syphilis:
- Syphilis transmitted non-venereally was endemic in many foci and was known by different names
- It has also been reported from India
- Disease is caused by *T. pallidum*
- It is common in young children
- No primary chancre seen
- Produces mucous patches and skin eruptions.

Yaws

Caused by *Treponema pertenue:*
- Occurs in hot, humid countries
- The primary lesion is an ulcerating papule
- Occurs usually on the arms or legs
- Transmission is by person to person contact in children less than fifteen years of age. Yaws represents a variant of syphilis adapted to transmission by non-sexual means.

Pinta

- It is caused by *Treponema carateum.*
- Disease appears to be restricted to dark skinned races.
- Occurs mostly in Mexico, Central and South America, Philippines, etc.
- The primary lesion is a non-ulcerating papule
- It occurs on exposed areas.
- Depigmentation and hyperkeratosis can take place after years.
- Pinta is transmitted by non-sexual means.

Rabbit Syphilis

Treponema cuniculi infection is a natural sexually transmitted infection of rabbits that produces minor lesions of the genitalia.

OTHER SPIROCHAETAL ORGANISMS

Borrelia Recurrentis

- It is an irregular spiral organism 10 to 30 µm long and 0.3 µm wide. The distance between turns varies from 2 to 4 µm.
- It causes relapsing fever. Relapsing fever is transmitted by ticks.

Borrelia Burgdorferi

- It causes Lyme's disease.
- The illness is named after the town of Lyme, Connecticut where a cluster of cases were identified.
- It is transmitted to humans by the bite of a small tick.
- The clinical illness involves a skin lesion and later arthralgia and neurological complications.
- Borrelia has been isolated from blood, cerebrospinal fluid and skin lesions.

Leptospira

Morphology

Tightly coiled, thin flexible spirochaetes. One end of the organism is often bent forming a hook. Very delicate spirochaete.

Culture

Leptospirae grow best under aerobic conditions at 28 to 30°C in protein-rich semisolid media (**Fletcher's**) where they produce round colonies (1 to 3 mm) in diameter in 6 to 10 days. Leptospirae also grow on chorioallantoic membranes of embryonated eggs.

Growth

Leptospirae derive energy from oxidation of long chain fatty acids.

Pathogenesis and Clincial Findings

The human infection is called Leptospirosis results usually from ingestion of water or food contaminated with leptospirae. Rarely the organisms may enter through mucous membranes or breaks in the skin. After an incubation period of one-to-two weeks there is a phase of fever during which leptospires are found in the blood. After this, they set up a multiorgan disease involving the liver, kidneys and meninges.

Diagnostic Laboratory Tests

- *Specimens*: — Blood
  — Serum
- *Microscopic examination*: Dark field examination of blood or thick smears stained by Giemsa technique often show leptospirae. Dark field examination of centrifuged urine may be positive.
- *Culture*: Whole fresh blood or urine can be cultured in Fletcher's semisolid or Tween 80 albumin medium. Growth is slow.
- *Animal inoculation*: Intraperitoneal inoculation of young hamsters or guinea pigs with fresh plasma or urine. Within a few days, spirochaetes become demonstrable in the peritoneal cavity. On the death of the animal (8 to 14 days) hemorrhagic lesions with spirochaetes are found in many organs.
- *Serology*: Agglutinating antibodies attaining high titres (1:10,000) or higher develop in leptospiral infection reaching a peak 5 to 8 weeks after infection. Leptospiral antibody can be detected by macroscopic agglutination of live organisms.

Passive hemagglutination of red blood cells with adsorbed leptospirae is sometimes used.

Treatment

In very early infection, antibiotics (doxycycline penicillin, etc.) has an effect.

Prevention and Control

The leptospiroses are essentially animal infections. Human infection is only accidental following contact with water or other materials contaminated with excreta of animal hosts. Rats mice, wild rodents, dogs and cattle are the principal sources of human infection.

Leptospirae remain viable in stagnant water for several weeks. Drinking, swimming, bathing or food contamination may lead to human infection.

FUSOSPIROCHAETAL DISEASE

A number of spirochaetes occur in every normal mouth, e.g. *Borrelia vincenti*. It is a motile spirochaete, easily stained with dilute carbol fuchsin and is gram-negative.

Under some adverse circumstances like injury to the mucous membranes of the mouth, nutritional deficiency or concomitant infection (e.g. with herpes simplex virus) of the epithelium, the normal spirochaetes of the mouth (*Borrelia vincenti*) together with anaerobic fusiform bacilli (fusobacteria) find suitable conditions for vast increase in numbers. When this occurs in ulcerative gingivostomatitis (trench mouth) it is called Vincent's stomatitis. When this type of process produces ulcerative tonsillitis and massive tissue involvement it is called Vincent's angina. In all these conditions necrotic tissue provides the anaerobic environment required by the fusospirochaetal flora. Antibiotics are given for treatment.

Section 4

Virology

- General Virology
- Specific Viruses
  - HIV
  - SARS
  - H1N1 Virus

VIROLOGY

INTRODUCTION

Viruses are tiny microorganisms that form the boundary between the living and the non-living microorganisms, and lack a cellular organization of their own. They are completely dependent on the host cell machinery for their survival and use it to their maximum advantage.

They are the cleverest of microorganisms, rapidly changing their appearance and eluding scientists. With the hunt for an ideal AIDS vaccine still going on, and the SARS virus epidemic recently, we are still far from understanding the complexities of the viruses. As of now, we have only half understood their mechanisms of survival, attack and defense. Viral research reveals new details every day and we hope that man will be able to control these small invaders in the near future.

As per the constraints of the MLT syllabus, two chapters have been included in this section. The first one deals with General Virology—the basic morphology, metabolism and replication of viruses as also their interaction with the human host.

The classification of the DNA and RNA viruses helps us to get a bird's eye view into the various viruses. The second chapter deals with HIV and AIDS which is of immense concern today. A small section has been added on the SARS virus as it is of current interest. The other viruses have not been taken up in detail keeping in mind the requirements of the MLT students.

In this second edition of the book a small chapter has been added about H1N1 as it started in 2009 and has been around for almost few years now.

CHAPTER

36

General Virology

LESSON PLAN

- Introduction
- General Properties of Viruses
- Morphology of Viruses
  - Size
  - Structure and Shape
  - Chemical Properties
- Resistance of Viruses
- Viral Multiplication
- Cultivation of Viruses
  - Animal Inoculation
  - Embryonated Eggs
  - Tissue Culture
- Detection of Growth of Viruses in the Cell Culture
- Classification of Viruses
  - DNA Viruses
  - RNA Viruses
- Laboratory of Viral Diagnosis Infections
- Virus-Host Interactions

INTRODUCTION

As we know, microorganisms are classified into eukaryotes and prokaryotes.

Eukaryotes include protozoa and fungi.

Prokaryotes include bacteria, mycoplasmas, rickettsiae and chlamydiae.

Viruses do not fall strictly into any category of microorganisms as they do not possess a cellular organization.

Definition of Viruses

Viruses are obligate intracellular parasites that do not have a cellular organization, and are totally dependent on their host cell for survival and multiplication.

GENERAL PROPERTIES OF VIRUSES

1. Viruses form the boundary between the living and non-living. Viruses are living chemicals.
2. They do not have a cellular organization.
3. They contain only one type of nucleic acid either DNA or RNA, never both.
4. They are obligate intracellular parasites.
5. They do not have any enzymes that are necessary for protein and nucleic acid synthesis and are dependent for replication on the host cells.
6. They multiply by a complex process and not by binary fission.
7. They are not affected by antibiotics.
8. As the smallest living units, viruses are the best models for understanding the chemistry of life.
9. Viral illnesses can be non-serious like common cold to highly fatal diseases like rabies or yellow fever.
10. Control of bacterial diseases has exposed the various viral infections present.
11. It is difficult to make drugs against viruses because they are intracellular.

12. It is difficult to make vaccines against viruses because their antigenic structure keeps on changing.

MORPHOLOGY OF VIRUSES

Size

The extracellular infectious virus particle is called virion.

They are too small to be seen under the light microscope. Viruses have different sizes:

The largest is poxvirus (300 nm) and the smallest virus is the foot-and-mouth disease virus (20 nm).

How Can we Measure the Size of the Virus?

1. Earlier membranes with pores were used which permitted the passage of the viruses and the pore diameter of the finest filter gave an estimate of the size of the virus.
2. The rate of sedimentation of a virus (using an ultracentrifuge) is dependent on its size and could provide indirect evidence of size.
3. Electron microscopy gives us an accurate idea.

Structure and Shape

The structure of the virus includes:

- Nucleocapsid
- Envelope.

Nucleocapsid

The virion consists of a nucleic acid core surrounded by a protein coat, the capsid. The capsid is made up of capsomeres. The capside with the enclosed nucleic acid is known as nucleocapsid (Fig. 36.1).

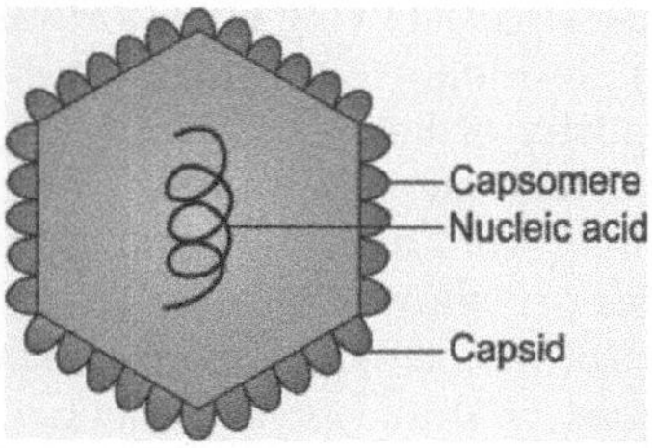

Fig. 36.1: Showing the viral nucleocapsid

Function of capsid

- The capsid is composed of a large number of capsomeres which form its morphological units.
- Chemical units of the capsid are polypeptide molecules which are arranged symmetrically to form a shell around the nucleic acid core.
- It protects the nucleic acid from inactivation by nucleases.
- It introduces the viral genome into host cells by adsorbing on to cell surfaces.

Envelope

- Virions may be enveloped or nonenveloped (naked). The envelope is the outer covering of the virus and is derived from the host cell membrane when the virus is released by budding. The envelope is lipoprotein in nature. Lipid is obtained from the host cell, while the protein is virus coded.
- The protein subunits project from the surface of the envelope. These structures are called peplomeres (may be one or greater than one).
- Function of the envelope is to give chemical, antigenic and biological properties to viruses. Enveloped viruses are susceptible to the action of lipid solvents like ether, chloroform and bile salts.
- Neutralization of virus infectivity depends on antibodies to the surface antigens.
- Biological properties such as hemagglutination depend on the envelope.

Shape of the virus is different in different groups of viruses. Most animal viruses are round, some are irregular and some are pleomorphic.

Rabies virus is bullet-shaped and Pox viruses are brick-shaped. TMV virus (Tobacco Mosaic Virus) is rod-shaped.

Chemical Properties

Viruses contain only one type of nucleic acid either single or double stranded DNA or RNA. No where in nature is genetic information solely carried by RNA as in some viruses.

Viruses also have protein which makes the capsid. Viral protein besides protecting the nucleic acid also determines the antigenic specificity of the virus.

Viruses do not have any enzymes for synthesis of viral components or for energy production but have other enzymes, e.g. neuraminidase and haemagglutinin found in influenza virus which serve as virulence factors.

RESISTANCE OF VIRUSES

With few exceptions, viruses are very heat sensitive. They are inactivated within seconds at 56°C, minutes at 37°C and days at 4°C.

They are stable at low temperatures. For long term storage they are kept frozen at-70°C. For prolonged storage, we use lyophilization or freeze drying (drying the frozen virus under vacuum). Some viruses (e.g. polio virus) do not stand freeze drying.

Inactivation of Viruses

Viruses are inactivated by heat, sunlight, UV rays and ionizing radiations.

Active antiviral disinfectants are hydrogen peroxide, potassium permanganate, hypochlorites, organic iodine compounds and chlorine.

Some viruses (e.g. hepatitis and polio viruses) are relatively resistant to chlorination.

Formaldehyde and Beta propiolactone are actively virucidal. Antibiotics are ineffective.

VIRAL MULTIPLICATION

The genetic information necessary for viral replication is contained in the viral nucleic acid but it does not have biosynthetic enzymes and so depends on the synthetic machinery of the host cell for replication (Fig. 36.2).

The viral multiplication cycle can be divided into six phases.

1. Adsorption or attachment.
2. Penetration.
3. Uncoating.
4. Biosynthesis.
5. Maturation.
6. Release.

Adsorption

The virus attaches to specific receptor sites on the host cell surface. Depending upon the presence or absence of receptors on host cells, the viruses differ in their susceptibility to cause disease.

Penetration

The whole virus cannot penetrate into bacterial cells and only the nucleic acid is introduced intracellularly by a complex mechanism. Animal cells do not have rigid cell walls and the whole virus can enter into them. Virus particles are engulfed by a mechanism like phagocytosis a process known as viropexis. Alternatively in the case of enveloped viruses, the viral envelope fuses with the plasma membrane of the host and releases the nucleocapsid into cytoplasm.

Uncoating

This is the process of stripping the virus of its outer layers and capsid so that the nucleic acid is released into the cell.

Biosynthesis

This phase includes synthesis of the viral nucleic acid, capsid protein and enzymes necessary in various stages of viral synthesis, assembly and release.

Also, certain regulator proteins are synthesized that shut down the normal cellular metabolism and direct the production of viral components.

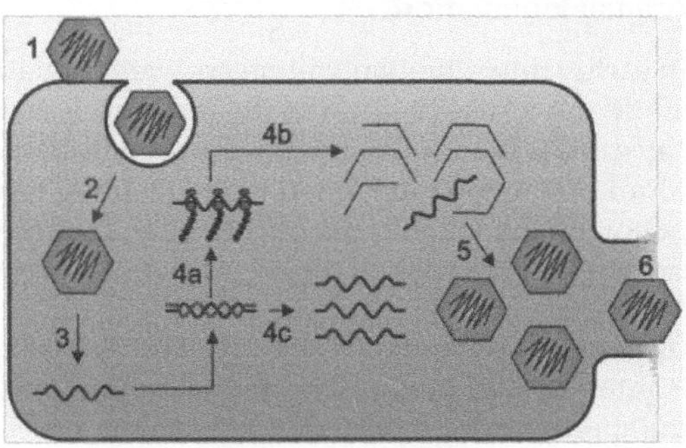

Fig. 36.2: (1) Adsorption, (2) Penetrations, (3) Uncoating, (4a to 4c) Biosynthesis, (5) Maturation, (6) Release

Steps of Biosynthesis

1. Transcription of mRNA from viral nucleic acid.
2. Translation of mRNA into early proteins. These are early or non-structural proteins which initiate and maintain synthesis of virus components. They may also induce shutdown of host protein and nucleic acid synthesis.
3. Replication of viral nucleic acid.
4. Synthesis of late or structural proteins which are the components of daughter virion capsids.

Maturation

Assembly of daughter virions occurs in the host cell nucleus or cyloplasm.

Envelopes are derived from the host cell membrane during the process of budding.

Release

In case of bacterial viruses, the release of virions takes place by the lysis of infected bacterium. But in the case of animal viruses, release usually occurs without cell lysis. An exception to this is the polio virus which is released by cell lysis.

CULTIVATION OF VIRUSES

As viruses are obligate intracellular parasites, i.e. they can only grow inside the cells, they require special techniques of cultivation. They cannot grow on any artificial culture medium. The methods commonly used are:

Animal Inoculation

In earlier times, human volunteers were used to study the viruses causing human diseases. But since this is harmful, animals were used instead. Monkeys were used for the isolation of the poliovirus by Landsteiner and Popper. But due to their cost and risk to handlers, monkeys find only limited use in virology. Mice are the most commonly used animals in diagnostic virology. Routes of inoculation can be subcutaneous, intraperitoneal or intranasal. Other animals such as guinea pigs, rabbits and ferrets can also be used. The growth of the virus may be indicated by death, disease or visible lesions.

The disadvantages of animal inoculation are that their immunity may interfere with viral growth. Also animals may have hidden viruses in them which may interfere with the growth of the desired virus.

Embryonated Eggs

The embryonated hen's egg was first used for the cultivation of viruses by Goodpasture in 1931 and the method was further developed by Burnet. The embryonated egg has several sites for the cultivation of viruses (Fig. 36.3).

Inoculation on the chorioallantoic membrane (CAM) produces visible lesions (pocks). Variola and vaccinia viruses also forms pocks.

Inoculation into the amniotic sac is used for the primary isolation of influenza virus. Yolk sac inoculation is used for the cultivation of some viruses, chlamydiae and rickettsia. Allantoic inoculation is employed for growing influenza virus for vaccine production. The vaccines prepared in the embryo are yellow fever, 17D strain and rabies (Flury strain).

Tissue Culture

Tissue culture means to culture the virus on live tissues. Steinhardt and his team used tissue culture in virology for the first time in 1913 when he maintained vaccinia virus in fragments of rabbit cornea. The discovery that poliovirus could be grown in a tissue culture of non-neural origin by Enders, Weller and Robbins in 1949 led to the cultivation of almost every virus in tissue culture.

Three types of tissue culture are available:

1. *Organ culture*: Viruses were grown in small bits of organ which could be maintained in vitro for days or weeks. Organ cultures are useful for the isolation of some viruses which appear to be highly specialized parasites of certain organs. Example: The tracheal ring organ culture is employed for the isolation of the coronavirus, a respiratory pathogen.

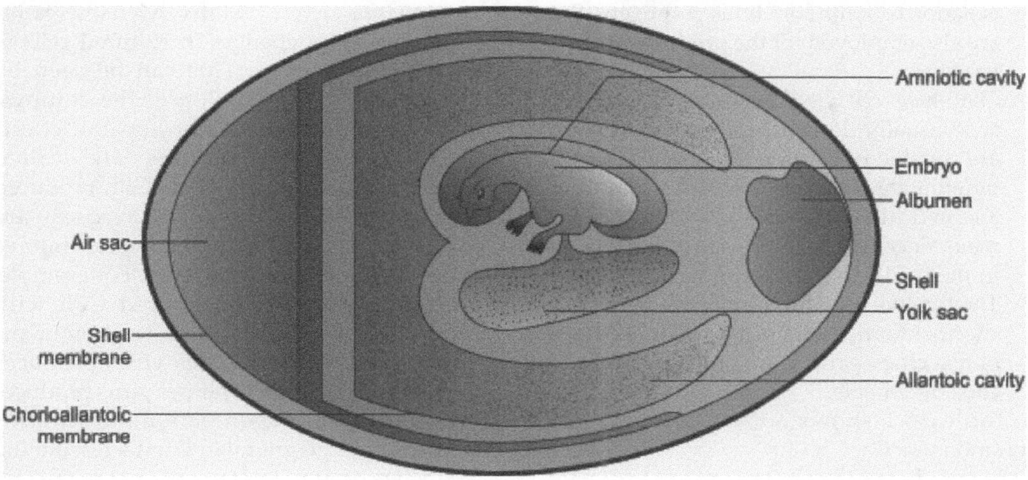

Fig. 36.3: The embryonated egg

2. *Explant culture*: Fragments of minced tissues can be grown as explants embedded in plasma clots. This method is not in use now.
3. *Cell culture*: This is the type of culture routinely employed for growing viruses. Tissues are broken down into component cells by the action of proteolytic enzymes such as trypsin and mechanical shaking. The cells are washed, counted and suspended in a growth medium.

The constituents of the growth medium are:
1. Thirteen essential amino acids.
2. Nine vitamins.
3. Salts.
4. Glucose.
5. Buffering system.
6. Five percent fetal calf serum.
7. Antibiotics are added to prevent the growth of contaminants.
8. Phenol red is an indicator.

This mixture is dispensed in bottles, tubes or petri dishes. The cells adhere to the glass surface and on incubation divide to form a confluent monolayer sheet of cells covering the surface within about a week. Most cell types multiply within 24 to 48 hours and form a sheet within a week.

Based on their origin, chromosomal characters and the number of generations through which they can be maintained, cell cultures are classified into three types.

a. *Primary cell cultures*: These are normal cells freshly taken from the body and cultured. They are capable of only limited growth in culture and cannot be maintained in serial culture. Examples:
   - Monkey kidney.
   - Human embryonic kidney.
   - Human amnion.
   - Chick embryo cell cultures.

   Primary cell cultures are useful for the isolation of viruses and their cultivation for vaccine production.
b. *Diploid cell strains*: These are cells of a single type that retain original diploid chromosome number and karyotype during serial sub-cultivation for a limited number of times. After about 50 serial passages they die. Diploid strains developed from human fibroblasts are susceptible to a wide range of human viruses and are very useful for the

isolation of some fastidious pathogens. They are also employed for the production of viral vaccines.

c. *Continuous cell lines*: These are cells of a single type usually derived from cancer cells that are capable of continuous serial cultivation indefinitely. Examples are HeLa, HeP-2, and KB cell lines. These cell lines can be maintained by serial sub-cultivation or stored in the cold (–70°C) for use when necessary. They are not used for the manufacture of viral vaccines for human use as the administration of vaccines grown in cancer cells is not considered safe.

Table 36.1 shows some cell cultures in common use.

Table 36.1: Some cell cultures in common use

a. *Primary cell cultures*	
1. Rhesus monkey kidney cell culture	
2. Human amnion cell culture	
3. Chick embryo fibroblast cell culture	
4. Human embryonic kidney cell culture	
b. *Diploid cell strains*	
1. WI-38	Human embryonic lung cell strain
2. HL-8	Rhesus embryo cell strain Foreskin fibroblasts cell strain
c. *Continuous cell lines*	
1. HeLa	Human carcinoma of cervix cell line
2. HeP-2	Human epithelioma of larynx cell line
3. KB	Human carcinoma of naso-pharynx cell line
4. McCoy	Human synovial carcinoma cell line
5. Detroit-6	Sternal marrow cell line
6. Chang C/I/L/K	Human conjunctiva (C) Intestine (I), Liver (L) and Kidney (K) cell lines
7. Vero	Veret monkey kidney cell line
8. BHK-21	Baby Hamster kidney cell line

DETECTION OF GROWTH OF VIRUSES IN CELL CULTURE

The growth of viruses can be detected by the following methods:

1. *Cytopathic effect*: Many viruses cause morphological changes in cultured cells in which they grow. This can be seen by microscopic examination of the cultures. These changes are called cytopathic effects (CPE) and the viruses are called cytopathogenic viruses. The CPE produced by different groups of viruses are characteristic and help in the presumptive identification of virus isolates. For example, enteroviruses produce rapid CPE with crenation of cells and degeneration of the entire cell sheet, measles virus produces syncytium formation, herpes virus produces discrete focal degeneration, adenovirus produces large granular clumps resembling bunches of grapes, etc.
2. *Metabolic inhibition*: In normal cell cultures, the medium turns acid due to cellular metabolism. When viruses grow in cell cultures, cell metabolism is inhibited and there is no acid production. This can be made out by the color of the indicator (phenol red) incorporated in the medium.
3. *Hemadsorption*: When hemagglutinating viruses (such as influenza and para-influenza viruses) grow in cell cultures, their presence can be indicated by the addition of guinea pig erythrocytes to the cultures. If the viruses are multiplying in the culture, the erythrocytes will adsorb on to the surface of the cells. This is known as hemadsorption.
4. *Interference*: The growth of a non-cytopathogenic virus in cell culture can be tested by the subsequent challenge with a known cytopathogenic virus. The growth of the first virus will inhibit infection by the second virus by interference.
5. *Transformation*: Tumor forming (oncogenic) viruses induce cell transformation and loss of contact inhibition so that growth appears in a piled-up fashion producing microtumors.
6. *Immunofluorescence*: Cells from virus infected cultures can be stained by fluorescent conjugated antiserum and examined under the UV microscope for the presence of virus antigen. This gives positive results faster.

CLASSIFICATION OF VIRUSES

I. Earlier viruses were named on the basis of the diseases they caused or the place from where they were isolated.
Dermotropic: Those viruses producing skin lesions, e.g. smallpox, chickenpox, measles.
Neurotropic Those viruses affecting the nervous system (poliomyelitis, rabies).
Pneumotropic: Those affecting the respiratory tract (influenza, common cold).
Viserotropic (those affecting visceral organs, e.g. yellow fever, hepatitis)

II. From the early 1950's viruses began to be classified in groups based on their physico-chemical and structural features. Now the classification of viruses is the official responsibility of the International Committee on Toxonomy of viruses. Viruses are classified into two main divisions depending on the type of nucleic acid they have:
Riboviruses are those containing RNA and Deoxyriboviruses are those containing DNA. Further classification is based on properties like symmetry of nucleocapsid, presence of envelope, size and shape of virion and number of capsomeres.

DNA Viruses

1. *Poxviridae Family*
   - Large brick-shaped virus or ovoid viruses.
   - They are enveloped.
   - Carry a single molecule of double stranded DNA.
   - The family includes the following important genera:
     - Orthopox virus (Variola, vaccinia).
     - Avipox virus (Fowl pox subgroup).
     - Capripox virus (Sheep pox subgroup).
     - Leporipox virus (Myxoma subgroup).
     - Entomopox virus (Insect poxvirus).
     - Parapox virus (Orf subgroup).
2. *Herpesviridae Family*
   - Medium-sized viruses.
   - Carry linear double stranded DNA.
   - They are enveloped.
   - Shape is icosahedral.
   - There is only one genus called herpes virus.
3. *Adenoviridae Family*
   - Medium sized viruses.
   - Carry single molecule of double stranded DNA.
   - Non-enveloped.
   - Icosahedral viruses.
   - Members have been classified into two genera.
     - Mastadenovirus (Mammalian adenovirus).
     - Aviadenovirus (Adenoviruses of birds).
4. *Papovaviridae Family*
   - Small viruses.
   - Carry double stranded DNA molecule.
   - Non-enveloped.
     - Two genera have been recognized-
     - Papillomavirus
     - Polyomavirus
5. *Parvoviridae Family*
   - Very small non-enveloped viruses.
   - They contain single stranded DNA molecule.
     - Three genera have been described.
     - Parvovirus
     - Adenosatellovirus
     - Densovirus
6. *Iridoviridae Family*
   - These are medium-sized enveloped viruses.
   - Carries a linear double stranded DNA.

RNA Viruses

1. *Picornaviridae Family*: These are small non-enveloped icosahedral viruses with single stranded RNA genome.
   Two genera have been seen.
   a. *Enterovirus*: This includes polio, coxsackie, echo and related viruses.
   b. *Rhinovirus*: This includes human, bovine and equine rhinovirus and foot-and-mouth disease virus.

2. *Orthomyxoviridae Family*
   - These are medium sized, spherical or elongated enveloped viruses carrying haemagglutinin and neuraminidase peplomers.
   - Genome consists of single stranded RNA in 8 pieces.
   - It has only one genus Influenza virus.
3. *Paramyxoviridae Family*
   - These are pleomorphic virions with lipid envelope having surface projections.
   - Genome is unsegmented single stranded linear DNA.

     Three genera have been recognized:

     Paramyxovirus—It consists of Newcastle disease virus.
   - Mumps virus.
   - Parainfluenza virus.
   - *Morbillivirus*—Contains measles and related viruses.
   - *Pneumovirus*—Contains respiratory syncitial virus.
4. *Togaviridae Family*
   - These are spherical viruses.
   - They have a lipoprotein envelope.
   - They have a single stranded RNA genome
   - Most members multiply in arthropods as well as vertebrates.

   Four genera have been described:
   - Alpha virus.
   - Flavivirus.
   - *Rubivirus*—consisting of rubella virus.
   - Pestivirus.
5. *Bunyaviridae Family*
   - These are spherical-enveloped virions.
   - All are arthropod borne viruses.
   - Only 1 genus *Bunyavirus* has been recognized.
6. *Arenaviridae Family*
   - These are spherical or pleomorphic viruses which contain a number of electron dense ribosome like particles giving a sandy appearance (Hence the name; arena meaning sand in Latin).
   - Members are generally rodent parasites causing persistent infection in the natural host but capable of infecting man rarely leading to severe haemorrhagic illness.
   - Only 1 genus—*Arenavirus* has been recognized. Species include lymphocytic cho-riomeningitis virus and Lassa virus.
7. *Rhabdoviridae Family*
   - These are bullet-shaped virus.
   - They are enveloped.
   - This includes two genera.
     - *Vesiculovirus*—containing vesicular stomatitis virus, Chandipura virus, etc.
     - *Lyssa virus*—containing rabies virus and related viruses.
8. *Reoviridae Family*
   - Icosahedral non-enveloped viruses 60 to 80 nm in size and has double layered capsid.
   - Genome consists of double stranded RNA in 10 to 12 pieces. Three genera have been recognized.
   - *Reovirus*
   - *Orbivirus*
   - *Rotavirus*
9. *Coronaviridae Family*
   - Pleomorphic enveloped viruses with unique club-shaped peplomers projecting as a fringe from the surface resembling the solar corona.

     Only 1 genus *Coronavirus* has been recognized. Members include human corona viruses causing respiratory disease.
10. *Retroviridae Family*
    - These are RNA tumor viruses.
    - They are enveloped.
    - Virions are icosahedral with lipoprotein envelopes.
    - It has RNA dependent DNA polymerase (reverse transcriptase) within the virus. Three subfamilies are recognized.

      Oncovirinae—the RNA tumor virus group.

      Spumivirinae—the foamy virus group.

      Lentivirinae (Lenti-slow) Visna and maedi viruses of sheep belonging to the slow virus group. AIDS virus belongs to this group.

11. *Calciviridae*—These are naked spherical particles which are non-enveloped.

Unclassified Viruses

Some viruses have not been classified yet as sufficient data is not available. Examples include hepatitis viruses (type A which may be a picornavirus and type B which may belong to a new family Hepadnaviridae and some viruses causing slow infections.

LABORATORY DIAGNOSIS OF VIRAL INFECTIONS

Laboratory diagnosis of viral infections is difficult because:

1. There are technical difficulties in isolation of virus.
2. It is time consuming and expensive.

But recently, with the development of rapid techniques of diagnosis of many virus infections, diagnostic virology is becoming easier.

Diagnosis in virology as to which virus has caused the infection is important in certain cases

1. For treatment of rubella in pregnant women.
2. For early specific therapy as in herpetic lesions of the eye.
3. To define upper respiratory tract infection
4. For the detection and prediction of epidemics and the identification of antigenic variation in viruses.
5. To diagnose and control outbreaks.

For good diagnosis of viral infections we should collect proper specimens. The various samples collected are as follows (Table 36.2).

The following methods are used for the diagnosis of viral diseases:

1. Microscopic demonstration of the virus or its inclusion body.
2. Demonstration of virus antigen.
3. Isolation and identification of the virus.
4. Detection of specific antibody.

Table 36.2: Types of specimens to be sent for virus diagnosis

System	*Specimens required*		
	For isolation	For direct examination	For serology
Respiratory	Throat swab, nasopharyngeal aspirates	Nasopharyngeal aspirate (IF) [throat washings (EM)]	Paired sera
Central nervous system	Faeces, blood (for arbovirus isolation), CSF (brain biopsy, throat swab, rectal swab)	Brain biopsy (IF and EM); CSF (EM and IF) corneal impression smears IF[3]	Paired sera
Cardiovascular system	Feces	Nil	Paired sera
Skin	Macular/papular scrapings, vesicular/pustular fluid, ulcer scrapings, crust, feces, throat swab	Vesicular/pustular fluid (EM and ID), Ulcer scrapings (EM), crusts (EM and ID)	Paired sera
Eye	Conjunctival scrapings or swabs	Conjunctival scrapings, as smears on microscope slides (LM and IF)	Paired sera
Liver	Blood (for yellow fever)	Serum (faeces)	Serum
General; congenital infections	Throat swab (products of conception)	Nil	Single sera (mother and baby)
General; PUO	Heparinized blood (arbovirus and arenavirus infections) throat swabs, feces (fresh urine)	Nil	Paired sera

Microscopy

- The detection of the rotavirus by electron microscopy is being used to diagnose viral diarrheas.
- Demonstration of inclusion body is a routine diagnostic method for rabies in dogs. Inclusion bodies are structures with distinct size, shape, location and staining properties that can be demonstrated in virus infected cells under the light microscope.

  They may be present in the cytoplasm (e.g. poxviruses), nucleus (herpes virus) or both (measles virus). The inclusion bodies are acidophilic and can be seen as pink structures when stained with Giemsa's or eosin methylene blue stains. Demonstration of inclusion bodies helps in the diagnosis of viral infections. The presence of intracytoplasmic eosinophilic inclusions (negri bodies) in the brain cells of animals suggests rabies. Inclusion bodies may be crystalline aggregates of virions or made up of virus antigens present at the site of virus synthesis. Some inclusions represent degenerative changes produced by virus infection which give altered staining properties.

  Direct and indirect fluorescent antibody techniques are used to diagnose diseases such as rabies.

Demonstration of Viral Antigen

In cases where virus antigen is abundant in the lesions, its demonstration by serological methods such as precipitation in gel or immunofluorescence offers a rapid method of diagnosis. Other tests are counter immunoelectrophoresis, radioimmunoassay and enzyme linked immunosorbent assay.

Isolation of Virus

Isolation of virus can be used as a diagnostic technique if the laboratory set up permits. The specimens should be properly collected. As most viruses are heat-labile, refrigeration is very important during transport. The viruses are inoculated into animals, eggs or tissue culture after the specimen is processed to remove bacterial contaminants. The results of isolation are interpreted along with clinical data.

Serological Diagnosis

The demonstration of a rise in titer of antibodies against a virus antigen during the course of disease indicates that the virus is the causative agent. For this it is important to examine paired sera. The acute sample is collected early in the course of the disease and the convalescent sample collected 10 to 14 days later.

Examination of a single sample of serum for antibodies may not be meaningful.

The serological techniques would depend on the virus but those in general use are neutralization, complement fixation, ELISA and hemagglutination inhibition.

Drugs Against Viruses

As viruses are strict intracellular parasites, we cannot use drugs that damage the host cell as well. But it is now known that there are many target areas available for attack on viruses. Viral infection may be checked at the level of:

1. Attachment.
2. Transcription of viral nucleic acid.
3. Translation of viral mRNA.
4. Replication of viral nucleic acid.
5. A number of virus specific enzymes have been identified which can be inhibited selectively thereby preventing viral multiplication without affecting the host cells.

   Interferon is able to differentiate between viral and cellular mRNA.

   There are effective drugs against viruses.

VIRUS-HOST INTERACTIONS

Pathogenesis of Virus Infection

Depending on the clinical features, virus infection may be classified as:

a. Inapparent (subclinical).
b. Apparent (clinical or overt).

Clinical infections may be acute, subacute or chronic. Some virus infections are latent. Recurrent herpes simplex and herpes zoster are examples of latent infections in which the clinical manifestations appear after a long time during which the virus remains hidden in the nerve root ganglia. The viruses which cause tumors also belong to this group.

Entry of the virus into the body.

Viruses enters the body through any of the following routes:
1. Respiratory tract.
2. Alimentary tract.
3. Skin.
4. Conjunctiva.
5. Genital tract.

The respiratory tract offers the most important portal of entry for viruses. Examples are small pox and chickenpox, influenza and rhinovirus. The alimentary tract is another important route of entry. Enteroviruses, adenoviruses, reoviruses, hepatitis virus and viruses causing gastroenteritis are able to set up intestinal infection. Some remain confined to the gut causing local disease. Others are transported to further sites of multiplication. Of the viruses that enter through the skin, only a few produce local lesions. The examples of viruses that produce dermal lesions are papilloma, vaccinia, cowpox, molluscum contagiosum, and orf.

Conjunctiva may also act as a portal of entry for viruses. This may lead to local disease (e.g. adenovirus) or to systemic spread (e.g. measles). Some viruses (e.g. herpes virus) may enter through the genital tract.

Spread of Viruses in the Body

The virus after entering into the body multiplies at site of entry and then goes along the lymphatics to the local nodes. After multiplication in the lymph nodes the virus enters the bloodstream (primary viremia) and is transported to the spleen and liver which act as central foci for viral multiplication. After extensive multiplication in the central foci virus reenters into the blood stream which is secondary viremia. This starts the onset of clinical symptoms and forms the prodromal phase. Then the virus reaches the target organs (skin in eruptive fevers) through the blood stream (Fig. 36.4). This Figure shows the spread of the virus in the body.

What is Incubation Period?

The incubation period is the time taken for the virus to spread from the site of entry to the organs of viral multiplication and then to the target

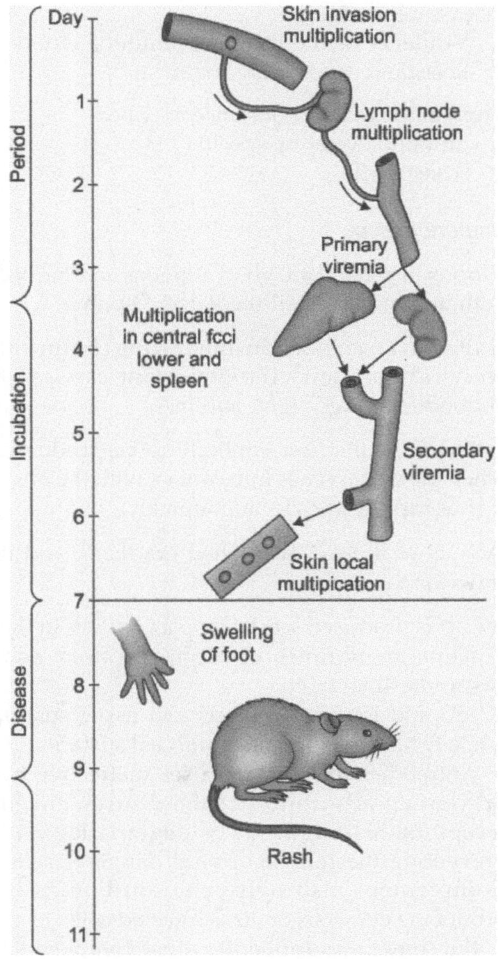

Fig. 36.4: Spread of viruses in the body

organs for the production of lesions. When the site of entry and site of lesion are the same, the incubation period is short, e.g. 1 to 3 days as in respiratory virus infection and in gastroenteritis. In systemic diseases where the virus enters through the respiratory and alimentary tracts and produces lesions in remote target sites the incubation period is long, e.g. 10 to 20 days as in smallpox or chickenpox.

Host Response

Whether a virus infection would produce clinical disease depends on:
1. Virulence of the infecting strain of virus.
2. Resistance offered by the host.

Mechanism of host resistance may be:
1. Immunological or specific
2. Nonspecific.

Immunological

Virions in general are good antigens and induce both humoral and cell-mediated response.

Humoral responses: In mediating humoral antiviral immunity the important classes of antibodies are IgG, IgM, and IgA.

IgM: This is the first antibody to be produced when the virus comes into contact with the host. It rises rapidly and declines quickly.

IgG: Its peak level is reached gradually and it stays for a long time.

IgA: It is produced locally by plasma cells in the mucous membranes of the respiratory and gastrointestinal tract.

IgG and IgM act in blood and tissue spaces while IgA is active against mucosal surfaces.

Antibodies make the viruses ineffective by preventing adsorption of the viruses to cell receptors, helping in virus degradation and preventing the release of viral daughter cells. Complement also helps the antibodies in producing cytolysis of virus infected cells.

But sometimes antibodies cause complement dependent damage. In infancy, the respiratory syncytial virus infection is more severe due to the presence of passively acquired maternal antibodies. In older children who have no antibody the virus causes a milder disease.

Cell-mediated immune response: This immunity is considered to play a major role in recovery from viral infections due to viruses that do not have a prolonged phase of viraemia.

Duration of Immunity: A prolonged immunity is characteristic of infections where there is an extensive viraemic phase and where the virus is antigenically stable. In infections such as measles, mumps, varicella, smallpox and yellow fever, the immune state persists for many years and second attacks of these diseases are extremely rare.

Limited immunity occurs where there has been no phase of viraemia and when there are frequent variations in the antigenic structure of the virus.

Nonspecific Responses

Phagocytosis: Polymorphonuclear leucocytes do not play any significant role in defense against virus infections. In fact more viral infections show leukopenia. Macrophages phagocytose viruses and are important in clearing viruses from the blood stream.

Body temperature: Fever acts as a natural defense mechanism against virus infections as most viruses are inhibited by temperatures above 39°C.

Hormones: Corticosteroids enhance most virus infections because they depress the immune response and inhibit interferon synthesis.

Malnutrition: Some virus infections such as measles produce a much higher incidence of complications and a higher case fatality rate in malnourished children than in well-fed patients.

Age: Most viral infections are more common and more dangerous at the two extremes of age.

Interferon: It was discovered by Isaacs and Lindenmann.

Interferons are glycoproteins produced by cells on induction by viral or non-viral inducers which make cells refractory to viral infection, i.e. they cannot be infected by the virus.

This is because on exposure to interferon, cells produce a protein [(translation inhibiting protein TIP)] which inhibits translation of viral mRNA without affecting cellular mRNA. It also inhibits viral transcription.

Properties of Interferons

- Interferons are species specific i.e. interferon produced by one species can protect only cells of the same or related species against viral infections.
- Activity of interferon is not virus specific.
- Viruses vary in their susceptibility to interferon.
- Viruses vary in their capacity to induce interferon.
- Interferon production is increased by increasing the temperature, and is inhibited by steroids.
- Interferons are divided into three types: alpha, beta and gamma.

  Alpha interferon (IFN) is produced by B lymphocytes or macrophages on stimulation by suitable viruses.

  Beta interferon is produced by fibroblasts or epithelial cells on stimulation by viruses or polynucleotides.

  Gamma interferon is produced by T lymphocytes on stimulation by antigens or mitogens.
- Many properties of interferons make it a very good candidate for use in the treatment of viral infections. It is non-toxic, non-antigenic and diffuses freely in the body; It has a very wide spectrum of antiviral activity. The only drawback initially was its species specificity so that interferon produced by non-human cells was not clinically useful. Interferon is produced from buffy coat and leukocytes from blood bank using viral inducers.
- Although interferon was originally thought of as an antiviral agent it influences many other functions like humoral and cellular immunity, phagocytosis and antitumor activity.

Local application of high doses of interferon show some benefit against upper respiratory infections, limited success against herpes infection and some results as an anticancer agent.

CHAPTER

37

Specific Viruses

LESSON PLAN

HUMAN IMMUNODEFICIENCY VIRUS

INTRODUCTION

AIDS means acquired immune deficiency syndrome caused by *Human Immunodeficiency virus (HIV)*. In this disease syndrome, there is a deficiency in the immune system of the individual due to which he becomes very susceptible to infections with relatively less virulent microorganisms and can die because of these infections. This deficiency is acquired and not present since birth so it is named acquired immune deficiency. These individuals also become more susceptible to lymphoid and other malignancies.

AIDS is increasing at a very rapid pace and it is a great challenge for doctors, scientists and public health workers.

It was in the summer of 1981 that the first indication of this syndrome came from New York and California. There was a sudden increase in the incidence of two very rare diseases—Kaposi's sarcoma and *Pneumocystis carinii* pneumonia in young adults who were homosexuals or addicted to heroin or other infected narcotics. They lost their ability to fight microorganisms. This condition was found in some hemophiliacs, sexual partners of patients and babies born to infected women. The syndrome was given the name acquired immune deficiency syndrome and was thought to be transmitted by sexual contact or transfer of blood or other body fluids.

Then began the search for the aetiological agent. Luc Montagnier in 1983 isolated a retrovirus from a West African patient with persistent generalized lymphadenopathy and called it the lymphadenopathy associated virus (LAV). In 1984, Robert Gallo and colleagues from the National Institute of Health, USA reported isolation of a retrovirus from AIDS patients and called it the human T cell lymphotropic virus-III (HTLV-III). Other similar isolates from AIDS cases were reported. Serological analysis and molecular coning established the common origin of these viruses and in 1986 the International Committee on Virus Nomenclature decided on the name *Human Immunodeficiency Virus (HIV)* for these viruses.

In 1984, the 1st serological test became available for detection of anti HIV antibodies. Serological screening of high risk groups, revealed a very large reservoir of HIV in patients and carriers all over the world.

STATISTICS

World

The true statistical figures of AIDS cannot be known because of the gross under reporting. Till the end of 2002 there were an estimated 42 million people living with the AIDS virus worldwide, with 2,201461 confirmed AIDS cases. In 20 years AIDS has killed 22 million people. Out of a total of 42 million, 3.2 million are less than 15 years and 19.2 million are women. The total number of people newly infected with HIV in the year 2002 was 5 million out of which 4.2 million were adults and 0.8 million were children less than 15 years of age. Of the 4.2 million, 2 million were women. The total number of deaths due to AIDS in the year 2002 was 3.1 million with women comprising 1.2 million and children (less than 15 years of age) 610,000.

In 1995 women represented only 7 percent of new AIDS cases and in 2000 women represented 24 percent of new cases.

Although much progress has been made in stemming the tide of the pandemic, the fact remains that, according to the United Nations, approximately 33 million people worldwide are living with HIV. Women and girls still account for nearly 60% of these worldwide, and in some regions, girls aged 15–24 years are infected at a rate five times higher than boys. Only 28% of pregnant women in sub-Saharan Africa receive

HIV testing, and only 45% of HIV-infected mothers and 32% of infants receive ART to prevent mother-to-child transmission (Table 37.1).

Note

- Adults are defined as men and women aged 15 or above, unless specified otherwise.
- Children orphaned by AIDS are defined as people aged under 18 who are alive and have lost one or both parents to AIDS.
- All the statistics on this page should be interpreted with caution because they are estimates.

India

The HIV/AIDS epidemic represents the most serious public health problem in India. HIV is prevalent in all parts of the country with over 3.8 million Indians infected with the virus, including 1.5 million women. The prevalence rate is reported to be 0.7 percent. This figure could be low due to under reporting. Ninty percent of the patients are in the 15 to 44 age group. Eighty five percent of the infections are from the sexual route, 4 percent from blood transfusion and 7 percent through injecting drug abuse. There are a total number of 42,947 cases reported of which females are 10786. One in every four cases reported is a woman.

The first AIDS case was reported in Delhi in 1998. Till April 2002 nearly 182 people have died of AIDS. The states very heavily infected are Maharashtra, Tamil Nadu and Manipur which make up 75 percent of the total infections in the country. The Delhi State AIDS control society is working hard to reduce the rate of transmission in AIDS.

There are five components for the control of AIDS:

- Awareness of STD/HIV/AIDS.
- Treatment of STD.
- Promotion and distribution of condoms.
- Counseling.
- Creating an environment in which awareness can be spread.

It takes the help of NGO's who work with street children, sex workers, truck drivers, migrant laborers, and intravenous drug users, etc. They provide information on various aspects of HIV/AIDS. (Eleven) STD clinics are functioning in Delhi to provide medicines and checkup. A school AIDS awareness program has been developed. To reduce transmission of HIV through blood, several steps have been taken to modernize the blood banks for effective quality control. Training for doctors has been done.

In 2006 UNAIDS estimated that there were 5.6 million people living with HIV in India, which indicated that there were more people with HIV

Table 37.1: Regional statistics for HIV and AIDS at 2008 year end by UNAIDS

Region	*Adults and children living with HIV/AIDS*	*Adults and children newly infected*	*Adult prevalence**	*Deaths of adults and children*
Sub-Saharan Africa	22.4 million	1.9 million	5.2%	1.4 million
North Africa and Middle East	310,000	35,000	0.2%	20,000
South and South-East Asia	3.8 million	280,000	0.3%	270,000
East Asia	850,000	75,000	<0.1%	59,000
Oceania	59,000	3900	0.3%	2,000
Latin America	2.0 million	170,000	0.6%	77,000
Caribbean	240,000	20,000	1.0%	12,000
Eastern Europe and Central Asia	1.5 million	110,000	0.7%	87,000
North America	1.4 million	55,000	0.4%	25,000
Western and Central Europe	850,000	30,000	0.3%	13,000
Global Total	33.4 million	2.7 million	0.8%	2.0 million

* Proportion of adults aged 15–49 who were living with HIV/AIDS

in India than in any other country in the world. In 2007, following the first survey of HIV among the general population, UNAIDS and NACO agreed on a new estimate—between 2 million and 3.1 million people living with HIV.

In 2008 the figure was confirmed to be 2.5 million, which equates to a prevalence of 0.3%. While this may seem a low rate, because India's population is so large, it is third in the world in terms of greatest number of people living with HIV. With a population of around a billion, a mere 0.1% increase in HIV prevalence would increase the estimated number of people living with HIV by over half a million.

The national HIV prevalence rose dramatically in the early years of the epidemic, but a study released at the beginning of 2006 suggests that the HIV infection rate has recently fallen in southern India, the region that has been hit hardest by AIDS. In addition, NACO released figures in 2008 suggesting that the number of people living with HIV has declined.

The average HIV prevalence among women attending antenatal clinics in India is 0.48%. Much higher rates are found among people attending STD clinics (3.6%), female sex workers (5.1%), injecting drug users (7.2%) and men who have sex with men (7.4%). NACO has not produced estimates of the number of people living with AIDS and the number of people who have died from AIDS, for some time. Some of the last figures produced were from 2005, that showed that by the end of 2005 the total number of reported AIDS cases in India was 116,905, of which 34,177 were women. Around a third of these were among people younger than 30 years.

Note: These figures significantly under-represent the actual number of people living with AIDS. Many AIDS deaths go unreported in India, due to unprecedented levels of stigma and discrimination. In many situations a patient dies without HIV having been diagnosed, and with the death attributed to an opportunistic infection, such as tuberculosis.

Virus

HIV, the causative agent of AIDS belongs to the lentivirus subgroup of the family Retroviridae. Retroviruses are those viruses which have a RNA dependent DNA polymerase (reverse transcriptase) in them.

Retroviruses are divided into three subgroups:

I. *Spumiviruses*—Foamy viruses found in primary cell culture not associated with disease.
II. *Oncoviruses*—RNA tumor viruses.
III. *Lentivirus.*
   a. Causing degenerative neural disease in animals.
   b. Causing immunodeficiency.
      1. HIV
      2. Simian immunodeficiency virus
      3. Feline T lymphotropic virus causing feline AIDS.

Structure

- HIV is an enveloped virus, 90 to 120 nm in diameter (Fig. 37.1).
- It has a nucleoprotein core containing single stranded RNA genome and proteins.
- In association with the viral RNA is the reverse transcriptase enzyme. When the virus infects a cell, the viral RNA is transcribed by the enzyme, first into single stranded DNA and then into double stranded DNA (**provirus**), which is integrated into the host cell chromosome. The provirus can remain latent for long periods but sometimes in response to viral promoters the provirus initiates viral replication by directing synthesis of viral RNA and other components.
- The virus core is surrounded by a protein shell.
- During viral replication when the naked virus buds out through the host cell surface membrane it acquires a lipoprotein envelope which consists of lipid derived from host cell

membrane and glycoproteins which are virus coded. The major virus coded envelope proteins are the projecting spikes on the surface and the anchoring transmembrane pedicles. The spikes constitute the major surface component of the virus which binds to the CD4 receptors on susceptible host cells.

Viral Genes and Antigens

The genome of HIV contains the three structural genes (gag, pol, and env) which is characteristic of all retroviruses and other non-structural and regulatory genes specific for the virus. The product of these genes act as antigens. Sera of infected persons contain antibodies to them. Detection of these antigens and antibodies is of great value in diagnosis and prognosis of HIV infections. Table 37.2 shows the major antigens of HIV.

The principal core antigen is p24 which can be detected in serum during the early stages of HIV infection before antibodies appear.

The *gag gene* **determines the core and shell of the virus.** It is expressed as a precursor protein p55. The proteins and glycoproteins are indicated by their mass expressed in kilo Daltons.

This protein is broken down into:

p55 → p15, p18, p24

The env gene determines the synthesis of envelope glycoprotein. It is expressed as the precursor glycoprotein gp160 which is cleaved into two envelope components gp120, which forms the surface spikes and gp41 which is the transmembrane anchoring protein.

The spike glycoprotein gp120 is the major envelope antigen and antibodies to gp120 are the first to appear after infection.

The *pol gene* codes for the polymerase reverse transcriptase and other viral enzymes. It is expressed as a precursor protein p100 which is cleaved into p31, p51 and p64.

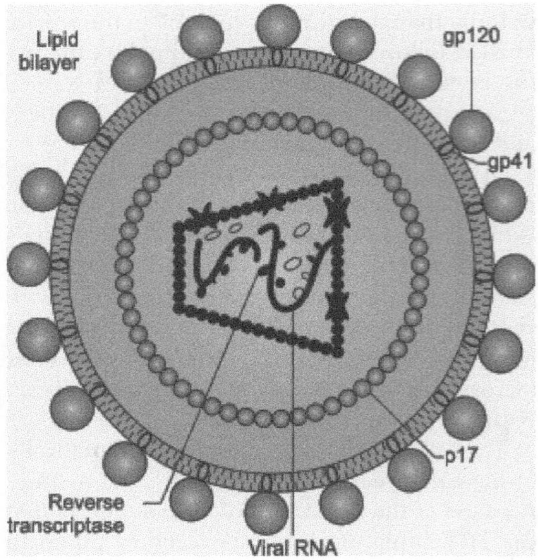

Fig. 37.1: Structure of HIV (a diagrammatic representation) A cross-section

Table 37.2: Major antigens of HIV
A. Envelope antigens.
1. Spike antigen-gp120 (principal envelope antigen).
2. Transmembrane pedicle protein gp41.
B. Shell antigen.
1. Nucleocapsid protein p18.
C. Core antigens.
1. Principal core antigen-p24.
2. Other core antigens-p15, p55.
D. Polymerase antigens-p31, p51, p64.

Types of HIV Virus

Two distinct antigenic types of HIV have been identified. HIV-1 is the original isolate and related isolates from America, Europe and other Western countries. HIV-2 represents isolates obtained in 1985 from West Africa which are only weakly reactive with HIV-1 antisera. HIV-2 is more closely related to Simian immunodeficiency viruses (SIV) than to HIV-1.

Cell Tropism

The receptor for the surface spike protein of HIV is the CD_4 antigen and hence the virus may infect all cells bearing CD_4. These are mainly the T_4 helper/inducer lymphocytes in which the virus induces a lytic infection. Some other immune cells also possess CD_4 on the surface and so can also be infected like 5 to 10 percent of B lymphocytes and 10 to 20 percent of monocytes and macrophages (the alveolar macrophages in the lungs and Langerhan's cells in the dermis). Glial cells and microglia in the central nervous system are also found infected.

Resistance

- HIV is a delicate virus.
- It is inactivated in 30 minutes at 56°C and in less than 1 sec at 100°C.
- HIV is susceptible to common disinfectants 70 percent ethanol, 35 percent isopropyl alcohol, 5 percent formaldehyde, 3 percent hydrogen peroxide, 5 percent lysol, 0.2 percent sodium hypochlorite (household bleach) and 2 percent solution of glutaraldehyde.

Pathogenesis

In an infected individual, HIV can be isolated from blood lymphocytes, cell free plasma, semen, cervical secretions, saliva, tears, urine and breast milk. Infection is transmitted when the virus enters the blood or tissues of a person and comes into contact with a suitable host cell–primarily the T4 lymphocytes. Infection is due to blood transfusion of infected blood or sexual contact.

A double stranded DNA transcript of the viral DNA is integrated into the genome of the infected cell causing a latent infection.

The primary pathogenic mechanism in HIV infection is the ***damage caused to the T4 lymphocytes***. This damage can be cell lysis or suppression of the function of the infected cell without causing structural damage. This reduces the cell mediated immunity. T4 lymphocytes called the helper T cells are essential for optimal B cell function. Therefore, AIDS patients cannot effectively deal with new antigens (**depressed B cell function**). An important feature in HIV infection is the polyclonal activation of B lymphocytes leading to **hypergammaglobulinaemia**. This is actually not helpful because the antibodies are against useless antigens and are auto antibodies. This may be responsible for allergic reactions due to immune complexes. The main immunological abnormalities in HIV are listed in Table 37.3.

The monocyte and macrophage function is also affected due to lack of secretion of activating factors by T_4 lymphocytes. As a result a lot of immune functions are affected.

The clinical features of HIV infection are:

1. Secondary to the failure of immune responses because of which the person is susceptible to opportunistic infections and malignancies.
2. Direct effect of HIV on the central nervous system causing dementia and other degenerative neurological lesions.

Families, Groups and Subtypes of AIDS Virus

There are currently two types of HIV virus—HIV-1 and HIV-2. Both HIV-1 and HIV-2 are transmitted by sexual contact, through blood and blood products and from mother to child and they appear to cause clinically indistinguishable AIDS. However, HIV-2 is less easily transmitted

Table 37.3: Immunological abnormalities in HIV infection
Major abnormalities
• Lymphopenia < 2000/cumm.
• Selective T cell deficiency—reduction in number of T4 cells (CD4) (Inversion of T4:T8 ratio).
• Decreased delayed hypersensitivity on skin testing.
• Hypergammaglobulinaemia—predominantly IgG and IgA and in children—IgM as well.
• Thrombocytopenia.
• Polyclonal activation of B cells and increased spontaneous secretion of Ig.
Minor abnormalities
• Decreased in vitro lymphocyte proliferative response to mitogens and antigens.
• Decreased cytotoxic responses by T cells and NK cells.
• Decreased antibody response to new antigens.
• Altered monocyte/macrophage function.
• Elevated levels of immune complexes in serum.

and period between initial infection and illness is longer in case of HIV-2.

HIV virus is a highly variable virus which mutates rapidly. HIV-1 is divided into two groups–M and O. Within gp M (Major) there are 10 genetically distinct subtypes of HIV-1. These are subtypes A-J. The O groups is named after outliers because they lie outside the usual subtypes. Out of the different subtypes, subtype B exists in US and Europe and subtypes A, C, D and E cause AIDS in the developing world. HIV-IC is the type now responsible for more than half the world's AIDS virus infection.

Distribution of the various subtypes:

B—It is mostly found in the Americas, Japan, Australia, Caribbean and Europe.

A-D—Predominate in Sub-Saharan Africa.

Subtype C—is found in South Africa and India.

Subtype E—Central Africa, Thialand and other countries of South East Asia.

Subtype F—Brazil, Romania.

GH—Russia, Central Africa.

I—Cyprus.

gpO—Cameroon.

Types C and E is transmitted through heterosexual contact while subtype B is transmitted through blood and blood products.

Considerable genetic diversity exists between viruses of different subtypes. To date most vaccines target subtype B. Yet to be fully effective worldwide, such vaccines must protect against other subtypes as well.

ACQUIRED IMMUNODEFICIENCY SYNDROME (AIDS)

The full blown AIDS syndrome is the last stage in the clinical spectrum of HIV infection. The Centre for Disease Control (USA) has classified the clinical course of HIV infection under various groups (Table 37.4).

1. **Acute HIV infection**
   Within a few weeks of infection with HIV, 10 to 15 percent people experience low grade fever, malaise, headache, lymphadenopathy with rash, or arthropathy resembling glandular fever. Spontaneous resolution occurs within weeks. HIV antibody tests are usually negative at the onset of illness but

Table 37.4: Summary of classification system of HIV infection (Center for Disease Control, USA)

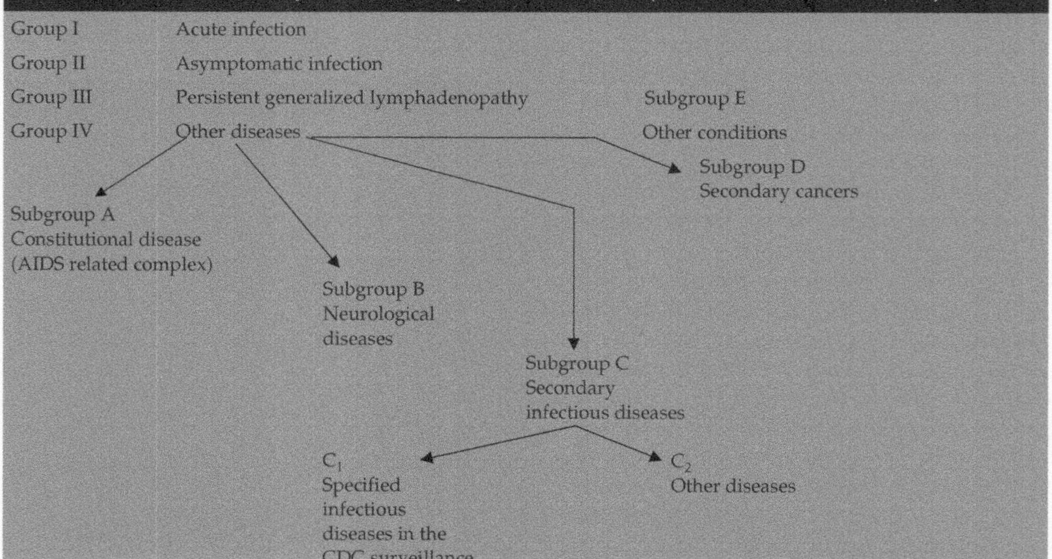

becomes positive during its course. Hence this is also called sero-conversion illness. At the beginning of this phase p24 antigenaemia may be demonstrated. The symptoms of seroconversion phase could be due to viral multiplication or due to immune complexes. Some people may not experience it.

2. **Asymptomatic infection**
   This is a stage in which the persons show positive HIV antibody tests and are infectious but they have no symptoms. This can last for many months to years. In some the infection does not progress any further and in some it leads to full blown AIDS or its other manifestations.
3. **Persistent generalized lymphadenopathy**
   This is defined as the presence of enlarged lymph nodes at least 1 cm in diameter in two or more non-contiguous, extra inguinal sites that persist for at least 3 months in the absence of any current illness or medication. A proportion of these patients progress to ARC or AIDS.
4. **AIDS-Related Complex (ARC)**
   In this group patients have **considerable immunodeficiency** and suffer from various constitutional symptoms or have minor opportunistic infections. The constitutional symptoms are fatigue, unexplained fever, diarrhea and weight loss of > 10 percent. The common opportunistic infections are oral candidiasis, herpes zoster, hairy cell leukoplakia, salmonellosis or tuberculosis. Generalized lymphadenopathy and splenomegaly are usually present. ARC patients are usually severely ill and many of them progress to AIDS in a few months.
5. **AIDS**
   This is the **end stage disease** representing the irreversible breakdown of immune defence mechanisms. The patient can get many opportunistic infections and malignancies. Most infections are endogenous and are caused by intracellular pathogens which have remained latent from previous infections.

The clinical severity varies with the disease present and malignancy present. In early AIDS, many patients are ill only during episodes of infection which may respond to specific treatment and they are well between the episodes.

The patients may live for a few months or years.

According to the system affected, patients present with the following complaints:

a. ***Respiratory***
   Dry cough, breathlessness and fever are the commonest presentations. In the developed countries, the usual pathogen is *Pneumocystis carinii* but in the developing countries it is *M. tuberculosis* or an atypical mycobacterium such as *M. avium intracellulare*. Pneumonia may also be viral (*Cytomegalovirus*) or fungal (*Histoplasma, Cryptococcus*).
b. ***Gastrointestinal***
   Mouth—thrush, herpetic stomatitis gingivitis, Kaposi's sarcoma
   Intestines—diarrhea, abdominal pain and distention.
   Pathogens may be cryptosporidium, salmonellae, mycobacteria, viruses such as *CMV or adenoviruses*. Chronic colitis is common in male homosexuals.
c. ***Neurological***
   The typical CNS opportunistic infections are toxoplasmosis and cryptococcosis. Infections are also seen with CMV, herpes simplex, papovaviruses, mycobacteria, aspergillus and candida. Lymphomas of the CNS are common.
d. ***Malignancies***
   Kaposi's sarcoma is the lesion seen in male homosexuals. It is a mucosal or cutaneous tumor of endothelial organ. The other tumors are lymphomas of both Hodgkin's and non-Hodgkin's types.
e. ***Cutaneous***
   Herpes lesions, candidiasis, seborrhoeic dermatitis, folliculitis, impetigo and

molluscum contagiosum are common cutaneous lesions.

6. **Dementia**
HIV may cause direct cytopathogenic damage in the central nervous system. It crosses the blood brain barrier and causes encephalopathy leading to loss of higher functions and progressing to dementia.
7. **Pediatric AIDS**
Fifty percent of babies born to infected mothers are infected with HIV. Many of them may not survive beyond a year. Infection can also be acquired from blood transfusions or blood products.

The common manifestations in paediatric AIDS is failure to thrive, chronic diarrhea, lymphadenopathy, tuberculosis and opportunistic bacterial infections.

OPPORTUNISTIC INFECTIONS AND MALIGNANCIES COMMONLY ASSOCIATED WITH HIV INFECTION

I. Parasitic
   1. *Pneumocystis carinii* pneumonia.
   2. Toxoplasmosis.
   3. Cryptosporidiosis.
   4. Isosporiasis.
   5. Generalized strongyloidiasis.

II. Mycotic
   1. Candidosis.
   2. Cryptococcosis.
   3. Aspergillosis.
   4. Histoplasmosis.

III. Bacterial
   1. Mycobacterial infections—Tuberculous and non-tuberculous infection.
   2. Salmonellosis.
   3. Campylobacter infection.
   4. Nocardia and Actinomycetes.
   5. Legionellosis.

IV. Viral
   1. CMV infection.
   2. Herpes simplex infection.

V. Malignancies
   1. Kaposi's sarcoma.
   2. Lymphomas-Hodgkin's and non Hodgkin's types.

LABORATORY DIAGNOSIS

Laboratory procedures for the diagnosis of HIV tests include tests for immunodeficiency as well as specific tests for HIV.

Nonspecific Tests

The following tests are usually done:
1. TLC-It shows leucopenia.
2. Total lymphocyte count < 2000/cu mm.
3. Absolute T4 cell count < 200/cu mm.
4. T4:T8 ratio reversed.
5. Platelet count-thrombocytopenia.
6. Raised IgG and IgA levels.
7. Low cell mediated immunity as shown by skin tests.

Specific Tests

- Antigen detection
- Virus isolation
- Antibody detection
- PCR.

Antigen Detection

If the infection is by blood transfusion and is a strong stimulus, the virus antigen (p24) may be detectable in blood after about two weeks of infection. If the infecting dose is small as following a needle stick injury the process may be delayed. Afterwards, the p24 antigen disappears from circulation and remains absent during the asymptomatic phase. It appears again only when clinical disease sets in. The IgM antibody appears in 4 to 6 weeks and is followed by IgG antibodies. Antigen detection tests are available only in specialized labs and cannot be done routinely.

Virus Isolation

- Once a person is infected with HIV, a person remains infected for life.

- The virus is present in the circulation and body fluids mostly within the lymphocytes but some are also cell free.
- Virus titers are high early in the infection about a week before antibodies start appearing. At this time the person is infectious but the antibody tests are negative and the case may not be detected in screening tests. Later the virus titers decrease and increase again when clinical disease sets in. The antibodies do not neutralize the virus and the two coexist.
- The virus is isolated most easily from the peripheral lymphocytes.
- The technique of isolation is by co-cultivation of the patients lymphocytes with uninfected lymphocytes in the presence of IL-2. Viral replication is indicated by demonstration of virus antigen as well as reverse transcriptase activity.

Antibody Detection

See Table 37.5 for Serological markers during HIV infection.

Sequence of appearance of antigens and antibodies after HIV infection is shown in Figure 37.2.

The demonstration of antibodies is the simplest and most widely used test for the diagnosis of HIV infection. But it takes several weeks to months for the antibodies to appear after infection and during the later part of this period, the individual may be infectious. For this reason antibody screening is not totally dependable for spotting infectious persons as for example blood donors.

After sexual exposure to HIV, antibodies appear within three to six months if infection has taken place. So antibody testing should be only done after six months.

IgM antibodies disappear in about 8 to 10 weeks, whereas IgG antibodies remain throughout life.

Serological tests for anti-HIV are of two types:

a. *Screening.*
b. *Confirmatory.*

Screening Tests: The screening tests have high sensitivity, are simple to perform and can be automated for handling a large number of samples at a time. They are not specific and give a few false positive results. All sera positive on screening tests are to be checked by a confirmatory test before the sample is taken as positive. The most widely used screening test is ELISA.

ELISA: The antigen is obtained from HIV grown in continuous T lymphocyte cell line or by recombinant technique. It is coated on microtiter wells or any other suitable solid surface. The test serum is added, and if the antibody is present, it binds to the antigen. After washing away the unbound serum, anti-human immunoglobulin linked to a suitable enzyme is added followed by a color forming substrate. If the test serum contains anti-HIV antibody, a visible detectable color is formed that can be read visually.

Advantages of ELISA

- It is simple and relatively inexpensive.

Disadvantages: False positive reactions are there with sera containing rheumatoid factor or stored for long periods. Some people in the world show nonspecific reaction due to cross-reacting antibodies.

Confirmatory Test

Western Blot: In this test, the HIV proteins are separated according to their electrophoretic mobility and molecular weight by polyacrylamide gel electrophoresis and blotted on to strips on nitrocellulose paper. These strips are reacted with test sera and then with an enzyme conjugated anti-human globulin. A suitable substrate is then added which produces a prominent color band where specific antibody has reacted with the separated viral protein. The position of the band on the strip indicates the antigen with which the antibody has reacted.

In a positive serum, bands will be seen with multiple proteins. A serum is considered positive if it shows antibody binding to at least 2 gene products of the 3 major HIV genes namely gag

Table 37.5: Serological markers during HIV infection

	Markers			
	p24 antigen	*anti HIV IgG*	*anti HIV IgM*	*WB*
Early infection	— → +	—	—	—
Acute sero conversion illness	+ → —	— → +	+	Partial p24 and /or gp120
Carrier, asymptomatic	—	+	—	Full pattern
PGL	+	+	—	Loss of p24/p55
AIDS	+	+	—	Absence of p24, loss of other reactivities

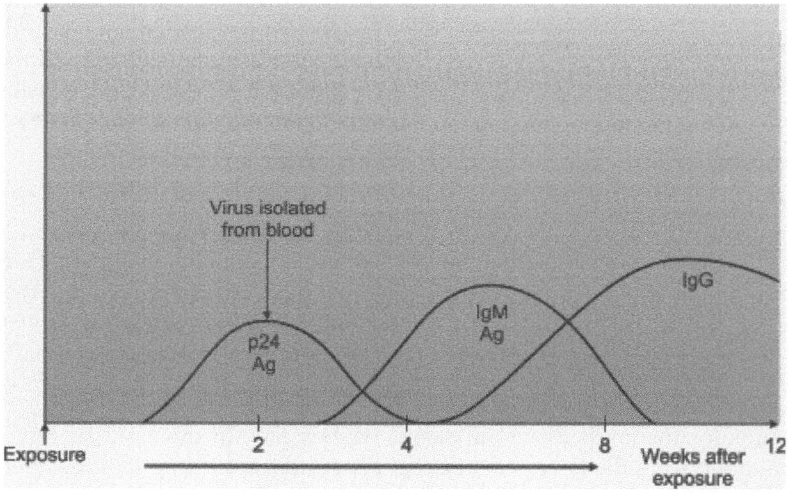

Fig. 37.2: Sequence of appearance of antigens and antibodies after HIV infection

(p17, p24, p55), env gene (gp 41, gp 120, gp 160) and pol (p31, p51, p66).

Interpretation becomes difficult when bands appear only at one or two sites as with p24 or gp120. This can happen in early infection but may also be non-specific. When in doubt a follow-up testing after 2 to 3 months is useful.

In AIDS there is immune deficiency, so the antibody formation is affected and serological diagnosis of infections may not be reliable.

Applications of Serological Tests

1. *Screening*—Screening is defined as the HIV testing either voluntary or compulsory of entire populations or selected target groups. These include donors of blood, blood products, semen, cells, tissues and organs, antenatal women, foreigners, etc. As antibody tests are negative during the early stage of HIV infection when the individual is infectious, screening may not detect all

dangerous donors but can still eliminate the large majority of them.

2. *Seroepidemiology*—Antibody surveys are very helpful in identifying the geographical extent of HIV.
3. *Diagnosis:*
   i. With clinical features of AIDS present—The antibody tests are positive.
   ii. In early illness—The antibody tests can be negative.
   iii. In very late cases—The antibody tests can be negative.
   iv. If there is infection with a different virus, e.g. HIV-2 and testing for another—The tests can be negative.

   In case of exposure such as sexual contact, blood transfusion or needle stick injury, one should get a serology after 2 months and repeat it at 6 months after exposure.
4. *Prognosis*—In a person infected with HIV, loss of detectable anti-p24 antibody indicates clinical deterioration. This is taken as an indication for active antiviral treatment. This is associated with HIV antigenaemia and increased virus titer in circulation.

PCR

The polymerase chain reaction can be used to directly detect disease specific sequences of either RNA or DNA from the tissue or body fluid of the patient. It is quite sensitive.

EPIDEMIOLOGY AND PREVENTION

Origin and Spread

AIDS was first seen in 1981 when it caused outbreaks in the USA. But it is now known that the virus was seeded in the USA as early as in the mid 1970's. It probably originated in Africa from a Simian immunodeficiency virus and spread to the USA, finally appearing as a first case in 1981. The virus may have spread to Europe from America or directly from Africa. The virus has spread to virtually all over the world. Prevalence rates in different countries are different. North America, Brazil, Western Europe, Australia, Central and West Africa have high prevalence, whereas Eastern Europe and Asia are only sparsely affected.

Common Modes of Transmission

Table 37.6 shows the common modes of transmission. HIV is primarily a sexually transmitted infection. It is more common in homosexuals than heterosexuals because of the increase in number of partners in homosexuals and more mucosal tears which are common in anal intercourse. The best method to prevent sexual transmission of infection is health education regarding safer sex practices and single partners.

The second mode of transmission is through blood and blood products. Screening of blood donors is now mandatory before blood donation even though it may not completely eliminate the danger (as the early infectious cases may be missed). The same situation applies for tissue and organ donation like semen, cornea, bone marrow, kidney, etc. Those individuals who have indulged in high risk practices are advised not to donate organs.

Contaminated needles can transmit the infection in case of drug addicts who share

Table 37.6: Common modes of transmission of HIV

I. Sexual intercourse
Anal
Vaginal
Oral
II. Blood and blood products
Blood transfusion, factor VIII, etc.
III. Tissue and organ donation
Semen, cornea, bone marrow, kidney
IV. Injections and injuries
Needles shared by drug addicts
Infections with unsterile syringes and needles
Needlestick and other injuries in health staff
Surgical wounds
V. Mother—Baby
Transplacental
At birth
After birth

syringes and needles. It can also happen in hospitals where sterilization methods are unsatisfactory. Use of disposable needles and syringes is mandatory.

The danger of needle stick injury is present in medical and paramedical personnel, though the chances of infection are much less than with HBV. The risk to medical and nursing personnel appears to be minimal provided they take adequate precautions. Medical and paramedical staff needs to be educated on caring for patients infected with HIV.

Guidelines for hospitals should be laid down regarding management of AIDS patients. They can be treated in same hospital but in a separate ward. Gloves, protective clothes and spectacles should be worn when there is danger of splashing of blood or fluids. Soiled materials should be sterilized before disposal. Blood or other fluids splashed on the skin, mouth or eyes should be washed thoroughly. Skin punctures should be encouraged to bleed and then washed.

Transmission of infection from the mother to baby can take place before, during or after birth. HIV may be present in breast milk and may rarely be transmitted through breastfeeding.

Normal social and domestic contact does not transmit the infection. Shaking hands, hugging, putting cheeks together or dry kissing is safe. Wet kissing is considered risky. The infection is not transmitted by mosquitoes, bed bugs or other blood sucking insects or transmitted through air, food, water or fomites.

Treatment

The treatment of AIDS includes:

1. Treatment and prophylaxis of infections and tumors.
2. General management.
3. Immunorestorative measures.
4. Specific anti-HIV agents.

Treatment and prophylaxis of infections is useful and the patient is able to resume a normal life between episodes of illness. General management involves making the patient feel comfortable at home or the hospital. Immunorestorative therapy has not been very successful namely administration of interleukin-2, thymic factors, leukocyte transfusion and bone marrow transplantation.

Antiviral Drugs

Zidovudine or Retrovir or AZT belongs to a group of drugs that are called nucleoside analogues or reverse transcriptase inhibitors. They inhibit an enzyme called reverse transcriptase. Other drugs belonging to this class are:

- ddI (didanosine or Videx).
  ddC (Zalcitabine or Hivid).

Other drugs in use are—Lamivudine or Epivir.
Stavudine or Zerit.
Nevirapine, Indinavir,
Ritonavir, Saquinavir,
Pentamidine, Viread.

SARS (SEVERE ACUTE RESPIRATORY SYNDROME)

INTRODUCTION

WHO calls SARS (Severe Acute Respiratory Syndrome) a new communicable disease that is a global health threat. It started in the late part of 2002 and early part of 2003 and caused an atypical pneumonia in patients. It was fatal in some. Untilmid April 2003 it had involved 26 countries, infecting 3864 people and killing 217. The figures were still rising (Table 37.7). There were conflicting theories on the causative agent of SARS. On April 16, 2003, WHO confirmed the culprit to belong to a family of viruses also

Table 37.7: Cumulative number of reported probable cases of severe acute respiratory syndrome (SARS) from 1st Nov. 2002 to 21 April 2003

	Cases	*Deaths*
Australia	3	0
Brazil	2	0
Canada	132	12
China	1959	86
Hong Kong	1402	94
China (Taiwan)	29	0
France	5	0
Germany	6	0
India	4	0
Indonesia	1	0
Italy	3	0
Japan	5	0
Kuwait	1	0
Malaysia	6	1
Mongolia	3	0
Philippines	2	1
Ireland	1	1
Romania	1	1
Singapore	178	16
S. Africa	1	0
Sweden	3	0
Switzerland	1	0
Thailand	7	2
UK	6	0
US	39	0
Vietnam	63	5
Total	**3863**	**219**

responsible for common cold (*Coronaviruses*). SARS virus is thought to be a mutated *Coronavirus* and has probably jumped from animals to man becoming more virulent in the process.

ORIGIN

It originated in the Guandong province in Southern China. Cases of pneumonia had been reported there as early as November 2002 and this has been linked to the current SARS outbreak. Scientists in Hong Kong and of WHO suspected that the virus most likely originated in animals, (pigs or poultry) mutated and crossed species. It could also be that human *Coronavirus* acquired genes from another more virulent virus by capturing a part of their genetic material (recombination).

SPREAD

The virus originated in China, but spread rapidly to neighboring areas—Hong Kong, Singapore, Vietnam, Thailand, Taiwan, Malaysia, Toronto and Canada. The last two were by a passenger who had flown from Hong Kong. Slowly most of the countries of the world were involved.

ORIGINAL VIRUS

Coronavirus is a **single stranded RNA virus,** 80 to 160 nm in diameter with a fringe of club-shaped projections about 20 nm long. It is enveloped.

The *Coronaviruses* are not harmful. They infect animals and in humans cause 1/3rd of mild to moderate respiratory illnesses such as common cold. The name *Coronavirus* refers to the spiky protein molecules surrounding the virus making it look like a crown (corona-crown). There are 5–6 polypeptides spikes associated with the virion. The group of *Coronavirus* includes three types of human respiratory common cold virus the viruses of avian and rodent infectious bronchitis and that of murine hepatitis and related though distinct viruses causing gastroenteritis in pigs, calves and probably man.

The **SARS virus** resembles *Coronavirus* family. The *Coronavirus* mutates easily and each mutation triggers off an epidemic of respiratory illness. A new mutation which arose in Gaungdong is suspected to have caused SARS.

METHOD OF TRANSMISSION

1. Most frequent method of transmission of SARS virus is by **close person to person contact.** If the sick person coughs or sneezes the virus can be carried in saliva droplets to people nearby infecting them. This usually involves **close contacts** (healthcare workers and family members).
2. Air borne transmission is questionable but it is a likely cause of transmission of the SARS virus too. It is possible that SARS virus like

other *Coronaviruses*, may have the property of surviving in dry air or surfaces for up to 3 hours in which condition it crystallizes and can float in air like dust. People who may be carrying more of the infectious virus within themselves are more likely to transmit it to others and are called superspreaders. Scientists now feel that the virus is usually spread by droplet infection but from time to time it reaches superspreaders who may spread the virus through air borne transmission.

3. **Fomites** are thought to be an important mode of transmission such as elevator and light buttons, taps, surfaces, mail boxes, etc.
4. Other modes of transmission like **cockroaches, contaminated water** flowing through sewage pipes, rodent feces, pets, etc. are also relevant. These modes of transmission become important when one considers the outbreak in the high rise buildings in Hong Kong where people unrelated to each other also developed the disease. It is possible that a patient's virus—laden stool contaminated the apartment sewage system and through faulty plumbing, somehow found a way into drinking water.

INCUBATION PERIOD

After the virus enters the body, it requires 3 to 10 days incubation period before the disease appears. According to current data, infected people do not pass on the virus to others during the incubation period. They become infectious only when the first symptoms appear—cough, sneezing, etc. which spreads droplets containing virus particles.

Infectivity and Virulence

Infectivity means the ability of the virus to jump from one person to another.

The recipient must receive a dose large enough to cause disease. From epidemic reports it appears that SARS has low infectivity and requires a large dose to pass on the disease to the recipient. Other members of the *Coronavirus* family have high infectivity (SARS virus is less infectious than influenza virus). **Virulence** is the property of the virus to cause damage to the patients. The SARS virus is very virulent as opposed to the other members of the *Coronavirus*, once it is inside the human host.

PATHOGENESIS

The virus causes high fever and creates an inflammatory storm as the body's immune system attempts to fight it off.

It causes **atypical pneumonia** in which the tissues outside the alveoli gets swollen and collapses the alveoli. (As different from typical pneumonia in which the alveoli fill up with exudates).

The effect of the virus is generally more harmful in the elderly or those with preexisting medical conditions. A significant proportion gets ill and is shifted on the ventilator. The mortality ranges from 4 percent to 5.1 percent.

SYMPTOMS

- Higher fever (>39°C) or 100.4°C.
- Dry nagging cough, nasal congestion and sneezing.
- Severe muscle and joint pain, headache, and malaise.
- Difficulty in breathing, similar to asthma.
- Continuous localized pain in the chest which increases when taking a breath.
- In certain cases rashes, loss of appetite, diarrhoea and confusion may also develop.

DIAGNOSIS

The diagnosis at present is done by **Polymerase Chain Reaction Kits** imported from Germany via WHO and sent to all countries. This is done to detect the DNA of the virus from urine, blood sputum or throat swab samples.

USA, Canada, Hongkong and Singapore have sequenced the virus and better diagnostic tests and antiviral drugs may be developed in the future.

Antibody detection tests are also being developed. Immunofluorescence assay (IFA) can be used to detect infection in convalescent sera three weeks after infection.

In India—The National Institute of Virology, Pune and the National Institute of Communicable Diseases, Delhi have been designated as the diagnostic centers. AIIMS, Safdarjung and RML Hospitals in Delhi are the treatment centers.

The virus can be seen by a Transmission Electron microscope capable of magnifying it about 150,000 times. It looks like fuzzy balls that fills the screen and has little hooks sticking out of its body—tell tale characteristics that help classify the pathogens as members of the *Coronavirus* family.

TREATMENT

- Isolation of the patients, so that they cannot spread the disease to others.
- Rest, good nutrition and supportive therapy for respiratory symptoms.
- Hospital admission and intervention is a must.
- Two antiviral drugs and corticosteroids are being given to treat patients.

Combination or a cocktail of antivirals such as ribavirin, **immunosuppressant steroids** that stop the immune system from devouring itself and **serum containing antibodies** from recovered SARS patients is used for treatment of the patient.

PRECAUTIONS

- All incoming passengers' should be monitored by immigration officials at International airports and ports. Indian embassies have been told to warn those applying for visas that they would be denied entry if suspected of SARS.
- All hospital staff should be trained to treat SARS patients.
- Disembarking passengers to fill up prescribed from designated by Health Ministry.
- All patients or suspected patients to stay at home for 7 to 10 days in which minimum outside contact should be there.
- Protective masks to be worn by the patient as well as close contacts.

  There are various types of masks which are available:

  a. *Tissue or paper masks* forms a barrier but offer no real protection against droplets. The paper moistens within an hour becoming ineffective.

  b. *Gauze masks* next to useless. Particles can still make their way through.

  c. *Cotton masks* not adequate protection.

  d. *Surgical masks*

     i. Johnson and Johnson—These are disposable face masks extra guard (non-woven double-layered type).

     ii. Romsons—Disposable surgical masks.

     iii. Company called 3 M offers 3 types of imported disposable masks.

     3 M 9913

     3 M 9004

     N-95

     This is recommended by CDC. These are triple-layered masks for non-oily environments with 95 percent efficacy. It is effective but uncomfortable.

     The surgical masks have 80 percent efficacy because the 0.3 micron size of the pore is effective in blocking the SARS virus.

  e. There are certain high tech masks—These are air-positive respirators developed by DRDO. It is useful for people in close contact with body secretions of an infected person.

FUTURE OF SARS VIRUS

The future of SARS virus is uncertain.

- The chances of SARS becoming a **pandemic** cannot be ruled out because whole populations around the globe have no immunity against the disease. The new cases are increasing.

- SARS may be present in the world for a long time to come. It will either remain dormant or **alive in animal reservoirs**. The world now has a new viral enemy and we are just beginning to understand it.
- SARS-like viral infections and outbreaks are definitely going to increase in the next few years. They are certain factors promoting this:
  a. *Rapid deforestation* has brought humans in contact with viruses that have been hidden for centuries.
  b. Movement of people by air is very rapid and it is difficult to contain the virus.
  c. Modern intensive farming methods cluster many animals together. Pigs are the dangerous species because they can be infected by human viruses as well as rodents and fowls. They thus become mixing vessels in which pathogens mutate and jump from animal species to humans. Guangdong province in Southern China has the world's largest concentration of pigs, humans and fowls living in close proximity explaining why many influenza outbreaks can be traced to that region. Many more such viral breeding grounds can be created.

CASES IN INDIA

There was only one confirmed case in India, though suspected cases were many.

There is no local transmission in India yet and only people who are travelling through high-risk countries such as Hong Kong, China, Vietnam and Bangkok need to take precautions.

Meanwhile, the coordinated effort against SARS by many scientists show that global teamwork is effective. In a very short time, the etiology and the sequencing of the virus has been done and it could pave the way for a drug or a vaccine at a later date.

Whether this viral outbreak will burn out or continue will remain to be seen.

Note: This article was written in early 2003 and is more relevant to that period.

SWINE FLU (INFLUENZA A H1N1) VIRUS

INTRODUCTION

The 2009 flu pandemic is a global outbreak of H1N1, a new strain of Influenza A virus, often referred to colloquially as "swine flu". Swine flu is the common name for the H1N1 virus to distinguish it from the seasonal flu. Genetic sequencing shows a new sub type of influenza A (H1N1) virus with segments from four influenza viruses: North American Swine, North American Avian, Human Influenza and Eurasian Swine. Although the virus, first detected in April 2009, contains a combination of genes from swine, avian (bird), and human influenza viruses, it cannot be spread by eating pork or pork products. The current swine flu outbreak is the type of H1N1 virus as seen during the flu pandemic of 1918 when more than twenty million people died.

STATISTICS

World

Swine flu is considered a global pandemic. A pandemic is an epidemic that becomes so widespread that it affects a region, continent, or the world. As of April 2009, the H1N1 swine flu outbreak did not meet this definition. However, as of June 11, 2009, WHO officials determined that H1N1 2009 influenza A swine flu reached WHO level 6 criteria (person-to-person transmission in two separate WHO-determined world regions) and declared the first flu pandemic in 41 years. The flu has reached over 74 different countries on every continent except Antarctica in about three month's time; fortunately, the severity of the disease has not increased.

Total Confirmed Cases of Influenza A H1N1 reported Worldwide are more than 622482 and Total Deaths Worldwide are at least 14142 affecting more than 209 countries.

India

Consolidated status of Influenza A H1N1 as on 27 Jan 2010 (By Press Information Bureau, India and WHO) shows that samples from 122209 persons have been tested for Influenza A H1N1 in Government Laboratories and a few private Laboratories across the country and 28665 (23.45%) of them have been found positive which includes 1206 deaths.

VIRUS

Infuenza A H1N1 virus belongs to the orthomyxovirus group. Though there are several serotypes of influenza virus causing swine flu like H1N1, H1N2, H3N1, H3N2, and H2N3. But now a days H1N1, H3N2, and H1N2 subtypes are creating terror. In earlier days it was H1N1 subtype as the main cause prior to 1998 and the role of pig was demonstrated after 1998 when H3N2 subtypes was isolated in them.

Structure

The (H1N1) virion (as the infectious particle is called) is roughly spherical (Fig. 37.3). It is an enveloped virus—that is, the outer layer is a lipid membrane which is taken from the host cell in which the virus multiplies. Inserted into the lipid membrane are 'spikes', which are proteins—actually glycoproteins, because they consist of protein linked to sugars—known as HA (hemagglutinin) and NA (neuraminidase). These are the proteins that determine the type of Influenza virus (A, B, or C) and the subtype (A/H1N1, for example). The HA and NA are given subtype numbers. They are important in the immune response against the virus; antibodies against these spikes may protect against infection. The NA protein is the target of the antiviral drugs Relenza and Tamiflu. Also embedded in the lipid membrane is the M2 protein, which is the target of the antiviral adamantanes—amantadine and rimantadine.

Beneath the lipid membrane is a viral protein called M1, or matrix protein. This protein, which forms a shell, gives strength and rigidity to the lipid envelope. Within the interior of the virion are the viral RNAs—8 of them for influenza A viruses. These are the genetic material of the virus; they code for one or two proteins. Each RNA segment, as they are called, consists of RNA joined with several proteins shown in the diagram: B1, PB2, PA, NP. These RNA segments are the genes of influenza virus. The interior of the virion also contains another protein called NEP.

Resistance

- The virus is thermosensitive and gets destroyed above 70° C. Thus, a well-xcooked pork is absolutely safe and can be eaten. However, raw and undercooked pork may be at risk.

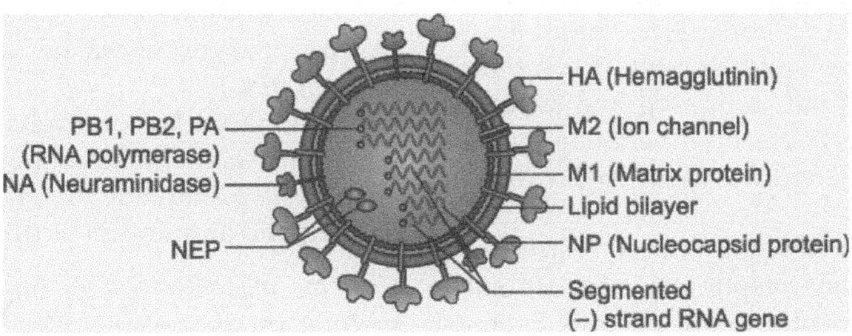

Fig. 37.3: Structure of H1N1 virus

- The climate ideal for the virus is at the beginning of cold but the recent outbreak has turned out to break this rule and even summer season is not spared.

Pathogenesis

When influenza virus is introduced into the respiratory tract, by **aerosol** or by **contact with saliva** or other respiratory secretions from an infected individual, it attaches to and replicates in epithelial cells. The virus replicates in cells of both the upper and lower respiratory tract. Viral replication combined with the immune response to infection leads to destruction and loss of cells lining the respiratory tract. As infection subsides, the epithelium is regenerated, a process that can take up to a month. Cough and weakness may persist for up to 2 weeks after infection.

Transmission

The transmission is by droplet infection and fomites.

Incubation Period

One to seven days.

Symptoms

The swine flu is most contagious disease especially in the early days that is first 7 days which is generally the incubation period and the disease is not manifested. Swine flu symptoms are similar to other strains of flu. The person suffering from Swine flu may be febrile and the temperature may be high above 100–102°F. There may be malaise and body ache, nausea and vomiting can occur. Upper respiratory symptoms including sore throat, coughing and sneezing may be present. There may be early sign of fatigueness and dehydration due to diarrhea in later stage.

Some patients develop severe respiratory symptoms and need respiratory support (such as a ventilator to breathe for the patient). Patients can get pneumonia (bacterial secondary infection) if the viral infection persists, and some can develop seizures. Death often occurs from secondary bacterial infection of the lungs; appropriate antibiotics need to be used in these patients.

With increased diarrhea, people should take extra care to stay hydrated—drink lots of fluids, eat clear soups and broths and take fever-reducing medicines. It's also important to be very strict with hygiene practices, especially caregivers who come in contact with bodily waste.

Clinical Diagnosis

Swine flu is presumptively diagnosed clinically by the patient's history of association with people known to have the disease and their symptoms listed above.

Diagnostic Criteria for H1N1

In general the investigation for Swine flu should be done for each suspected case which is defined as a person with acute febrile respiratory illness with onset within 7 days of close contact with a person who is a confirmed case of swine influenza A (H1N1) virus infection.

A close contact means a contact with an infected person within about 6 feet of an ill person who is a confirmed case of swine influenza A virus infection.

Laboratory Diagnosis

What Sample to be Collected?

Respiratory specimens including:

1. Bronchoalveolar lavage.
2. Tracheal aspirates.
3. Nasopharyngeal washes or oropharyngeal aspirates.
4. Nasopharyngeal ororopharyngeal swabs.

Swab specimens should be collected only on swabs with a synthetic tip (such as polyester or Dacron) and aluminium or plastic shaft.

When to Collect Respiratory Specimens?

- As soon as possible after symptoms begin
- Before antiviral medications are administered

- Even if symptoms began more than one week ago
- Multiple specimens on multiple days could be collected if you have access to the patient.

Specimen: before initiating collection of sample a full complement of PPE should be worn.

Personal Protective Equipment

- Masks (N-95)
- Gloves
- Protective eye wear (goggles)
- Hair covers
- Boot or shoe covers
- Protective clothing (gown or apron).

The samples are to be tested in BSL-3 (biosafety level three) laboratory.

Demonstration of Viral Antigen

Rapid influenza antigen detection test is a rapid test performed to see if the patient is infected with influenza A or B virus. In this, the patient's sample (either a throat swab or a nasopharyngeal swab) is mixed with the extraction buffer and few drops of the preparation are added to the sample wells in the card containing separate sections for influenza A and B. The result is available as a band indicating the positivity in the respective section along with the control band. This test can distinguish between A and B types of Influenza virus.

Interpretation

- If the test is negative, there is no flu infection.
- If the test is positive for type B, the flu is not likely to be swine flu (H1N1).
- If it is positive for type A, the person could have a conventional flu strain or swine flu (H1N1).

However, the accuracy of these tests has been challenged, and the US Centers for Disease Control and Prevention (CDC) has not completed their comparative studies of these tests.

Viral Culture

The throat swab is generally taken to culture virus from the suspected cases. Though if it is not detected, it doesn't rule out the disease.

Detection of Antibodies

This is a sensitive test and there is four-fold rise in swine influenza A (H1N1) virus-specific neutralizing antibodies.

Thus a timely detection and confirmation of the case can not only save the life of the sufferer but can also be helpful in restricting the spread of the disease.

Reverse Transcriptase-Polymerase Chain Reaction (RT-PCR)

In this detection of mRNA of H1N1 virus is done. This is a specific test for swine flu which involves the detection of genes originated from birds, swine and human influenza virus. The reverse transcription PCR (RT-PCR) method for the detection of novel influenza A(H1N1) virus targeting the haemagglutinin and neuraminidase genes is followed. The results showed that the RT-PCR methods were suitable for sensitive and specific detection of novel influenza A(H1N1) RNA in human samples.

TRANSMISSION

Influenza viruses can be directly transmitted from pigs to human and from human to pigs. Primarily the disease occurs in pigs and the respiratory tracts of pigs are the reservoir for this virus. Human infection with H1N1 virus from pigs is most likely to occur when people are in close proximity to infected pigs, such as in pig barns and livestock exhibits housing pigs at fairs. Once a human being gets infected then coughing and sneezing spreads the virus from one to another. Human-to-human transmission of swine flu can also occur. It may also be transmitted through fomites. The human being is infective upto 7 to 10 days after getting infected and can spread infection during that period even by being in close contact as the infection is transmitted through air.

Swine flu is not transmitted through food. But always be safe when serving pork and be sure the internal temperature is at least 160°F to kill all possible germs.

Any person suffering from fever, cough and coryza should immediately attend the hospital and get himself investigated and diagnosed as it has been declared as a medical emergency in many countries.

TREATMENT

The guiding principles are:

- Early implementation of infection control precautions to minimize nosocomical/ household spread of disease.
- Prompt treatment to prevent severe illness and death.
- Early identification and follow-up of persons at risk.
  Infrastructure/manpower/material support
- Isolation facilities: Patient is kept in isolation with negative pressure.
- *Manpower*: Dedicated doctors, nurses and paramedical workers.
- *Equipment*: Portable X-ray machine, ventilators, large oxygen cylinders, pulse oxymeter.
- *Supplies*: Adequate quantities of PPE, disinfectants and medications (Oseltamivir, antibiotics and other medicines).
- Reinforce standard infection control precautions, i.e. all those entering the room must use high efficiency masks, e.g. N95 respirator, gowns, goggles, gloves, cap and shoe cover.
- Restrict number of visitors and provide them with PPE and showed keep a distance of 6 feet from patient.
- Hand hygiene by all is most important aspect in prevention of spread of infection.
- Social distancing, e.g. giving a call to patient rather than visiting him.
- Staying at home if one is sick.
- Covering of mouth and nose while coughing and sneezing.
- Provide antiviral prophylaxis to health care personnel managing the case and ask them to monitor their own health twice a day.
- Dispose waste properly by placing it in sealed impermeable bags labeled as bio-hazard.

Medication

- **Oseltamivir** is the recommended drug both for prophylaxis and treatment.
- *Dose for treatment is as follows:*
  - *By Weight:* For weight <15 kg 30 mg BD for 5 days:
    15–23 kg 45 mg BD for 5 days.
    24 -< 40 kg 60 mg BD for 5 days.
    > 40 kg 75 mg BD for 5 days.
- *For infants:*
  < 3 months 12 mg BD for 5 days.
  3–5 months 20 mg BD for 5 days.
  6–11 months 25 mg BD for 5 days.
  It is also available as syrup (12 mg per mL)
  If needed, dose and duration can be modified as per clinical condition.

Adverse Reactions

Oseltamivir is generally well-tolerated, gastrointestinal side-effects (transient nausea, vomiting) may increase with increasing doses, particularly above 300 mg/day. Occasionally it may cause bronchitis, insomnia and vertigo. Less commonly angina, pseudo membranous colitis and peritonsillar abscess have also been reported. There have been rare reports of anaphylaxis and skin rashes.

In children, most frequently reported side-effect is vomiting. Infrequently, abdominal pain, epistaxis, bronchitis, otitis media, dermatitis and conjunctivitis have also been observed. There is no recommendation for dose reduction in patients with hepatic disease.

Though rare reporting of fatal neuro-psychiatiric illness in children and adolescents has been linked to oseltamivir, there is no scientific evidence for a causal relationship.

Supportive Therapy

The Centers for Disease Control and Prevention recommended two antiviral agents which have been reported to prevent or reduce the effects of swine flu. They are zanamvir (Relenza) and oseltamivir (Tami flu), both of which are found to be effective in preventing or reducing influenza A and B symptoms. These drugs should not be used indiscriminately, because viral resistance to them can and has occurred. Also, they are not recommended if the flu symptoms already have been present for 48 hours or more, although hospitalized patients may still be treated past the 48-hour guideline.

The Centers for Disease Control (CDC) have issued serious warnings for pregnant women and are strongly recommending they be vaccinated. People who receive early treatment recover more quickly and have fewer complications.

DISCHARGE POLICY

- Adult patients should be discharged 7 days after symptoms have subsided.
- Children should be discharged 14 days after symptoms have subsided.
- The families of patients discharged earlier are educated on personal hygiene and infection control measures at home; children should not attend school during this period.

Chemoprophylaxis

- All close contacts of suspected, probable and confirmed cases. Close contacts include household/social contacts, family members, workplace or school contacts, fellow travelers, etc.
- All health care personnel coming in contact with suspected, probable or confirmed cases.
- Oseltamivir is the drug of choice.
- Prophylaxis should be provided till 10 days after last exposure (maximum period of 6 weeks)
  - *By Weight:*
    For weight <15 kg 30 mg OD
    15–23 kg 45 mg OD
    24–< 40 kg 60 mg OD
    > 40 kg 75 mg OD
- *For infants:*
  <3 months not recommended unless situation judged critical due limited data on use in this age group
  3–5 months 20 mg OD
  6–11 months 25 mg OD

Quarantine

Close contacts of suspected, probable and confirmed cases should be advised to remain at home (voluntary home quarantine) for at least 7 days after the last contact with the case. Monitoring of fever should be done for at least 7 days. Prompt testing and hospitalization must be done when symptoms are reported.

PREVENTION

Prevention of Pig to Human Transmission

The transmission of swine flu from swine to human is believed to occur mainly in swine farms where farmers are in close contact with live pigs. Although strains of swine influenza are usually not able to infect humans this may occasionally happen, so farmers and veterinarians are encouraged to use a face mask when dealing with infected animals. The use of vaccines on swine to prevent their infection is a major method of limiting swine to human transmission. Risk factors that may contribute to swine-to-human transmission include smoking and not wearing gloves when working with sick animals.

Prevention of Human to Human Transmission

Good hygiene is the most important part of prevention. Washing hands, use of alcohol-based hand gel, cleanliness of surfaces and bathrooms, use of a tissue to sneeze or cough and use of a simple surgical mask when caring for sick children or others also helps to prevent airborne spread of the virus.

VACCINE

Vaccines are available for different kinds of swine flu. The US Food and Drug Administration (FDA) approved the new swine flu vaccine for use in the United States on September 15, 2009. Studies by the National Institutes of Health (NIH) show that a single dose creates enough antibodies to protect against the virus within about 10 days.

There are two kinds of 2009 H1N1 vaccines: a nasal spray flu vaccine and a flu shot that is given with a needle, usually in the arm. The first vaccine released in early October 2009 was the nasal spray vaccine. It is approved for use in healthy individuals ages 2 through 49. This vaccine consists of a live attenuated H1N1 virus and should not be used in anyone who is pregnant or immunocompromised. The injectable vaccine, made from killed H1N1, became available in the second week of October. This vaccine is approved for use in ages 6 months to the elderly, including pregnant females. Both of these vaccines have been approved by the CDC only after they had conducted clinical trials to prove that the vaccines were safe and effective. However, caregivers should be aware of the vaccine guidelines that come with the vaccines, as occasionally, the guidelines change.

CDC recommends influenza vaccination as the first and most important step in protecting against the flu. As the supplies of 2009 H1N1 vaccines are ample, CDC is now encouraging everyone to get vaccinated, including people 65 years and older. Vaccination of people with certain health conditions is especially important because they are more likely to get serious flu-related complications. Health conditions that increase the risk of being hospitalized with 2009 H1N1 include lung disease like asthma or chronic obstructive pulmonary disease (COPD), diabetes, heart, or neurologic disease, and pregnancy.

Section 5

Parasitology

- Protozoology
- Helminthology

PARASITOLOGY

INTRODUCTION

Parasitology deals with the study of parasites which live in the human body and cause them harm. The body in turn mounts an immune response against them.

This section is divided into two parts—Protozoology which deals with the study of the unicellular protozoa and Helminthology which deals with the study of the multicellular helminths. Each parasite is discussed under the headings of geographical distribution, habitat, morphology, life cycle, clinical disease it causes and laboratory diagnosis. The focus is on the diagnostic aspects and unnecessary details have been avoided for simplification.

We shall begin by understanding certain basics about Parasitology.

When two living organisms interact, one of the following situations may develop:

- ***Symbiosis**—An association between two living organisms in which both are dependent upon each other and none of them suffers any harm.*
- ***Commensalism**—An association between two living organisms in which only one of them is benefitting from the other. The former is called a commensal and the latter the host. The commensal however does not cause any injury to the host. The commensal can lead an independent life too.*
- ***Parasitism**—An association between two living organism in which one of them (called the parasite) gets full support from the other (called the host) but the host suffers from injury and tries to fight the parasite.*

*A **parasite** can then be defined as a living organism who receives nutrition and shelter from another organism (host) on or in whom it lives. In this section we shall be dealing with small animals that parasitize the human body.*

*A **host** is an organism that supports the parasite. There are two kinds of hosts:*

- ***Definitive host**—It harbors the adult stage of the parasite where the parasite utilizes the sexual method of reproduction. In the majority of human parasitic infections, man is the definitive host but in malaria and hydatid disease man acts as an intermediate host.*
- ***Intermediate host**—It harbors the larval stages of the parasite. In some cases larval development is completed in two intermediate hosts called first and second intermediate host.*

We shall now attempt to study a few parasites. The scheme that shall be followed is:

1. ***History**—When was the parasite identified?*
2. ***Geographical distribution**—Where is the parasite found?*
3. ***Habitat**—Where does the parasite stay inside the human host?*
4. ***Morphology and life cycle***
5. ***Modes of infection***
6. ***Effect of the parasite on the human body***
7. ***Diagnosis in the laboratory***
8. ***Treatment and prevention***

Medical Parasitology includes three main groups.

***Phylum Protozoa**—Medical Protozoology*

Phylum Platyhelminthes and Phylum Nemathelminthes—Medical Helminthology

Phylum Arthropoda—Medical Entomology

CHAPTER

38

Protozoology

LESSON PLAN

- Definition
- Classification
  - Pseudopodia
  - Flagella
  - Cilia

Rhizopoda: *Entamoeba Histolytica*

- *Entamoeba*
- Endolimax
- Iodamoeba
- Dientamoeba

- Classification
  - Pathogenic
  - Nonpathogenic
- *Entamoeba Histolytica*
  - History
  - Geographical Distribution
  - Habitat
  - Morphology
  - Life Cycle
  - Clinical Features
  - Amoebic Liver Abscess
  - Source of Infection
  - Mode of Infection
  - Incubation Period
  - Pathological Lesions Caused by *E. Histolytica* (Optional)
  - Laboratory Diagnosis

Mastigophora: *Giardia Lamblia, Trichomonas Vaginalis* and *Leishmania Donovani*

- Intestinal Oral and Genital Flagellates
  - *Giardia Lamblia* (Intestinalis)
- Blood and Tissue Flagellates
  - *Leishmania Donovani*

Sporozoa: *Plasmodium*

- Classification
  - Intestinal Sporozoa
  - Blood Inhabiting Sporozoa
- Geographical Distribution
- Life Cycle of the Malarial Parasite
  - Human Cycle
  - Mosquito Cycle
- Method of Transmission of Malaria
  - Incubation Period
- Clinical Features of Malaria
  - Fever
  - Types of Fever
  - Anemia
  - Splenomegaly
- Complications of Falciparum Malaria
  - Pernicious Malaria
  - Black Water Fever
- Laboratory Diagnosis of Malaria
  - Other Methods in Diagnosis
- Life Cycle
  - Enteric Cycle (Intestinal Phase)
  - Exoenteric Cycle (Extraintestinal Phase)

Sporozoa: Toxoplasma

- Morphology
- Staining Reaction
- Cultivation
- Pathogenicity
- Mode of Infection
  - Congenital
  - Acquired
- Clinical Features
- Incidence
- Immunology
- Changes in Blood and CSF
  - Blood
- CSF
- Laboratory Diagnosis
  - Direct Evidence
  - Indirect Evidences
  - Treatment
  - Prophylaxis

Contd...

Sporozoa: *Cryptosporidum*
- History
- Habitat
- Species
- Life Cycle
- Morphology of Oocyst
- Mode of Infection
- Clinical Features
- Laboratory Diagnosis
- Treatment

Ciliata: *Balantidium Coli*
- Geographical Distribution
- Habitat
- Morphology
  - Trophozoite Stage
  - Encysted Stage
- Cultivation
- Life Cycle and Method of Reproduction
- Pathogenicity
- Lesions
- Diagnosis
- Treatment
- Prophylaxis

DEFINITION

A protozoan parasite consists of a single cell-like unit that is complete in itself and performs all the functions.

CLASSIFICATION

The phylum Protozoa has been divided into four classes based on the organs of locomotion.

Class	Organ of locomotion
• Rhizopoda	Pseudopodia
• Mastigophora	Flagella
• Sporozoa	None
• Ciliata	Cilia

Pseudopodia

These are extensions of the ectoplasm seen in class Rhizopoda. It is a false foot-like structure.

Flagella

These are long delicate thread-like filaments seen in Mastigophora.

Cilia

These are fine needle-like filaments covering the entire surface of the body as seen in Ciliata.

Flow chart 38.1 shows the classification of protozoa.

Flow chart 38.1: Classification of protozoa

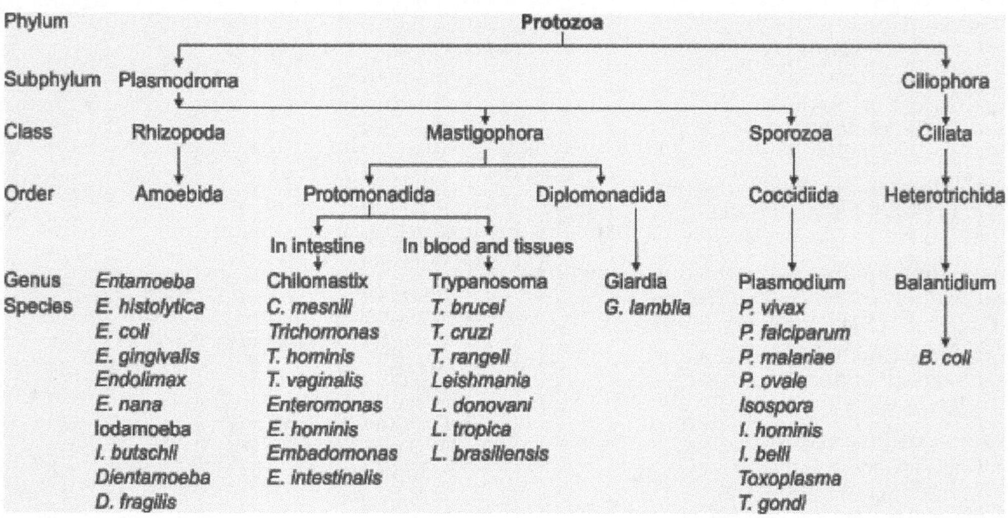

RHIZOPODA: *ENTAMOEBA HISTOLYTICA*

INTRODUCTION

The protozoan parasites belonging to this group while in motion throw out ectoplasm called pseudopodia that represent organs of locomotion. The genera included in the order Amoebida are:

1. *Genus Entamoeba—E. histolytica, E. coli and E. gingivalis*
2. *Genus Endolimax—E. nana*
3. *Genus Iodamoeba—I. bütschlii*
4. *Genus Dientamoeba—D. fragilis*

The four genera are distinguished by the structure of the nucleus (Fig. 38.1).

Entamoeba

The nuclear membrane is lined with chromatin granules and the compact karyosome is either centrally or eccentrically-placed.

Endolimax

The karyosome is an irregular mass situated peripherally. It may be connected with another small mass.

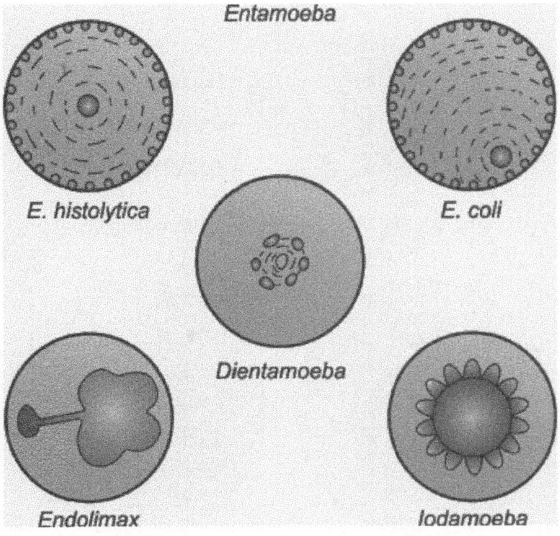

Fig. 38.1: Nuclear character of various genera under Amoebida

Iodamoeba

The karyosome is a large circular mass surrounded by refractile globules.

Dientamoeba

The karyosome consists of 6 chromatin granules. There are 2 nuclei.

CLASSIFICATION

The amoeba infecting man may be classified according to their pathogenicity and habitat as follows:

Pathogenic

Intestinal amoeba—*E. histolytica*

Nonpathogenic

(Harmless commensal)

1. Mouth amoeba—*E. gingivalis*
2. Intestinal amoebae—*E. coli, E. nana, I. bütschlii, D. fragilis.*

ENTAMOEBA HISTOLYTICA

History

Lambl in 1859 first discovered the parasite.

Losch in 1875 proved its pathogenic nature and Schaudinn differentiated pathogenic and non-pathogenic types of amoebae.

Geographical Distribution

Worldwide. More common in tropics and subtropics than in temperate zone.

Habitat

Trophozoites of *E. histolytica* live in the mucus and submucus layers of the large intestine of man.

Morphology

There are three morphological forms that have been described (Figs 38.2A to D).

A. Trophozoite
B. Precystic stage
C. Cystic stage.

Trophozoite

- This is called the growing stage.
- The parasite shows a slow gliding movement with the ectoplasm showing a jerky movement followed by endoplasm. This movement is enabled by the pseudopodia.
- The shape is not fixed because of constantly changing position.
- Size ranges from 18 to 40 µm.
- Cytoplasm is divided into two portions—a clear translucent ectoplasm and a granular endoplasm. RBCs, occasionally leucocytes and tissue debris are found inside endoplasm. The RBC's appear yellowish-green and the endoplasm bluish in unstained preparations.
- The nucleus is visible only faintly when the trophozoite is moving. When we use iodine for staining, the nucleus shows a central dot-like karyosome surrounded by a fine thread-like network having a spoke-like radial arrangement. The nuclear membrane is delicate and lined with a single layer of uniformly distributed fine chromatin granules (Fig. 38.2A).

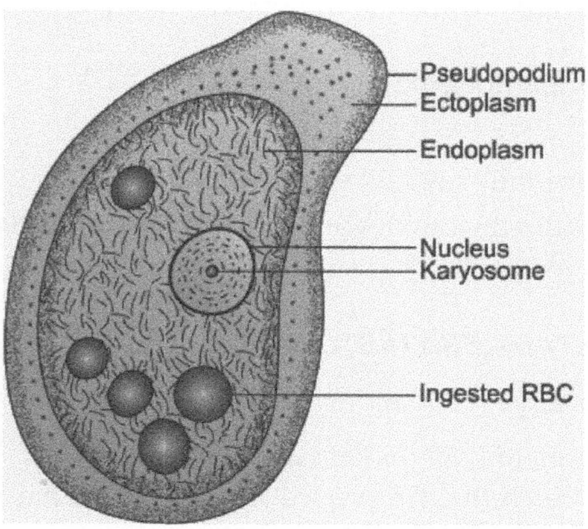

Fig. 38.2A: Trophozoite of *E. histolytica*

Precystic Stage

- Smaller in size
- No red blood cells seen inside the endoplasm
- It becomes oval with a blunt pseudopodium projecting from the periphery (Fig. 38.2B).

Cystic Stage

The parasite becomes completely round and is surrounded by a highly refractile membrane called cyst wall. The cyst has 1 to 4 nuclei depending on its stage of development (Figs 38.2 C and D). In the early stages of development the following are seen.

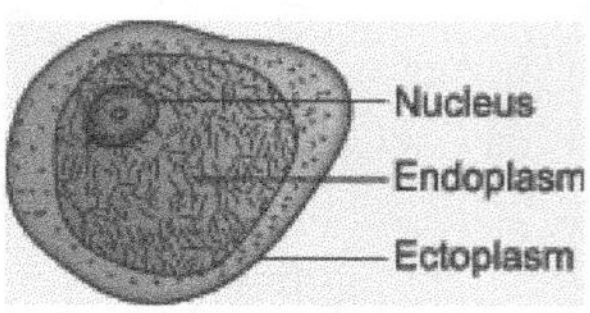

Fig. 38.2B: Precystic stage of *E. histolytica*

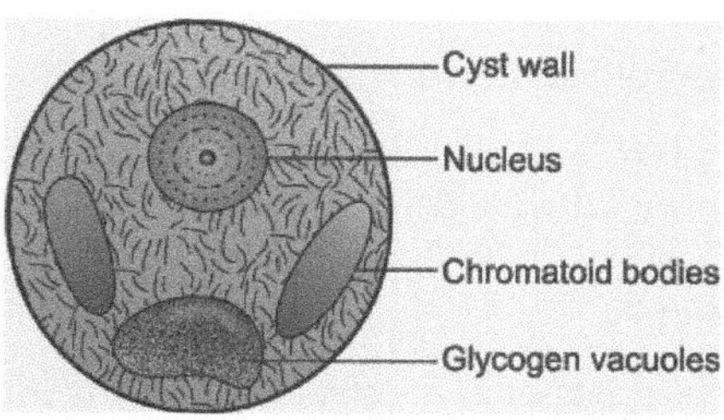

Fig. 38.2C: Uninucleate cyst of *E. histolytica*

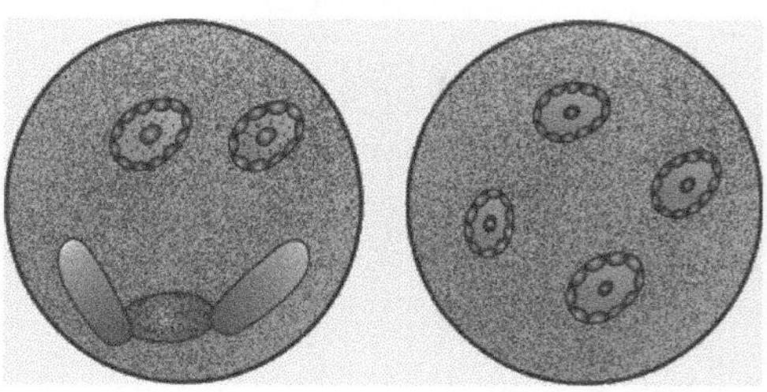

Fig. 38.2D: Binucleate and quadrinucleate cysts of *E. histolytica*

Chromatoid bars: They are seen as refractile oblong bars with rounded ends in unstained preparations and are also not stained in iodine preparations. They stain black in iron hematoxylin preparations. Number varies from 1 to 4 and size varies from 1/2 to 2/3 the diameter of the cyst.

Glycogen mass: This stains brown with iodine but is not visible in unstained preparations.

Life Cycle (Fig. 38.3)

E. histolytica passes its life cycle in only one host the man. The infective forms of the parasite are the mature quadrinucleate cysts. When these cysts are swallowed along with contaminated drink or food they go through the stomach unaffected because they are not acted upon by gastric juice. When they reach the intestine, caecum or lower part of ileum, they are acted upon by trypsin. Here, in alkaline pH, excystation occurs and body retracts and loosens itself from the cyst wall. Vigorous amoeboid movements cause a crack to appear in the cyst wall through which the body of the amoeba comes out. Each cyst liberates a single amoeba with four nuclei (a tetra nucleate amoeba), which eventually forms eight amoebulae by the division of nuclei and fission of cytoplasm. The young amoebulae lodge in the submucous tissue of the large gut. They grow and multiply by binary fission. These dividing trophozoites produce the lesions of amoebiasis. During growth, these amoebae secrete a proteolytic chemical which breaks down tissues and gives the parasite nourishment. After this the outcome may be different. The amoeba may be carried to the liver through the portal veins. Secondary involvement in the other organs like spleen, skin, brain or lungs may also occur. More often, the parasites remain in the intestine itself. They cause an attack of acute dysentery in which many trophozoites are discharged along with the slough. After sometime of acute illness, the resistance of the host increases and the lesions calm down. The person then enters a chronic amoebiasis state. The parasite begins to change into cysts which are passed out into the stool. Sometimes, if the parasite enters a resistant host, the injuries produced are very less. The *E. histolytica* remains in the trophozoite stage in the acute phase of the illness changes to cystic form later. These persons can infect others.

Clinical Features

Here, we shall basically discuss clinical features of amoebic dysentery and amoebic liver abscess.

Amoebic Dysentery

This is a condition in which the infection is confined to the intestinal canal and is characterized by the passage of blood and mucus in the stool. This is because of extensive ulcerations in the intestine due to the active trophozoites. Amoebic ulcerations are found in the large gut. They may be generalized or localized.

Generalized: The whole length of the gut as far down as the internal anal sphincter is involved.

Localized: There are two levels of involvement:

A. Ileocaecal region—Here the caecum, ascending colon, ileocecal value and appendix are involved.
B. Sigmoidorectal region—Here the sigmoid colon and rectum are involved.

The earliest lesions are characterized by the formation of scattered areas of small nodular elevations having an opening at the center with hyperemia and edema. Later, the base of the ulcer is filled with blackish slough and a hyperemic zone.

Amoebic Liver Abscess

The clinical features of amoebic liver abscess are pain and tenderness in the right hypochondrium due to stretching of the capsule of the liver. Referred pain in the right shoulder may be felt. The necrosed liver cells give rise to fever. The general health of the patient falls down.

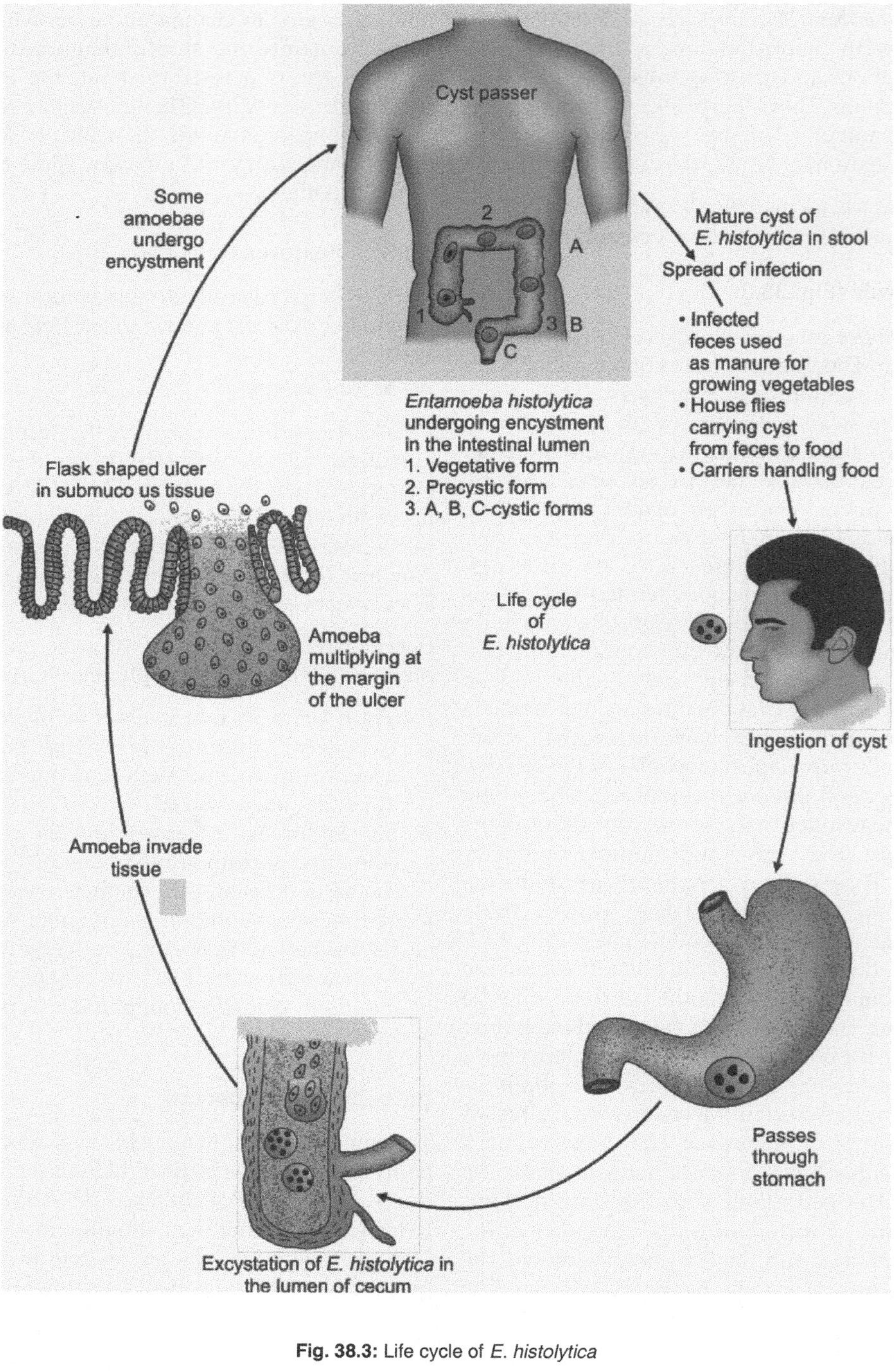

Fig. 38.3: Life cycle of *E. histolytica*

Source of Infection

Natural infection of *E. histolytica* is seen among man and monkeys. Man is the commonest source of infection. He can be a patient or a carrier.

Carriers are of two types—contact and convalescent.

Contact carriers are healthy and have never suffered from the disease. Convalescent carriers have first recovered from the disease.

Mode of Infection

- Mature quadrinucleate cysts are the infective forms of the parasite.
- Fecal contamination of drinking water, vegetables and food leads to infection. Eating of uncooked vegetables and fruits which have been fertilized with infected human feces has led to the occurrence of this disease. Drinking water contaminated with infected feces leads to epidemics.

Incubation Period

The incubation period is generally 4 to 5 days.

Pathological Lesions Caused by *E. histolytica* (Optional)

Amoebiasis means all those conditions that are produced in the human host by infection with *E. histolytica*. Amoebiasis can include intestinal lesions and secondary or metastatic lesions. The secondary sites where the trophozoites can migrate and produce lesions are liver, lungs, brain, spleen and skin.

Intestinal Lesions

Involve the gut only

1. *Acute amoebic dysentery*: Multiple ulcers, deep, extensive. Complications that may arise are pericaecal and pericolic abscess, amoebic appendicitis, perforation and generalized peritonitis.
2. *Chronic intestinal amoebiasis*:
   - Single latent ulcer in the caecum
   - Multiple small superficial ulcers scattered through the large gut
   - Thickened cecum and colon with occasional stricture formation.

Extraintestinal or Metastatic Lesions

1. *Liver*—In amoebic liver abscess
   a. Multiple small abscesses involving the whole organ.
   b. A large solitary abscess in the postero-superior surface of the right lobe.
2. *Pulmonary amoebiasis*
   a. *Primary*—It is a rare condition occurring independently even without the presence of any hepatic abscess. In these cases trophozoites of *E. histolytica* gain entrance from the gut wall via the portal circulation into pulmonary capillaries. These are usually multiple abscesses. They may be in one or both the lungs.
   b. *Secondary*—It arises as a complication of the liver abscess by direct extension through the adhesion formed with the diaphragm, the liver and the base of the right lung. In such cases a single abscess, varying in size may form in the lower lobe of the right lung.
3. *Cerebral amoebiasis*: It is one of the rare varieties of metastatic amoebiasis. Amoebic brain abscess arises a complication of either hepatic or pulmonary abscess or both. The abscess is generally single and of small size and is located most commonly in one of the cerebral hemispheres.
4. *Splenic abscess*: It is found in association with hepatic abscess. Transmission of the trophozoites of *E. histolytica* occurs directly through an adherent splenic flexure of the colon.
5. *Cutaneous amoebiasis*: Amoebic invasion of the skin is usually found over the region which is along a visceral lesion such as in the areas of drainage of liver abscess. Extensive necrosis and sloughing of the skin and subcutaneous tissues are caused by the trophozoites of *E. histolytica* in these areas.
6. *Urogenital tract*: Amoeba gain entrance either through a rectovesical fistula or a recto-vaginal fistula.

Laboratory Diagnosis

This can be divided into:

1. Diagnosis of intestinal amoebiasis
2. Diagnosis of hepatic amoebiasis.

Diagnosis of Intestinal Amoebiasis

This includes a symptomatic group and an asymptomatic group.

Symptomatic Group: The symptomatic group is of acute amoebic dysentery.

We try to distinguish between amoebic dysentery and bacillary dysentery on the basis of macroscopic and microscopic findings (Table 38.1) (Figs 38.4 and 38.5).

Table 38.1: Difference between amoebic dysentery and bacillary dysentery

	Amoebic dysentery	*Bacillary dysentery*
Macroscopic		
Number	6-8 motions a day	Over 10 motions a day
Amount	Copious	Small
Odour	Offensive	Odourless
Color	Dark-red	Bright-red
Nature	Blood and mucus mixed with faeces	Blood and mucus not mixed with faeces
Reaction	Acid	Alkaline
Consistency	Not adherent	Adherent
Microscopic		
RBC's	RBC's are in clumps & reddish-yellow in color	Discrete, bright-red in color
Pus cells	Scanty	Numerous
Macrophages	Very few	Large and numerous. Many of them contain RBC. Hence mistaken for *E. histolytica*
Eosinophils	Present	Few
Pyknotic bodies	Very common	Nil
Parasite	Trophozoites of *E. histolytica*	Nil
Bacteria	Many motile Bacteria	Nil
Charcot-Layden crystals	Present	Nil

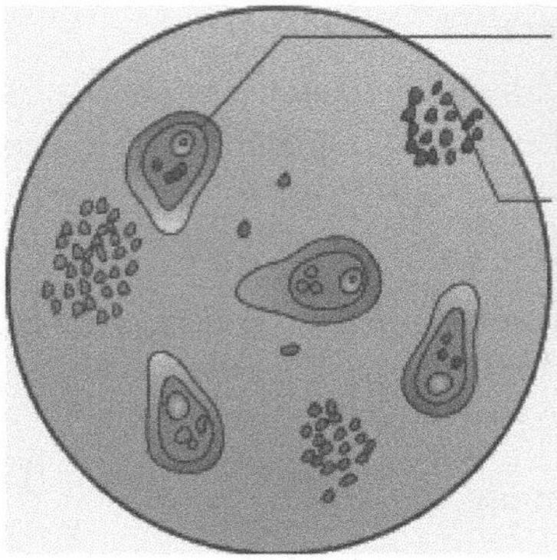

Fig. 38.4: Stool in acute amoebic dysentery

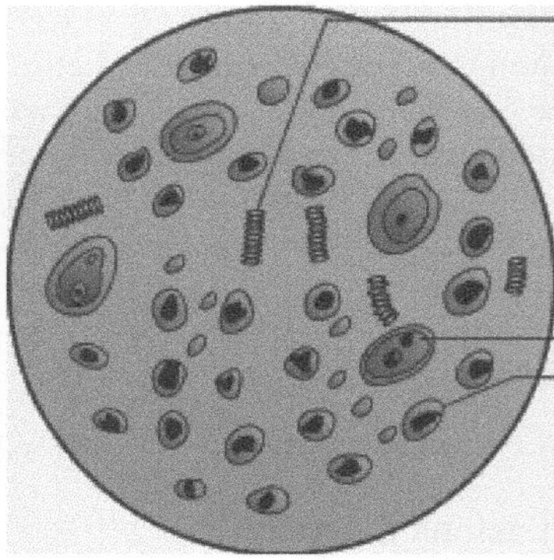

Fig. 38.5: Stool in acute bacillary dysentery

1. *Examination of Stool*
   - Macroscopic appearance
   - Bad smelling
   - Dark brown
   - Semifluid
   - Acidic in reaction
   - Mixed with blood, mucus and much faecal material
     - Microscopic appearance (Fig. 38.4)
   - Presence of less of cells
   - Pyknotic bodies (only nuclear masses of pus cells)
   - Clumped red blood cells reddish yellow in color
   - Charcot-Leyden crystals
     - The appearance is the same as calcium oxalate crystals in urine.

- Demonstration of *E. histolytica*
  - The amoebic trophozoites can be recognized by their movement and the presence of ingested RBC.

2. *Examination of peripheral blood film*: Shows moderate leukocytosis.
3. *Serology*: In early cases the serological tests are negative.

Asymptomatic Group

- *Cyst passers or cyst carriers*
  - Examination of the stool for cysts.
  - *Blood examination*: Not characteristic.
  - *Serological tests*: Mostly negative.

Diagnosis of Hepatic Amoebiasis

1. *Diagnostic aspiration*: Exploratory puncture is used for confirming the diagnosis of amoebic liver abscess. The pus is a mixture of sloughed liver tissue and blood. It is chocolate-brown in color and thick in consistency. The pus is bacteriologically sterile. Microscopical examination of the pus shows degenerated liver cells, a few red blood cells and occasional pus cells. The trophozoites of *E. histolytica* are not found in freshly aspirated liver pus but appear in the pus 4 to 5 days after initial evacuation, because they are attached to the walls of the cavity.
2. *Liver biopsy*: *E. histolytica* trophozoites may be seen in cases of amoebic hepatic abscess.
3. *Examination of stool*: Cysts of *E. histolytica* are present in < 15 percent of cases of amoebic liver abscess.
4. *Examination of blood*: Shows leucocytosis varying from 15000 to 30,000 per mm^3 of blood with neutrophil leukocytosis.
5. *Radiological examination*: Helps in diagnosis.

Very often students confuse Entamoeba coli with Entamoeba histolytica. Let us see the differences (Table 38.2). *E. coli* is a non-pathogenic species whereas *E. histolytica* is usually pathogenic.

Figure 38.6 shows the stages of *Entamoeba coli*.

Table 38.2: Difference between *Entamoeba coli* and *Entamoeba histolytica*

	Entamoeba histolytica	*Entamoeba coli*
Trophozoite		
Fresh preparation		
Trophozoite size	20-30 µm	20–40 µm
Motility	Very active	Sluggish
Cytoplasm	Clearly defined into ectoplasm and endoplasm	Not defined, ectoplasm scarcely seen
Cytoplasmic inclusions	Red blood cells, leucocytes and tissue debris but no bacteria	Bacteria and other materials but never red blood cells
Nucleus	Not visible in unstained preparation	Visible in unstained preparation
Stained with Iodine		
Nuclear character	Central karyosome. Fine chromatin granules line the delicate nuclear membrane	Eccentric karyosome. Coarse chromatin granules line the thick nuclear membrane
Cyst		
Fresh preparation		
Chromatoid bars	Rounded	Filamentous thread-like with square or pointed ends
Stained with Iodine		
Size	6–15 µm	15–20 µm
Nucleus	1–4, central karyosome	1–8, eccentric karyosome
Glycogen mass	Visible in uninucleate stage	Large and visible in binucleate stage

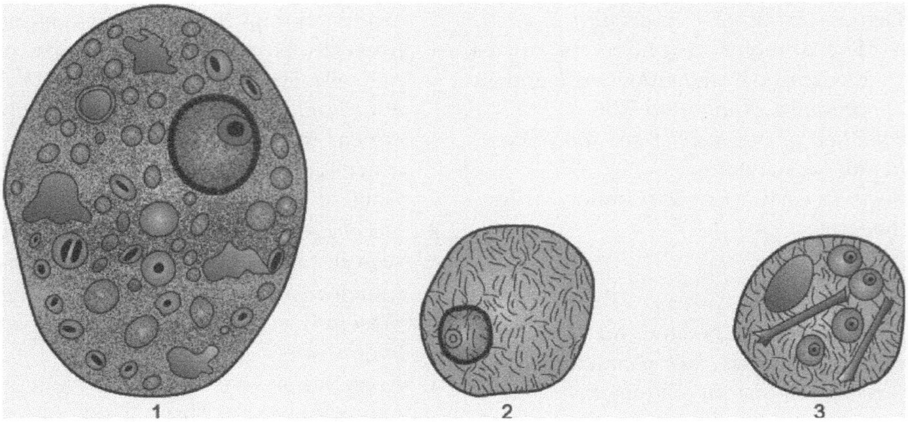

Fig. 38.6: Three stages of *Entamoeba coli*; (1) Trophozoite; (2) Pre-cystic form; (3) Cyst form with one to eight nuclei

MASTIGOPHORA: *GIARDIA LAMBLIA, TRICHOMONAS VAGINALIS* AND *LEISHMANIA DONOVANI*

INTRODUCTION

The parasites belonging to this group of protozoa possess one or more flagella. They are classified into two groups:

1. *Intestinal, oral and genital flagellates*. These infect the intestinal canal, oral cavity and the genital tract. They are mostly non- pathogenic (except *G. lamblia* and *Trichomonas vaginalis*).
2. *Blood and tissue flagellates*: These infect the vascular system and various tissues of the body. These include two genera that are pathogenic to man:
   a. *Trypanosoma*
   b. *Leishmania*

INTESTINAL ORAL AND GENITAL FLAGELLATES

Out of these two are of pathogenic importance
1. *Giardia lamblia*
2. *Trichomonas vaginalis*

Giardia lamblia causes diarrhea and Trichomonas vaginalis causes inflammation of the vaginal mucosa.

Giardia Lamblia (Intestinalis)

History

First seen by Leeuwenhoek while examining his own stool.

Geographical Distribution

Worldwide.

Habitat

It stays in the duodenum and the upper part of jejunum of man.

Morphology

Exists in two phases—trophozoite and cyst phase (Fig. 38.7).

Trophozoite: When viewed flat, the shape of the trophozoite is like that of a tennis or badminton racket. The dorsal surface is convex and the ventral surface is concave with a sucking disc. The size of the trophozoite is 14 µm long and 7 µm broad. The anterior end is broad and

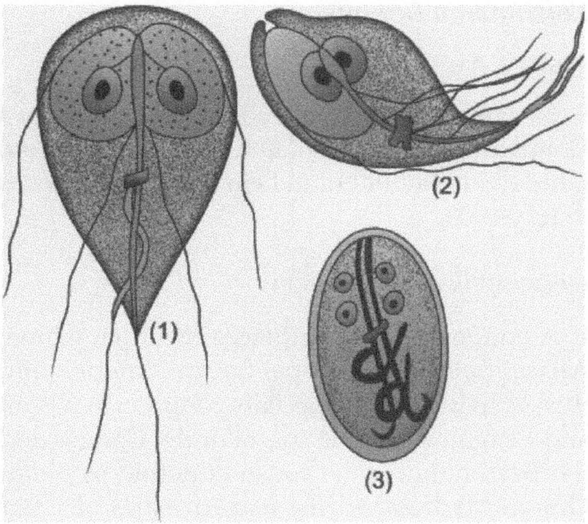

Fig. 38.7: Trophozoite and cyst of *Giardia intestinalis.* Surface view (1) and side (2) of a trophozoite; (3) cyst

rounded and the posterior end tapers to a sharp point. All the organs of the body are paired. Thus there are two axostyles, two nuclei and four pairs of flagella.

Cyst: The fully formed cyst is oval in shape and is 12 µm × 7 µm broad. The axostyles lie diagonally forming a sort of dividing line within the cyst wall. There are four nuclei which remain clustered at one end or lie in pairs at opposite poles. The remains of the flagella and the margins of the sucking disc may be seen inside the cytoplasm. An acid environment causes the parasite to encyst.

Life Cycle

In the trophozoite stage, the parasite multiplies in the duodenum of man by binary fission. When conditions in the duodenum are unfavorable encystment occurs in the large intestine. During encystment, a thick resistant wall is secreted by the parasite and the cell then divides into two within the cyst. Infection of man is brought about by ingestion of cysts. These cysts hatch out two trophozoites which then multiply and colonize the duodenum. To avoid the high acidity of duodenum, giardia localize in the gallbladder.

Pathogenicity

The sucking disc helps the parasite to attach on the epithelial cells in the intestine and leads to disturbance of intestinal function leading to malabsorption of fat. The clinical symptoms may be as follows:

1. Silent cases without any symptoms.
2. Intestinal cases—chronic enteritis and acute enterocolitis.
3. General symptoms—fever, anemia and allergic manifestations.
4. Chronic cholecystopathy.

Laboratory Diagnosis

1. A microscopic examination of a freshly passed stool for demonstration of giardia trophozoites and cysts.
2. Recovery of giardia trophozoites in bile drawn by duodenal intubation.

Trichomonas

- These are common flagellates of the tropics and are frequently observed in diarrheic stools.
- They have only the trophozoite phase and there is no cystic phase.
- The flagellates have pear-shaped bodies and measure 10 to 12 µm in length.
- The single ovoid nucleus is situated at the round anterior end and a cleft-like depression (cytostome) lies at its side.
- There are three to five anterior flagella that are free. A thicker flagellum passes backward along the side of the body forming the undulating membrane and comes out free at the posterior end.

These flagellates are of not much importance except, *T. vaginalis* that is found in large numbers in discharge of females and is the cause of inflammation of the vaginal mucosa.

In case of man, *T. vaginalis* infection is a sexually transmitted disease causing urethritis. Infection has been recorded in newborn females and female children.

Trichomonas can be classified into:

- *Trichomonas hominis* (8 µm): Inhabiting the ileocecal region.
- *Trichomonas tenax*: Inhabiting the oral cavity, being found around the tartar of the teeth and in pyorrhoeic sockets.
- *Trichomonas vaginalis*: (13 µm).

Inhabiting the female genital tract; also found in the urinary tract of both males and females. In this species the cytostome is less conspicuous (Fig. 38.8).

BLOOD AND TISSUE FLAGELLATES

These flagellates live in the blood or tissues of man or other animals. They pass through a cycle in the gut of insects which serve as intermediate hosts. The family includes two genera that are of pathogenic importance to man—Trypanosoma, Leishmania.

We will be studying *Leishmania donovani*, the causative agent of kala-azar in detail.

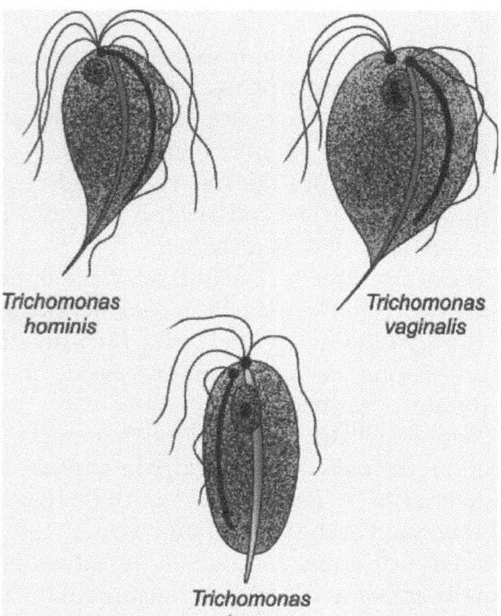

Fig. 38.8: Intestinal, vaginal and oral trichomonas

Leishmania Donovani

History

It is named after two people Leishman and Donovan. Leishman isolated the organism from London in May 1903 and Donovan from Madras in July 1903.

Geographical Distribution

It is endemic in many places in India, China, Africa, Southern Europe, South America and Russia. In India it is especially common in Assam and Bengal, along the coasts of the Ganges and the Brahmaputra. It is also endemic in Bihar, Orissa, Madras and the eastern parts of Uttar Pradesh as far as Lucknow.

Habitat

It is essentially a parasite of the reticuloendothelial system. Inside the vertebrate host (man) the parasite is always intracellular occurring in the amastigote form.

Morphology

The parasite exists in two stages:

1. *Amastigote stage* occurs in man
2. *Promastigote stage* occurs in:
   i. Gut of insect (sandfly)
   ii. Artificial culture.

Amastigote form: The parasite at this stage resides in the cells of the reticuloendothelial system of vertebrate hosts (Figs 38.9A and B).

The characteristics of the amastigote form are:

Shape and size: It is a round or oval body measuring 2 to 4 µm along the longitudinal axis. Cell membrane is delicate.

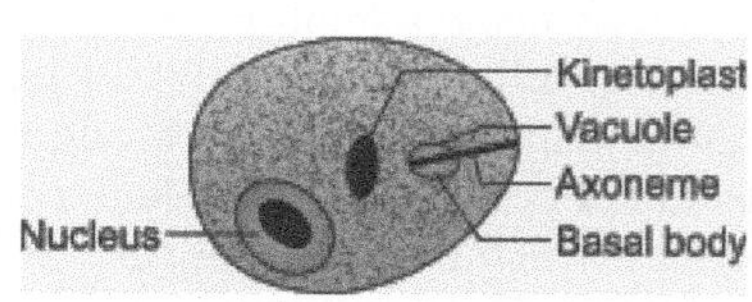

Fig. 38.9A: Diagrammatic representation of the morphology of amastigote form of *L. donovani*

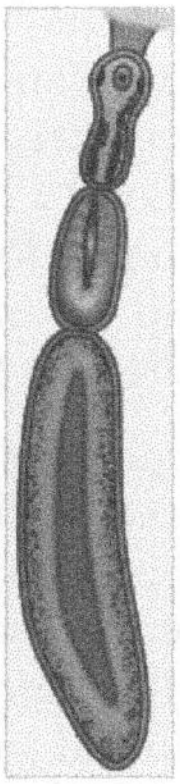

Fig. 38.9B: Diagrammatic representation of the morphology of promastigote form of *L. donovani*

Nucleus: It is < 1 μm in diameter. It is oval or round and is situated either in the middle or on the side.

Kinetoplast: It has a DNA containing body and a mitochondrial structure. It is at right angles to the nucleus.

Axoneme: This is a delicate filament from the kinetoplast to the margin of the body.

Vacuole: This is a clear unstained space lying along the axoneme.

Promastigote Stage: This is the flagellar stage (Fig. 38.9B).

This stage of the parasite is seen in cultures and in insect vectors (sandflies).

These are spindle-shaped bodies measuring 15 to 20 μm in length by 1 to 2 μm in breadth. The nucleus is situated centrally. Kinetoplast lies transversly near the anterior end. The flagella projects from the front.

Life Cycle

The parasite has two stages in its life cycle:

1. The amastigote form occurring in man.
2. The promastigote form occurring in sandfly.

The amastigote forms multiplies by binary fission till the cells become packed with parasites. The host cell is enlarged and ruptures releasing the amastigotes. These attack fresh cells and the cycle is repeated. In this way, the entire reticulo-endothelial system becomes infected. A blood sucking insect takes these free amastigote forms. In certain species of sandfly these amastigote forms develop into promastigote forms which again multiply by binary fission producing a large number of flagellates. Multiplication occurs in the midgut of the sandfly and the flagellates then spread to the anterior part of the alimentary canal. A heavy pharyngeal infection is seen between the 6th and 9th day of its infective blood meal. Transmission then occurs with the bite of a sandfly where the promastigotes enter the human body and change to amastigotes.

Reservoirs of Infection

In India, man is the main or only source of infection. In the Mediterranean region, China and Brazil, the dog is considered to be a reservoir.

Mode of Infection

It is transmitted by the bite of the sandfly Phlebotomus argentipes in India. In other countries the species are different. It has been seen that sandflies who have fed on plant juices before their second blood meal show a heavy infection and their buccal cavity becomes completely blocked by the flagellates. Bites of such blocked flies always lead to infection because it has to discharge some promastigotes before taking in a blood meal. Out of these some of the promastigote forms change into amastigote forms in the reticuloendothelial system. Some of the flagellates are destroyed.

Incubation Period

This is the period between the time of initial infection and the appearance of clinical symptoms. It generally varies from three to six months but may exceed one year.

Clinical Features

Infection with Leishmania donovani produces thedisease kala-azar or visceral leishmaniasis characterized by the following:

1. *Fever*: It may be continuous or become intermittent.
2. *Splenic enlargement*: Most important feature.
3. The *liver is also enlarged* but not as much as spleen.
4. *Lymphadenopathy* may be observed in African and Chinese form also.

In a fully-developed case, *anemia and weakness become prominent*. The skin over the entire body is dry, rough and harsh and it is often pigmented. The disease Kala-azar (black) gets its' name after the pigmentation. The hair tends to be brittle and falls out.

If left untreated, 75 to 95 percent of the patients die within a period of two years. Death is due to some complication such as amoebic or bacillary dysentery, pneumonia, pulmonary tuberculosis and other septic infections.

Laboratory Diagnosis of Kala-azar

There can be direct evidences or indirect evidences.

Direct evidences: These include all those evidences which directly show the presence of *L. donovani* in

1. Peripheral blood.
2. Blood culture.
3. Biopsy material obtained from lymph node, or sternal or iliac crest puncture.

Peripheral blood film: A microscopical examination of a stained blood film can demonstrate the presence of amastigote forms of the parasite in the peripheral blood. A thick blood film as in the detection of malarial parasite can be made. We should also produce a straight leucocyte edge. The citrated blood is centrifuged. The sediment at the bottom of the tube is withdrawn by means of a capillary pipette, smeared, dried and stained. This increases the yield of the parasite.

Blood culture: Disadvantage of this method is that it is slow and takes a long time (one month). About 1 to 2 mL of blood is taken aseptically from a vein and diluted with 10 mL of citrated saline solution (85 percent of normal saline containing 2 percent sodium citrate). The cells are then allowed to settle in a cool incubator (22°C) over night. The cellular deposit is then inoculated into water of condensation of NNN medium and incubated at 22° for one to four week. At the end of each week a drop of condensation fluid is examined for promastigote forms.

NNN medium: This medium was introduced by Novy and MacNeal, later modified by Nicolle and commonly referred to as NNN medium. This medium is composed of two parts of salt agar and one part of defibrinated rabbits blood. *L. donovani* can be cultured in this medium. The material for culture is inoculated into water of condensation of the medium and incubated at 22°C to 24°C.

In the NNN medium, the amastigote forms change into promastigote forms which then multiply to produce a large number of flagellates.

Spleen puncture: It is one of the most valuable methods for establishing the diagnosis. The amastigote forms are found in stained films and promastigote forms in culture.

Bone marrow biopsy: It is safer than spleen puncture but more painful.

Indirect evidences: Infection with Leishmania causes certain changes:

- *Blood count*: There is leucopenia with neutropenia but relative increase of lymphocytes and monocytes. The blood count can fall as low as 3000 per mm^3 of blood. The red blood cells are also decreased in number but not as much as leukocytes.
- *Serological tests*: In leishmaniasis, there is hypoalbuminaemia and hypergammaglobulinaemia. Based on this there are many serological tests (Aldehyde and Antimony Test). Also development of certain immune bodies takes place which is detected by the Complement fixation test.
  1. The Aldehyde (Formal gel test).
  2. Antimony test.
  3. Complement fixation test with WKK antigen.

Aldehyde test: About 1 to 2 mL of a serum is taken from a case of kala-azar in a test tube and to it is added a drop of 40 percent formalin.

A positive result is indicated by jellification of milk white opacity like the white of a hard boiled egg. If it occurs in the course of 2 to 20 minutes, the reaction is said to be strongly positive. The aldehyde test is positive after three months of disease.

Antimony test: This also depends upon a rise of gammaglobulin. When 4 percent urea stibamine solution in distilled water comes in contact with whole serum or serum diluted 1 in 10 from a kala-azar patient a profuse flocculent precipitate forms. A negative result is indicated when the two fluids mix without precipitation. Antimony test is less reliable than aldehyde test.

Complement fixation test: This test depends upon the presence of certain immune bodies in blood sera of Kala-azar patients. This test becomes positive within three weeks of the infection. WKK antigen was used. WKK stand for Witebsky, Klingenstein and Kuhn who were the scientists who prepared the antigen from human tubercle bacillus. *Leishmania* and *Mycobacteria* share a common antigen.

Now this test is carried out with an antigen prepared from Kedrowsky's acid fast bacillus.

Other Serological Tests

The immunofluorescence test has been found to be a valuable test for the diagnosis of visceral leishmaniasis. The antigen is prepared from promastigote forms in culture and smeared on slides. A specific complement fixation test may also be carried out with an antigen prepared from promastigotes of *L. donovani*, or with an antigen prepared from infected hamster spleen or liver. Figure 38.10 shows the methods of diagnosis of kala-azar.

Treatment

The specific chemotherapeutic drugs include:

A. Antimony compounds—Urea stibamine
B. Synthetic non-metallic compounds—Pentamidine isothionate.

Prophylaxis

The preventive measures include the following:

1. Attack on the parasite—By means of adequate treatment.
2. Attack on the vector—Measures against sandfly
3. Personal prophylaxis—Use of sandfly mosquito net, avoiding the ground floor for sleeping purposes and periodic fumigation.

Other Leishmania Lesions

1. Dermal Leishmanoid (Post-kala-azar Dermal Leishmaniasis)—Develops in about 10 percent kala-azar patients generally one or two years after completion of antimonial treatment.
2. Cutaneous Leishmaniasis or Oriental Sore This is caused by Leishmania tropica.
3. Espundia or Mucocutaneous Leishmaniasis caused by *Leishmania brasiliensis*.

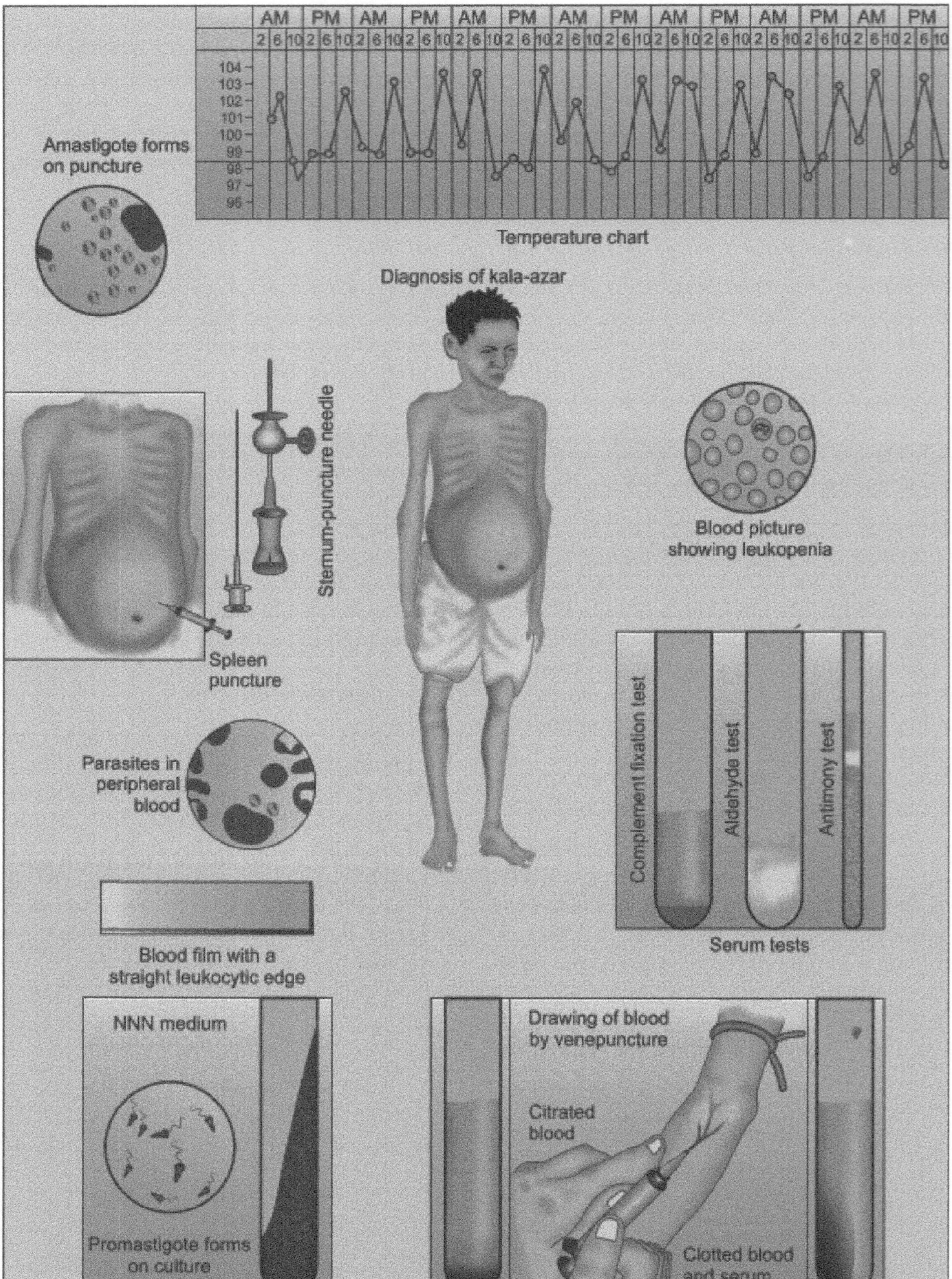

Fig. 38.10: Diagram showing the methods of diagnosis of kala-azar *(For color version see Plate 2)*

SPOROZOA: *PLASMODIUM*

INTRODUCTION

The parasites belonging to this class do not have any special organs of locomotion such as flagella or cilia. They show only slight change in form. They reproduce by two methods:

1. *Asexually by schizogony.*
2. *Sexually by sporogony.*

This is called alteration of generation. In genus *Plasmodium* this takes place in different hosts and so there is alteration of host as well as alteration of generation.

CLASSIFICATION

The sporozoa infecting man is divided into two main groups:

1. Intestinal sporozoa.
2. Blood inhabiting sporozoa.

Intestinal Sporozoa

Here after sexual union, the development of oocyst occurs in the passed feces on the soil and infection is transmitted by contamination. Example is genus *Toxoplasma* and *Cryptosporidium*.

Blood Inhabiting Sporozoa

Here the sexual union takes place inside the insect host and infection is transmitted by inoculation. Example is genus *Plasmodium*.

Genus *Plasmodium* has four species that can infect man:

1. *Plasmodium vivax.*
2. *Plasmodium malariae.*
3. *Plasmodium falciparum.*
4. *Plasmodium ovale.*

GEOGRAPHICAL DISTRIBUTION

Malarial parasites are found in all countries from 40°S to 60°N. Except for *P. ovale*, all species are found in India. Malaria is derived from two Italian words *mala* and *aria* meaning bad air. It was believed that the disease was transmitted by bad air. The parasites are mostly found in tropics. *P. malariae* is also found in the subtropical zone. *P. vivax* is also found in the temperate zone. P. *ovale* has been reported from East Africa, West Africa especially Nigeria and Philippines.

LIFE CYCLE OF THE MALARIAL PARASITE

The malarial parasite passes its life cycle in two hosts.

1. *In man*: Man is the intermediate host of the malarial parasite, i.e. the asexual cycle occurs in the liver cells and the red blood corpuscles.
2. *In female anopheline mosquito*: The female anopheles mosquito is the definitive host of the malarial parasite because the sexual cycle occurs inside the insect.

Human Cycle

The human cycle starts with the introduction of sporozoites by the bite of an infected anopheles mosquito. It ends with the formation of male and female gametocytes (Fig. 38.11).

The stages in the human cycle are as follows:

Pre-erythrocytic Schizogony

Pre-erythrocytic schizogony means the developmental phase before the erythrocytic schizogony. The sporozoites introduced by the bite of an infected female anopheles mosquito undergo a developmental phase inside the parenchymal cells of the liver before entering the erythrocytes. This cycle lasts for:

- Eight days in *P. vivax.*
- Six days in *P. falciparum.*
- Nine days in *P. ovale.*

No clinical symptom or damage is produced by the parasite while developing inside the liver.

Erythrocytic Schizogony

This is the most important phase for diagnosis.

During this phase, the parasite enters the red blood cells and passes through three stages:

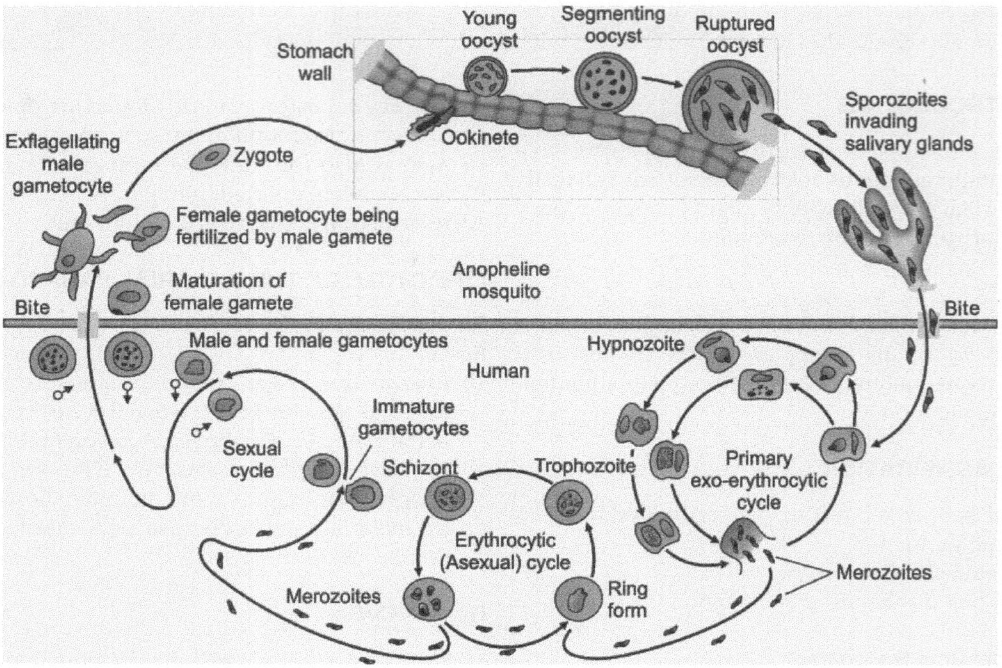

Fig. 38.11: Life cycle of malarial parasite

- Trophozoite
- Schizont
- Merozoite.

These forms can be seen in the peripheral blood thick smears 4 days after the completion of pre-erythrocytic schizogony, i.e. in *P. vivax* about 12 days and in *P. falciparum* about 9 to 10 days after exposure.

This erythrocytic phase takes place in cycles and when the schizont ruptures to release merozoites a rise in fever results. Each cycle takes 48 to 72 hours in *P. vivax*, *P. ovale* and *P. falciparum*, whereas in *P. malariae* it takes 72 hours. This cycle can continue for long time but in course of time, the infection tends to die out either due to exhaustion of asexual reproductive capacity or due to spontaneous destruction of parasites by the body's immune response.

Gametogony

After erythrocytic schizogony has gone on for sometime some of the merozoites instead of developing into trophozoite and schizont, give rise to forms which are capable of sexual function after leaving the human host. They are called gametocytes and their development occurs inside the red blood cells of the capillaries of internal organs (spleen and bone marrow). Once the mature gametocytes are formed, they come out in the peripheral blood. The maturation is completed in 96 hours (4 days). Gametocytes do not produce any fever. Table 38.3 shows the differences in the gametocytes of *P. vivax*. Table 38.4 shows the differences between the microgametocyte and macrogametocyte of *P. falciparum*.

Table 38.3: Differences between microgametocyte and macrogametocyte of *P. vivax*

	Microgametocyte	*Macrogametocyte*
Size	9-10 µm	10-12 µm
Cytoplasm	Stains light blue	Stains deep blue
Nucleus	Diffuse, lies laterally	Small compact lies peripherally

Table 38.4: Differences between microgametocyte and macrogametocyte of *P. falciparum*

	Microgametocyte	*Macrogametocyte*
Shape	Broader, shorter, ends are blunt	Longer narrower, ends are pointed
Size	8-10 µm × 2-3 µm	10-12 µm × 2-3 µm
Cytoplasm	Srains light blue	Strains deep blue
Nucleus mass	Scattered over a wider area in the form of fine granules	Condensed into a small compact at the center
Pigments	Scattered through the cytoplasm	Aggregate like a wreath around the nucleus

Exo-erythrocytic Schizogony

After the establishment of the blood infection, the pre-erythrocytic phase disappears completely in *P. falciparum*, whereas in *P. vivax*, *P. ovale* and in *P. malariae* it persists in the form of a local cycle. This is called exo-erythrocytic phase. These are responsible for relapses and form a continuous source of the parasites. Figure 38.12 shows the differential characters of the erythrocytic stages of malarial parasites of man.

Mosquito Cycle

The mosquito cycle starts with ingesting both the sexual and asexual forms of the parasite during its blood meal from an infected person. The asexual forms are not capable of further development and die off immediately. The sexual forms develop further.

For infecting the mosquito the blood of a human carrier must contain 12 gametocytes per mm^3 of blood and the number of female gametocytes must be in excess of males.

The first phase of development occurs in the midgut of the mosquito. From one male gametocyte 5 to 8 thread-like filamentous microgametes are developed. From one macrogametocyte (female gametocyte), only one macrogamete is formed. The gametes are then ready for fertilization and by a process of chemotaxis, microgametes are attracted towards macrogametes. Fusion takes place between male and female gametes and the resulting body is called a zygote. The zygote changes into an ookinete and that into an oocyst which lies now in the stomach wall. The number of oocysts in the stomach varies from few to more than 100. The oocysts has inside it many sporozoites (from a few 100 to 1000). When fully mature, the oocyst ruptures releasing sporozoites in the body cavity of the mosquito. These sporozoites have a special attraction towards the salivary glands and reach a greatest concentration in the ducts. The mosquito can transmit the infection to man at this stage.

Let us now discuss the blood forms of the two most commonly seen parasites in detail (Table 38.5).

METHOD OF TRANSMISSION OF MALARIA

The infection is transmitted by the inoculative method. During the act of biting the mosquito's proboscis pierces the skin and the salivary secretion is injected into the puncture wound.

The other ways in which malaria can be produced are:

- Transfusion
- Congenital malaria
- Malaia in drug addicts.

Incubation Period

The sporozoite after gaining entrance into the human hist undergoes a development cycle in the liver and then in the red blood cell. With the start of the erythrocytic schizogony, the parasite multiplies in geometric progression and on reaching a sufficient concentration in the blood brings about the onset of fever. This period of development is called the incubation period (time from infection with the sporozoite to the onset of fever).

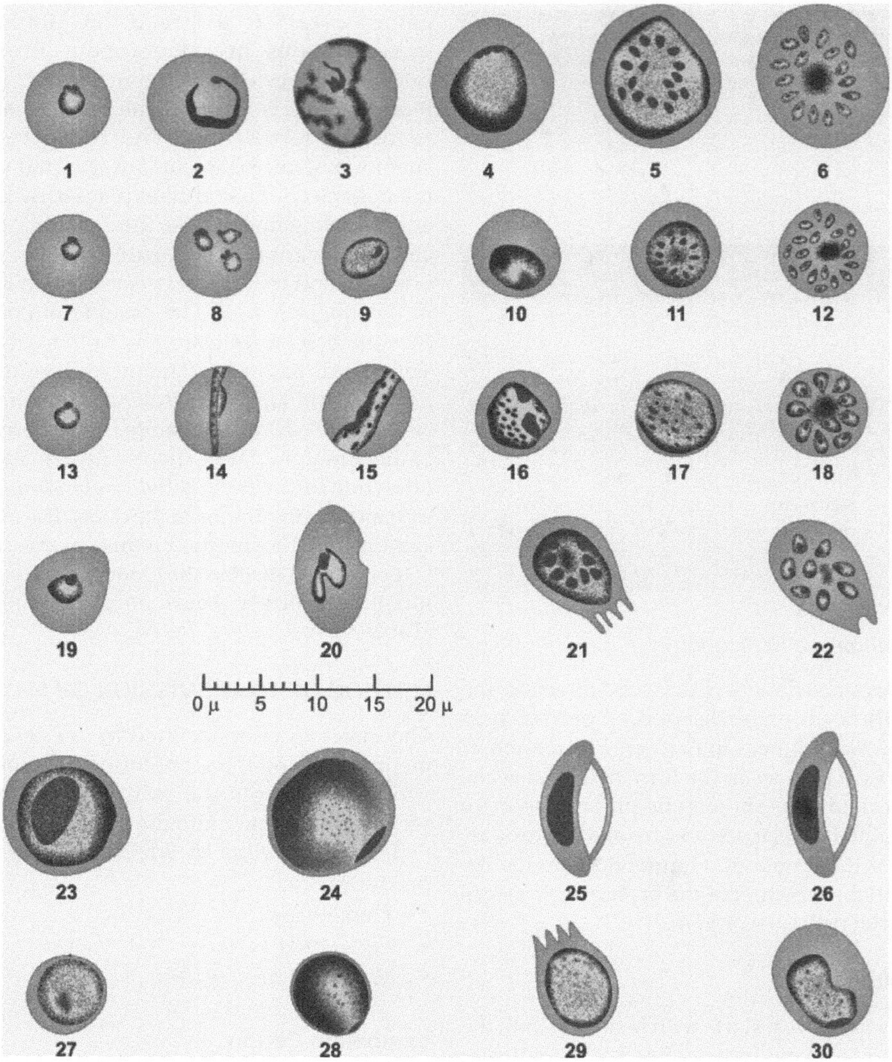

Fig. 38.12: Malarial parasites of man: Differential characters of erythrocytic phases (color) *(For color version see Plate 3)*

1,6, *P. vivax*, 1,2,3, trophozoites (1 early ring-form, 2 &3 larger ring-forms with Schüffiner's dots, 3 amoeboid form); 4,5,6, schizonts—early to mature (rosette) stage.

7 to 12, *P. falciparum*. 7,8,9, trophozoites; 10,11,12, growth of a schizont (inside the capillary of internal organ); 8, showing multiple infections with form "accole"; 9 & 10, showing Maurer's dots in the host-cell. Note the normal size of the infected cell.

13 to 18, *P. malariae*. 13, ring-form; 14,15, band-form; 16,17,18, growth of a schizont. Note the normal size of the host-cell and undotted erythrocytes.

19 to 22, *P. ovale*. 19, 20, trophozoites; 21,22, developing schizonts. Note Jame's dots in all the stages as also the irregular and oval shape of the enlarged host-cell.

23 to 30, mature gametocytes *P. vivax* (23 male, 24 female), *P. falciparum* (25 male, 26 female), *P. malariae* (27 male, 28 female) and *P. ovale* (29 male, 30 female).

Table 38.5: Differences between the blood forms of *P. vivax* and *P. falciparum*

	P. vivax	*P. falciparum*
Schizogony duration	48 hours	48 hours
Forms in peripheral blood	Trophozoites, Schizonts, Gametocytes	Rings and crescents only. Growing trophozoites and schizonts seen rarely
Trophozoites		
Ring forms	Size 2.5 µm Cytoplasm opposite the nucleus is thicker	Size 1.25 to 1.5 µm Cytoplasm fine and regular in outline. Often with 2 nuclei. Form accole. Multiple infection
Growing form	Irregular with vacuole Actively amoeboid	Assumes a compact form. Pigments collect into a single mass early
Schizont mature	Size 9–10 µm Regular, almost completely fills the enlarged red blood cell	Size, 4.5–5 µm. Fills two-thirds of a red blood cell which is not enlarged.
Merozoites	12-24. Arranged in an irregular grape like cluster	18-24. Arranged in a grape like cluster
Infected RBC (Host cell)	Enlarged pale. Schuffner's dots present	Usually unaltered. crenation, reddish violet colour and Maurer's dots present.
Gametocyte*	Spherical or globular Much larger than a red blood cell. Host cell enlarged.	Crescentic. Larger than a red blood cell. Host cell hardly seen.
Malarial pigments	Yellowish-brown fine granules	Dark-brown or blackish. One or two solid blocks.

* *Female* Cytoplasm stains blue, nucleus, small and compact
Male Cytoplasm stains pale blue or reddish, nucleus, large and diffuse

CLINICAL FEATURES OF MALARIA

Fever forms the most important symptom followed by anemia and splenic enlargement.

Fever

Each fever paroxysm has three stages:

- Cold stage which lasts for 20 minutes to one hour
- Hot stage (lasts 1 to 4 hours)
- Sweating stage (lasts 2 to 3 hours).

Types of Fever

The febrile paroxysm synchrinises with the erythrocytic schizogony.

1. With a 48 hours cycle, the fever recurs every 3rd day—Tertian fever.
2. With a 72 hours cycle the fever recurs every 4th day—Quartan fever.
3. Fever recurring at intervals of 24 hours (quotidian periodicity) has also been observed in infections with *P. vivax* or with *P. malariae*. This is due to the maturation of two generations of tertian parasites on two successive days.
4. The fever may not develop according to the above pattern because of many generations of parasite multiplying. In such cases the fever is continuous.

Anaemia

After a few paroxysms, anaemia develops as a result of breaking down of red blood cells during segmentation of parasites.

Splenomegaly

Enlargement of the spleen is one of the most important physical signs in malaria.

COMPLICATIONS OF FALCIPARUM MALARIA

Pernicious Malaria

The term "pernicious malaria" is referred to a series of phenomena occurring during the course of an infection with *P. falciparum*, which if not effectively treated, threatens the life of a patient within 1 to 3 days. The serious complications that may develop in pernicious malaria are the result of capillary blockage due to agglutination of parasitised erythrocytes. The various ways in which pernicious malaria can present is:

1. *Cerebral malaria*—manifested by hyperpyrexia, coma and paralysis.
2. *Algid malaria*—Characterized by cold and clammy skin with vascular collapse leading to peripheral circulatory failure.
3. *Septicaemic malaria* Characterized by high fever, pneumonia, etc.

The blockade of the capillary blood vessels of the internal organs arising from agglutination of the parasitised erythrocytes could be due to the fact that the asexual parasites of *P. falciparum* go to the capillaries of the internal organs to complete their schizogony. They have a stickiness, helping in agglutination. Vasoconstriction of the capillaries also adds to this. The blockage of the capillary blood vessels lead to the various symptoms.

Black Water Fever

Definition

It is a manifestation of falciparum malaria occurring in previously infected patients and is characterized by sudden intravascular hemolysis followed by fever and hemoglobinuria.

Why Does it Happen?

The exact mechanism of hemolysis in blackwater fever is not yet clearly known. There is some haemolytic agent involved which causes the red cells to undergo lysis and liberate a large quantity of oxyhaemoglobin into the blood stream.

In falciparum malaria, intravascular hemolysis occurs periodically at the time of schizogony. This stimulates the reticuloendothelial system to form antibodies (hemolysins). Whenever a precipitating factor is present such as heavy *P. falciparum* infection, administration of quinine, cold, exposure to the sun, fatigue, trauma, pregnancy, etc. an explosive output of haemolysin results which causes haemolysis. Individuals having glucose-6-phosphate dehydrogenase deficient red blood cells are particularly susceptible to such hemolysis.

Effects of Intravascular Hemolysis

When the red blood cells rupture, they release hemoglobin. This excess hemoglobin is either catabolized into methemalbumin or converted by reticuloendothelial system into bilirubin and haemosiderin or excreted through kidneys. The following effects are observed:

- Methemalbuminemia
- Hyperbilirubinemia
- Hemoglobinuria.

Clinical Features

The attack begins with fever and rigor followed by aching pain in the loins haemoglobinuria, jaundice, vomiting, circulatory collapse and acute renal failure.

Laboratory Diagnosis

- RBC count is 1 to 2 millions/mm^3
- Hemoglobin drops down to 10 mg/dL
- There may be normocytic anemia
- Neutrophil leucocytosis
- Blood urea is increased, blood cholesterol is lowered
- *Urine*: The color of the urine is red to dark brown and is acid in reaction. When allowed to settle, there is a heavy amorphous deposit at the bottom. Albumin is excreted in large amounts, urobilin test shows a marked reaction. Microscopical examination shows haemoglobin casts and haematin crystals.
- In the majority of cases *P. falciparum* parasites are not detected in the peripheral blood either during or after an attack as they are destroyed. The parasites reappear within a week or a fortnight after the haemolytic crisis.

Treatment

If the parasites are detected in the peripheral blood, antimalarial chemotherapy should be given and the drug of choice is chloroquine.

- Blood transfusion should be given
- Quinine should be avoided
- The patient of black water fever should leave the endemic area and must not return.

LABORATORY DIAGNOSIS OF MALARIA

A microscopical examination of a blood film is one of the most important diagnostic procedures in malaria. Both thick and thin films are recommended. The various stages of the malarial parasites are recognized and a species diagnosis is made.

Other Methods in Diagnosis

There are many other methods to diagnose malaria which are not routinely recommended.

- *Cultural examination*: This is not required for diagnosis except only in special circumstances, when there is a difficulty in differentiating the trophozoite (ring form of *P. vivax* from that of *P. falciparum*).

  Culture methods are used to study only one generation. Bass and John's technique with a slight modification is used for cultivation of malarial parasite in artificial culture media.
- *Blood count*: There is moderate leucopenia with monocytosis (15 to 20%).
- *Serological tests*: Not necessary for acute infection but are used for studying immunological aspects of populations living in highly endemic areas or for detecting latent infection in subjects who are blood donors.

INTRODUCTION

Toxoplasma is a small parasite discovered by Nicolle and Manceaux in 1908 in a small rodent, gondii (*Ctenodactylus gundi*) of Africa.

LIFE CYCLE

Toxoplasma gondii has an intestinal phase in its life cycle in the cat (*Felis catus*) and an extra-intestinal phase in mouse, man and other animals.

Enteric Cycle (Intestinal Phase)

The cycle takes place in the intestinal cells of the cat. Schizogony and gametogony occurs in the epithelium of the tips of the intestinal villi in the ileum but the whole intestine can be affected. This cycle starts when the cat is fed the mouse brain containing cysts (tissue cysts) of *T. gondii*. All the stages to schizogony and gametogony occur inside the epithelial cells of ileum. Micro- and macrogametocytes form micro- and macro- gametes and then the oocyst when they unite.

Exoenteric Cycle (Extraintestinal Phase)

The oocysts containing two sporocysts are excreted in cat's faeces for 1 to 2 weeks. The oocysts can be infective to man and other animals. After ingestion the oocysts liberate sporozoites which penetrate the mucosal cells of the intestine and are carried by the blood and lymph stream to the mesenteric lymph nodes (lymphoid-macrophage system) and then to the distant organs such as brain, eyes, liver, spleen lymph nodes, heart, skeletal muscles and placenta.

In all these places they form pseudocysts and the parasite inside the cyst is known as endozoite (the nucleus is central in position). The pseudocyst is the proliferative stage of the parasite and is responsible for causing extensive damage to the tissues in which it develops. Some of the sporozoites and the endozoites tend to localize in the central nervous system and musculature where they are transformed into tissue cysts which has inside it cystozoites (nucleus is situated at the rounded end). The tissue cyst is not associated with any symptoms and signs. Both the pseudocyst and tissue cyst are infective and animals can acquire infection by eating other animals (Fig. 38.13).

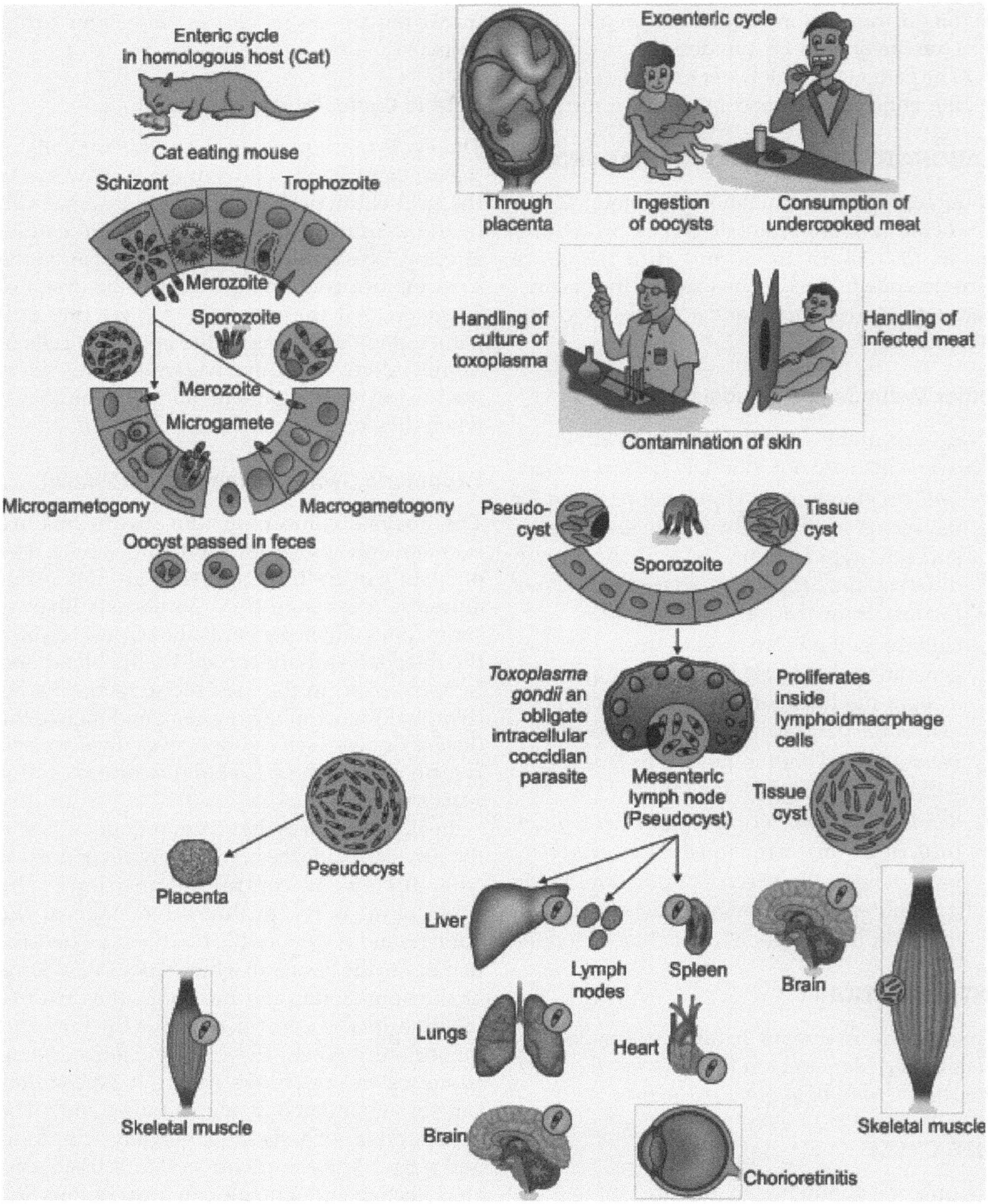

Fig. 38.13: Life cycle of *Toxoplasma gondii*

SPOROZOA: *TOXOPLASMA*

MORPHOLOGY

Two forms of toxoplasma are found in man (also mammals and birds):

- Pseudocyst (intracellular form)
- Tissue cyst (extracellular form).

Pseudocyst or intracellular form: It is found in the cells of the reticuloendothelial system and many nucleated cells. It can be found in the placenta, liver, lungs, brain, skeletal muscle, lymph nodes, heart and eye. It has endozoites which are crescent shaped but may be oval and the nucleus is central in position. It measures 4 to 6 μm in length × 2 μm in breadth.

Tissue cyst or extracellular form: It may be found free in tissue fluids. It is more often found in the CNS and muscles where it is surrounded by a tissue cyst wall. It has cystozoites which are slender crescent shaped organisms, one end rounded and the other pointed. The single nucleus is situated at the rounded end.

STAINING REACTION

It stains readily with alkaline methylene blue. When stained with Giemsa stain, the cytoplasm appears blue, the nucleus reddish-purple and the paranuclear body red.

CULTIVATION

It can be cultivated in association with living tissues (in chorioallantoic membrane of the developing chick embryo).

PATHOGENICITY

The pathological lesion is characterized by anarea of focal necrosis surrounded by inflammatory cells. A large number of parasites may be found inside the cell which is enlarged to form a pseudocyst.

MODE OF INFECTION

Human toxoplasmosis can occur in two ways:

Congenital

The fetus *in utero* is infected through the transplacental route. The organism is transmitted from the infected mother who may not show any symptom of the disease. Infection occurring in early months of pregnancy results in abortion or stillbirth. Infection in the later months of pregnancy results in signs of the disease which develop 2 to 3 months after birth.

Acquired

Infection may occur in children or in adults. The organism may enter by the following routes

A. By ingestion of underdone meat (containing pseudocyst), cows milk and eggs, contact with the oocysts discharged in the feces of the infected reservoir animal (cat).
B. By inhalation (droplet infection). The organisms are found in the bronchial secretions and sputum.
C. By inoculation (through skin) by contact with infected tissues of animals. *Toxoplasma* can penetrate through cracks and small abrasions in the skin.

CLINICAL FEATURES

- Congenital toxoplasmosis—It is fatal.
- Acquired toxoplasmosis—Signs and Symptoms.

  Cerebrospinal—Hydrocephalus, calcification of cerebral lesions, chiefly found in infants/ children.

  Eyes—Focal chorioretinitis.

  Lymphatic—Fever with generalized lymphadenitis (posterior cervical lymph nodes).

  Skin—Maculopapular rash resembling rashes of typhus fevers, chiefly found in adults.

  Lungs—Interstitial pneumonia resembling atypical virus pneumonia.

  Heart—Myocarditis.

  Liver and spleen—Enlarged.

INCIDENCE

Worldwide.

IMMUNOLOGY

Both cellular and humoral immunity develop after infection. Humoral antibodies which develop in toxoplasma infection are demonstrated by serological tests. Both the immunoglobulins IgG and IgM are present. A negative test is significant and a positive test is indicated when a rising titer is demonstrated in two samples of blood at 3 to 4 weeks interval.

CHANGES IN BLOOD AND CSF

Blood

Leucocytosis (12,000/mm^3) of blood with relative increase of lymphocytes and monocytes. In some cases eosinophilia can be seen.

CSF

Color is yellow, protein is increased. Leukocytes are present in large numbers.

LABORATORY DIAGNOSIS

Direct Evidence

A. Microscopical examination of stained smears of the material obtained from bone marrow puncture and splenic puncture or centrifuged deposit of CSF and smears made from any tissues removed by biopsy (lymph node or muscle).
B. By inoculation of the suspected material in mice, guinea pigs and hamsters.

Indirect Evidences

Based on serology:

1. Fluorescent stain for toxoplasma (Goldman's test). The organism appears brightly fluore scent when treated with fluorescein tagged globulin fraction of homologus antiserum. It can be used to find parasites in tissue smears and sections.
2. Methylene blue dye test of Sabin and Feldman. The principle of this test is to find out a cytoplasm modifying antibody in the patient's serum. If the patient's serum contains the specific antibody, less than 50 percent of free toxoplasma accept the stain and the cytoplasm appears colorless.

In a negative serum 90 to 100 percent of the free *Toxoplasma* accept the stain. The highest dilution of the serum in which 50 percent or more of the organism have unstained cytoplasm is taken as the titer. The dye test (due to persistent antibody) is positive early, persists longer and does not disappear completely. Titer of 1:128 is taken as diagnostic because it may give positive reactions with others too.

Other serological tests are:

- IHA (indirect haemagglutination test).
- IFA (indirect fluorescent antibody test).

Treatment

Pyrimethamine combined with sulphadiazine is an effective remedy.

Spiramycin may also be used.

Prophylaxis

The pathways of transmission should be blocked.

SPOROZOA: *CRYPTOSPORIDIUM*

INTRODUCTION

Cryptosporidium is a small coccidian parasite that is an important cause of acute and persistent diarrhoea. It was initially described by Tyzzer as a protozoan isolated from the gastric mucosa of asymptomatic mice in 1907. It belongs to class Sporozoa.

HISTORY

The first reported human case of cryptosporidiosis occurred in 1976 and was associated with exposure to farm animals. In the early 1980's most reported infections were in patients with acquired immunodeficiency syndrome. Cryptosporidium was considered to be an opportunistic pathogen. Recently the disease has been found in non-immunocompromised humans and it has been confirmed that cryptosporidium may be second only to viruses in the aetiology of acute diarrhea and persistent diarrhea in children.

HABITAT

The usual habitat of Cryptosporidium is the vertebrate host intestine, in which the protozoa grow attached to the epithelial cell membrane in the brush border. Both sexual and asexual forms are found in this area (Fig. 38.14). Whether this organism should be regarded as an intracellular or an extracellular parasite is not resolved.

Cryptosporidia have been found in a variety of mammals, birds, and reptiles since their discovery in 1907, but they were not reported to be associated with human disease until 1976. Until recently, they received little attention because few diagnosticians were aware of their existence, because they were considered not pathogenic, and because they are not likely to be encountered in routine stool examinations.

SPECIES

There are three species of Cryptosporidium:

- *C. parvum*
- *C. muris*
- *C. bialeyi.*

C. parvum is responsible for most cryptosporidial diarrheal diseases in humans and cattle.

LIFE CYCLE

The life cycle is very similar to the toxoplasma. Cryptosporidium oocyst excretion tends to follow the clinical course of diarrheal episode and usually terminates 1 to 2 weeks after the arrest of diarrhea.

MORPHOLOGY OF OOCYST

Thick-walled, 4 to 6 μ, with four sporozoites, which may or may not be visible on light microscopy. On modified Ziehl-Neelsen staining, they stain pink red against a green background.

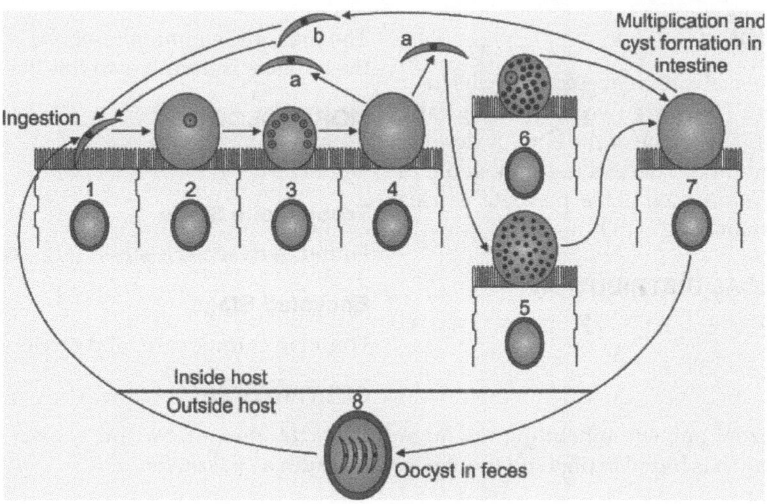

Fig. 38.14: Life cycle of *Cryptosporidium*

MODE OF INFECTION

- Zoonotic transmission
  - This was initially considered to be the principal source of human infection.
- Person-to-person transmission is likely by
  - Homosexual contact
  - Contaminated water
  - Air borne transmission

CLINICAL FEATURES

Incubation period ranges from 1 day to 2 weeks. The clinical signs and symptoms are watery diarrhea, abdominal pain, cramping, anorexia, malaise, weight loss, bloating and gas formation. Symptoms last for one to two weeks on the average but may continue for more than one to two months and usually resolve on its own. In immunocompromised individuals the symptoms are much more virulent and persistent.

LABORATORY DIAGNOSIS

- *Oocyst detection*: Oocyst detection in stool forms the standard procedure for routine identification of cryptosporidium. Concentration methods may increase diagnostic yield. Kinyoun's acid fast staining for stool smears is a good stain for the detection of cryptosporidium oocysts.
- *Serological detection*: An enzyme linked immunosorbent assay for the detection of cryptosporidium specific immunoglobulin G and IgM has been used.
- *Cultivation*: Sporozoites of *C. parvum* can grow in monolayers of the mouse fibroblast cell line L929.
- *Animal inoculation*: Definitive confirmation of the presence of cryptosporidium in a fecal sample can be obtained by oral inoculation into suckling mice.

TREATMENT

Most promising has been the use of spiramycin, a macrolide antibiotic in a class with erythromycin.

CILIATA: *BALANTIDIUM COLI*

INTRODUCTION

The body of the parasite is covered with cilia (hair like processes). There are two morphologically distinct nuclei. The shape of the body is defined by a cell membrane. The species pathogenic to man is *Balantidium coli*. This parasite causes dysentery in man.

GEOGRAPHICAL DISTRIBUTION

Worldwide.

HABITAT

Largest protozoal parasite inhabiting the large intestine of man. It is found in pigs and monkeys. The pig is the common reservoir of infection but the parasite is harmless to this host.

MORPHOLOGY

The parasite exists in two stages:

Trophozoite Stage

Found in dysenteric stools (Fig. 38.15A).

Encysted Stage

Found in chronic cases and carriers (Fig. 38.15B).

CULTIVATION

Balantidium coli can be grown in the same medium as *E. histolytica*.

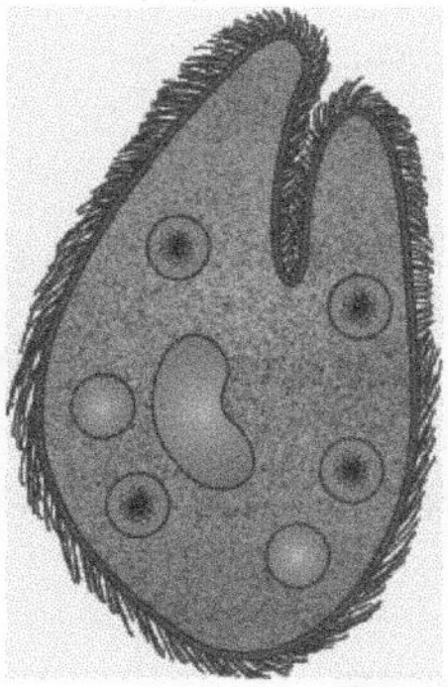

Fig. 38.15A: Morphology
Balantidium coli: Trophozoite stage

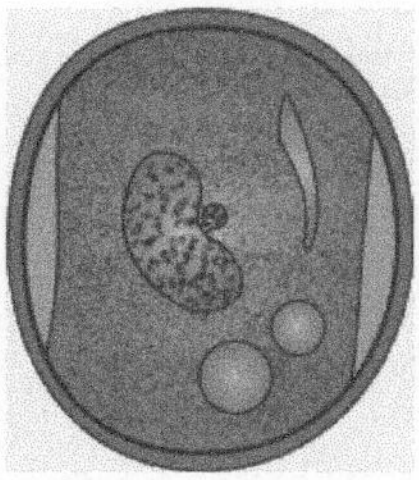

Fig. 38.15B: Cyst of *Balantidium coli*

LIFE CYCLE AND METHOD OF REPRODUCTION

Balantidium coli passes its life cycle in two stages but in one host only.

Pig—The natural host.

Man—This is the rare host.

Cyst—Infective stage of the parasite.

Portal of entry—Mouth, by ingestion.

Transmission occurs from pig to pig, pig to man, man to man and man to pig.

The cyst when ingested, liberates trophozoites in the large intestines and from each cyst a single trophozoite is formed. The trophozoites can enter into the submucus coat of the large intestine and divide. After a period of growth and multiplication, the trophozoite undergoes encystment when conditions are unsuitable for vegetative existence.

PATHOGENICITY

The pig is the usual source of infection to man. Persons having an occupational contact with these animals can get the infection. Transmission is effected through the ingestion of food contaminated by cysts obtained either from the faeces of a pig or man.

The parasite thrives mainly on starchy food found in abundance in pig's intestine. In the presence of abundant starchy food, the parasite does not invade the epithelial cells of the intestine. Therefore it is harmless in pig. The scarcity of starchy food in the human bowel explains why it causes lesions in man.

LESIONS

This consists of ulceration of the colon similar to amoebic ulcers.

The clinical manifestations include passage of blood and mucus in the stool. The condition is afebrile.

DIAGNOSIS

Clinically balantidial dysentery cannot be differentiated from often forms of dysentery. It can only be diagnosed by a microscopical examination of the stool showing the presence of the trophozoites of *Balantidium coli*. The technique for stool examination is the same as for other intestinal protozoa.

TREATMENT

Arsenical preparations.

PROPHYLAXIS

Protection against contamination of food and drink with pig or man feces containing cysts of *Balantidium coli*.

CHAPTER

39

Helminthology

LESSON PLAN

- Introduction
- General Characters of Cestodes
- Classification of Cestodes
  - Pseudophyllidean Cestodes
  - Cyclophyllidean Cestodes
- *Taenia Saginata*
  - Geographical Distribution
  - Habitat
  - Morphology
- *Taenia Solium*
  - Life Cycle
  - Larval Development of *T. Saginata* and *T. Solium*
  - Mode of Infection
  - Diagnosis
  - Treatment
  - Prophylaxis
- *Echinococcus Granulosus*
  - Geographical Distribution
  - Habitat
  - Morphology
  - Life Cycle
  - Mode of Infection
  - Hydatid Cyst
  - Clinical Features
  - Laboratory Diagnosis
  - Treatment
  - Prophylaxis
- Nematoda
  - General Characters
  - Life Cycle
  - Classification of Nematodes
  - Mode of Infection of Nematode Parasites

Individual Parasites: *Trichuris Trichiura*
- Geographical Distribution
- Habitat
- Morphology
- Life Cycle
- Clinical Features
- Laboratory Diagnosis
- Treatment
- Prophylaxis

Ancylostoma Duodenale
- Geographical Distribution
- Habitat
- Morphoglogy
- Life Cycle
- Mode of Infection
- Pathogenic Effects
- Laboratory Diagnosis
- Treatment
- Prophylaxis
- Species Diagnosis
- Specific Diagnosis

Ascaris Lumbricoides
- Geographical Distribution
- Habitat
- Morphology
- Life Cycle
- Mode of Infection
- Clinical Features
- Laboratory Diagnosis
- Treatment
- Prophylaxis

Enterobius Vermicularis
- Geographical Distribution
- Habitat
- Morphology
- Life Cycle
- Mode of Infection
- Clinical Features
- Laboratory Diagnosis
- Treatment
- Prophylaxis

Contd...

INTRODUCTION

The helminthic parasites are multicellular, bilaterally symmetrical animals having three germ layers. They can be divided into two main groups—Platyhelminthes and Nemathelminthes.

Platyhelminthes includes class Cestoda and Trematoda and Nemathelminthes the class Nematoda.

The table below shows us the differences between Cestodes, Trematodes and Nematodes (Table 39.1).

Platyhelminthes: Cestodes—Taenia Saginata and *Echinococcus Granulosus*

Platyhelminthes includes Cestodes and Trematodes.

GENERAL CHARACTERS OF CESTODES

1. The majority of cestodes are long, segmented and tape-like, hence they are called **tapeworms**. They are flattened.
2. The size varies from few mm to several meters.
3. Adult worms are found in the intestinal canal of man and animal.
4. Head is provided with suckers and sometimes with hooks which serve as organs of attachment.
5. There are three regions in an adult worm:
   a. Head (scolex).
   b. A neck.
   c. A strobila (body or trunk consisting of a series of segments) called *proglottides*.
6. The sexes are not separate, i.e. each individual worm is a *hermaphrodite*.
7. Body cavity is absent.
8. Alimentary canal is entirely absent. Excretory and nervous systems are present.
9. Reproductive system is highly developed and complete in each segment. Three types of segments can be seen:
   Immature: Male and female organs are not differentiated

Table 39.1: Differences between cestodes, trematodes and nematodes

	Cestode	*Trematode*	*Nematode*
Shape	Tape like, segmented	Leaf-like, unsegmented	Elongated, cylindrical, unsegmented
Sexes	Not separate (hermaphrodite) (monoecious)	Not separate	Separate
Head end	Suckers, often with hooks	Suckers, no hooks	No suckers, no hooks, well-developed buccal capsule may be seen in some species
Alimentary canal	Absent	Present but incomplete; no anus	Present and complete; anus present
Body cavity	Absent	Absent	Present

Mature: Male and female organs have become differentiated

Gravid: Uterus is filled with eggs (other organs atrophied or disappeared).

CLASSIFICATION OF CESTODES

Pseudophyllidean Cestodes

Possessing false or slit-like grooves called bothria.

1. ***Adult worms in intestine:***
   i. Genus-*Diphyllobothrium-D. latum (fish tapeworm).*
2. ***Larval stages (plerocercoid) in man:***
   i. *Sparganum mansoni.*
   ii. *Sparganum proliferum.*

Cyclophyllidean Cestodes

Possess cup-like and round suckers.

1. ***Adult worms in intestine:***
   i. Genus *Taenia—T. saginata* (beef tapeworm), *T. solium* (pork tapeworm).
   ii. Genus *Hymenolepis—H. nana* (dwarf tapeworm), *H. diminuta* (rat tapeworm).
   iii. Genus *Dipylidium—D. caninum* (double-pored dog tapeworm).
2. ***Larval stages in man:***
   i. Genus *Echinococcus*—Hydatid cyst of *E. granulosus* (dog tapeworm), *E. multilocularis.*
   ii. Genus *Taenia—Cysticercus cellulosae* of *T. solium.*
   iii. Genus *Multiceps—Coenurus cerebralis* of *M. multiceps* and *Coenurus glomeratus* of *M. glomeratus.*

TAENIA SAGINATA

Geographical Distribution

Worldwide. In India, it is particularly seen among muslim community because they are beef eaters. It is also called the beef tapeworm or the **unarmed tapeworm of man.**

Habitat

Adult worms live in the small intestine (upper jejunum of man).

Morphology

Adult Worm

- It is white and semitransparent, measuring 5 to 10 m in length but may be upto 24 m.
- The head measures 1–2 mm in diameter and has four suckers.
- The neck is fairly long.
- The segments can be from 1000 to 2000. The eggs are liberated by the rupture of the ripe proglottides.
- Life span of the adult worm may be up to 10 years (Fig. 39.1).

Eggs

The characteristics of the egg are as follows:

1. Spherical and brown in color (bile-stained).
2. Measure 31 × 43 μm in diameter.
3. The outer shell is thin and transparent.
4. The inner embryophore is brown, thick-walled and radially striated.
5. Contains an oncosphere with three pairs of hooklets.
6. Eggs are resistant and may remain viable for 8 weeks (Fig. 39.2).

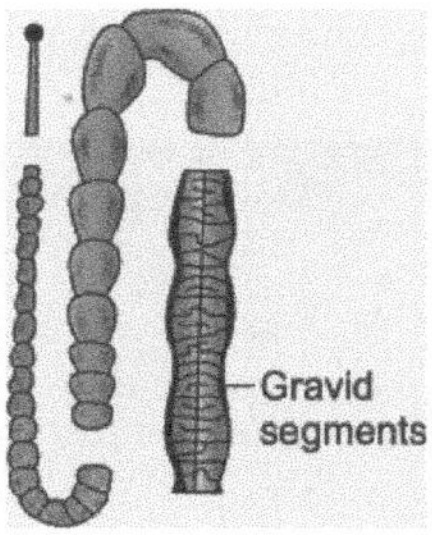

Fig. 39.1: Adult worm of *T. saginata*

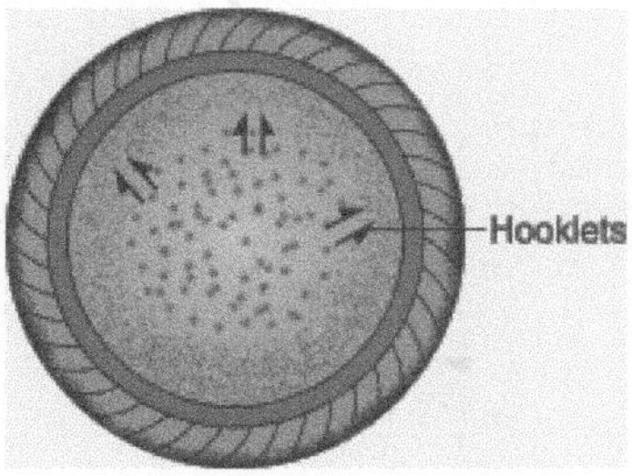

Fig. 39.2: Egg of *T. saginata*

TAENIA SOLIUM

- This is called **pork tapeworm** or the armed tapeworm of man.
- It is smaller than *T. saginata*, the head is smaller and the proglottids are fewer in number.
- The head is armed with a double layer of alternating large and small hooklets (rostellum).
- The pig is the intermediate host.

T. solium and *T. saginata* are very similar to each other and shall be considered together.

See Table 39.2 for the differences in the adult worms of *T. solium* and *T. saginata*. There is no difference in the eggs of *T. solium* and *T. saginata*.

Table 39.2: Differences between adult worms of *T. saginata* and *T. solium*

	T. saginata	*T. solium*
Length	5–10 metres	2–3 metres
Head	Large, without rostellum and hooks. Suckers may be pigmented	Small, globular with rostellum and hooks. Suckers are not pigmented
Proglottides (Segments)		
Number	1000–2000	< 1000
Expulsion	Singly and may put pressure on anal sphincter	Expelled passively in chains of 5 or 6
Uterus	Lateral branches 15–30 on each side	Lateral branches, 5–10 on each side
Vagina	Vaginal sphincter present	Vaginal sphincter absent
Ovaries	two in number, without any accessory lobe	two in number with an accessory lobe
Testis	300–400 follicles	150–200 follicles

Life Cycle

The worm passes its life cycle in two hosts:

1. The definitive host—Man—harbours the adult worm.
2. The intermediate host—Cattle (cow or buffalo) harbours the larval stage. In *T. solium*, the intermediate host is the pig.

The adult worm lives in the **small intestine** of man. The eggs or gravid segments are passed out with the feces on the ground. The animals (cow or buffalo) swallow these eggs while grazing in the field. When these eggs reach the alimentary canal of the intermediate host, the eggs are ruptured and the oncospheres are liberated. These penetrate the gut wall with the aid of their hooks and gain entrance into the portal vessels or mesenteric lymphatics finally reaching the systemic circulation.

The naked oncospheres are filtered out from the circulating blood into muscular tissues where they ultimately settle down to undergo further development. The muscles most commonly affected are tongue, neck, shoulder, ham. The oncospheres lose their hooks on reaching their destination. In about 8 days after infection each oncosphere forms an oval vesicle containing at its bottom the larva (scolex or the future head of the adult worm) referred to as cysticercus. Human beings are infected through the eating of undercooked beef containing the cysticerci (Measly beef). When it enters the alimentary canal of man, the scolex on coming in contact with bile exvaginates and anchors to the gut wall by means of its suckers and develops into an adult worm. The worm grows to sexual maturity in 2 to 3 months and starts producing eggs which are in turn passed in the feces along with the gravid segments, thereby repeating the cycle (Fig. 39.3).

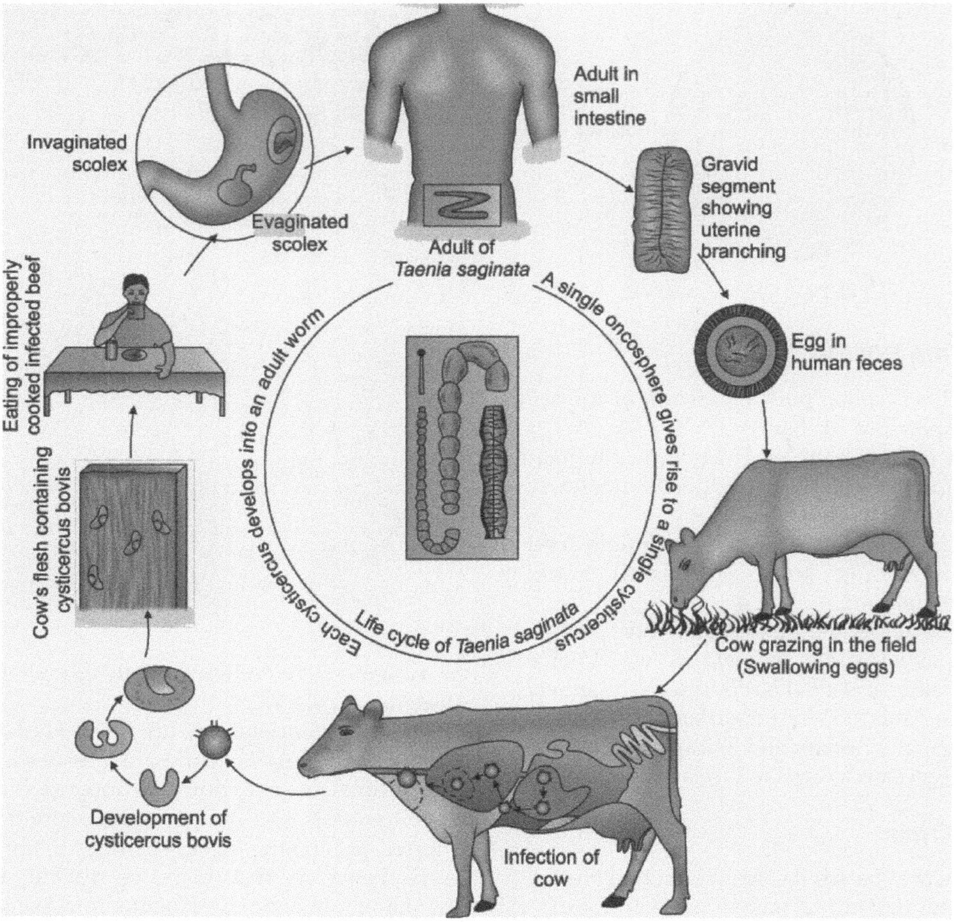

Fig. 39.3: Life cycle of *T. saginata*

Life cycle of *T. solium*, is the same as *T. saginata*. The intermediate host is the pig (Fig. 39.4).

Larval Development of *T. saginata* and *T. solium*

Cysticercus Bovis

This is the larval stage of *T. saginata* developing in the muscles of a cow or a buffalo. It measures 5 to 10 mm in breadth and 3 to 4 mm in length and contains an unarmed scolex (head of the adult worm) invaginated at one side. It can live for about 8 months in the flesh of cattle and can only develop further when ingested by man, its definitive host. *Cysticercus bovis* does not occur in man.

Cysticercus Cellulosae

This is the larval stage of *T. solium* developing in the muscles of pig. A mature cyst is an oval body and measures 8 to 10 mm in width by 5 mm in length. The long axis of the cyst is parallel to the muscle fiber. There is a dense milk white spot at the side where the scolex with its hookers and suckers remains invaginated. The cyst contains a fluid rich in salt and albuminous material. It can live for about 8 months in the flesh of pig

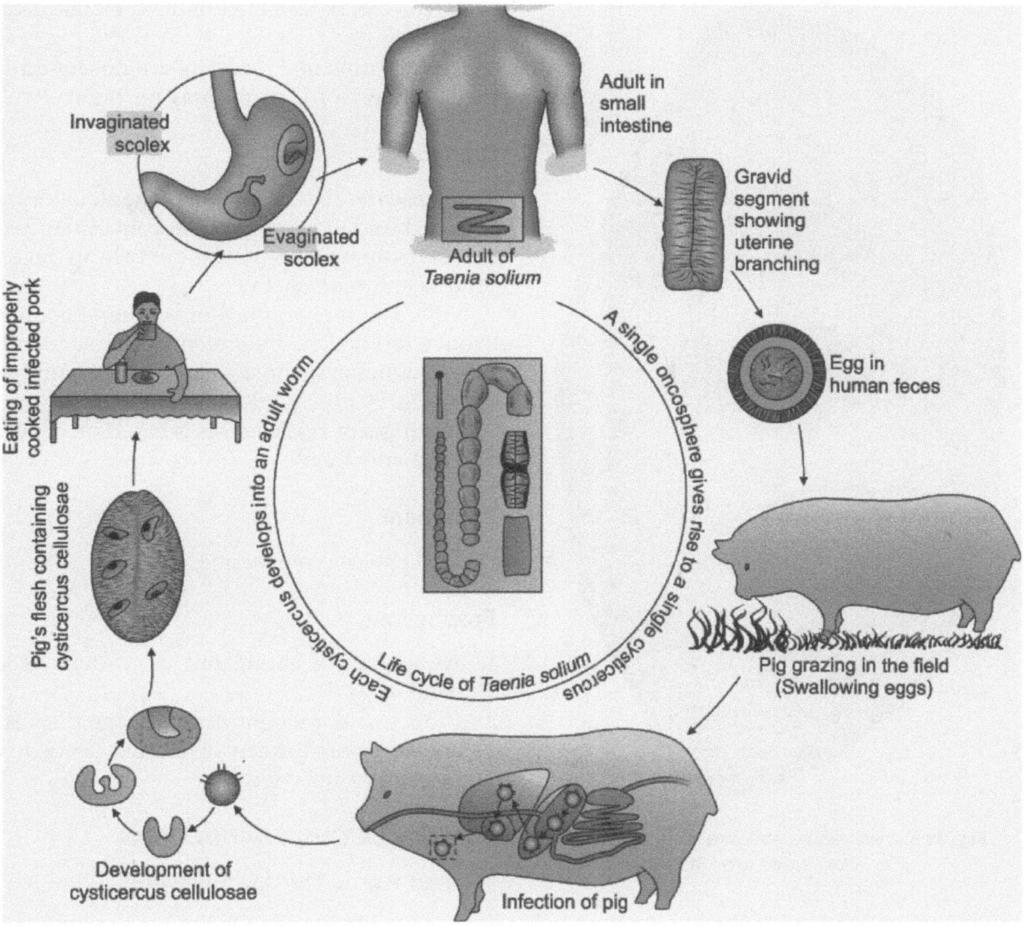

Fig. 39.4: Life cycle of *T. solium*

and can only develop further when ingested by man, its definitive host. Man, sometimes serves as the larval host of *T. solium* and he becomes infected in the same way as the pig, i.e. by drinking contaminated water or by eating uncooked vegetables infected with eggs. Sometimes a man harboring the adult worm may auto infect himself due to unclean and unhygienic personal habits or by a reversal of peristaltic movements of the intestine in which gravid segments are thrown back to the stomach equivalent to swallowing of thousands of eggs.

These cysticerci are usually found in tens of thousands but sometimes singly. They may develop in any organ and the effect produced depends upon the location of the cysticerci in the body. The distribution of these cysticerci is usually in the subcutaneous tissue and muscles causing palpable or visible nodules but may also be found in the brain leading to epileptic fits. Diagnosis is done by biopsy examination of a subcutaneous module, X-ray examination which may show calcified cysticerci, eosinophilia and serological examination of taeniasis (Fig. 39.5).

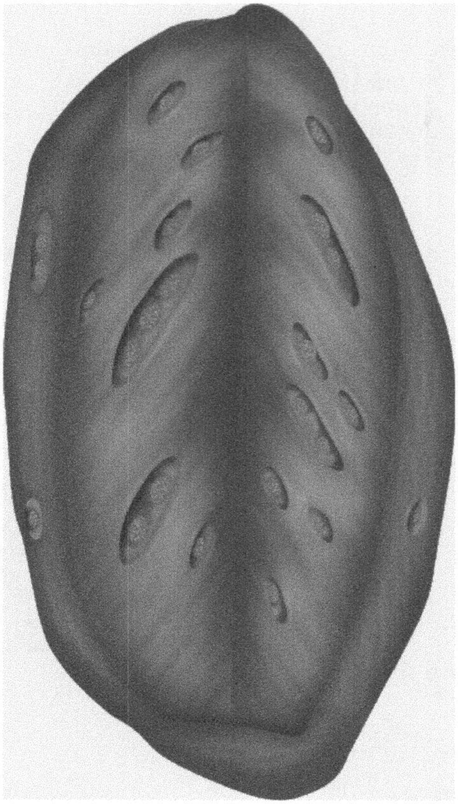

Fig. 39.5: Cysticercus cellulosae in pig's muscle *(For color version see Plate 4)*

Mode of Infection

By ingestion of undercooked meat of the intermediate hosts.

1. In *T. saginata* Beef, containing cysticercus bovis.
2. In *T. solium* Pork containing cysticercus cellulosae.

Adult worms while living in the intestine usually do not give rise to any symptom. Occasionally they may be responsible for vague abdominal discomfort, chronic indigestion, anaemia and intestinal disorders such as diarrhoea alternating with constipation. The segments can be detected on the persons body or clothing.

Larval forms of *T. saginata* are not found in man but those of *T. solium* may be found.

Diagnosis

A microscopical examination of the stool for the eggs of the adult worm is carried out by (i) direct smear preparation of the sample of feces, (ii) concentration of stool.

Naked eye examination of the specimen should be made for segments. The segments appear whitish against a dark background of feces (Fig. 39.6).

Diagnosis of cysticercosis is based on clinical findings and X-ray.

Treatment

Drug of choice is mepacrine.

Prophylaxis

1. Avoidance of eating raw or undercooked meat.
2. Proper sanitary control of sewage disposal and effective treatment of infected indivi-dual to prevent infection.

ECHINOCOCCUS GRANULOSUS

Hydatid worm. The dog tapeworm.

Geographical Distribution

Although the hydatid disease is worldwide in distribution, it occurs specially in those countries where there is a close association between man, sheep and dog.

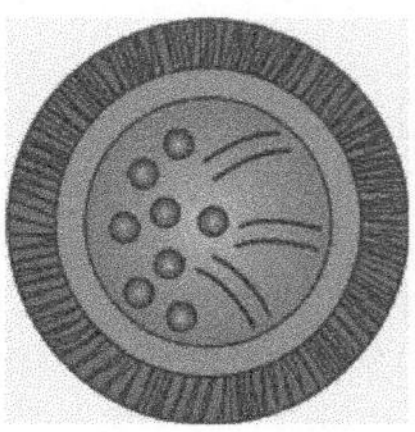

Fig. 39.6: Eggs of *T. solium* and *T. Saginata*

Habitat

Man harbors the **larval form** and not the adult worm.

Morphology

Adult Worm

It is a small tapeworm measuring 3 to 6 mm in length. It has a scolex (head), neck and strobila (consisting of 3 segments, occasionally 4). The first segment is immature, the second one is mature, and the last one and the fourth if present is gravid. The terminal segment is by far the biggest measuring 2 to 3 mm in length × 6 mm in breadth (Fig. 39.7).

Egg

The egg is ovoid in shape and resembles other eggs of *Taenia*. It measures 32 to 36 µm in length by 25 to 32 µm in breadth and contains a hexacanth embryo with three pairs of hooks. The egg is infective to man, cattle, sheep and other herbivorous animals.

Larval Form

This is found within the hydatid cyst developing inside the intermediate hosts. It represents the structure of the scolex of the future adult worm and remains invaginated within a vesicular body. On entering the definitive host, the scolex with 4 suckers and rostellar hooklets becomes evaginated and develops into an adult worm.

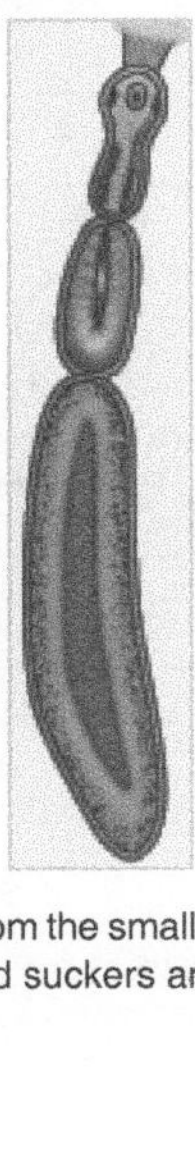

Fig. 39.7: Adult worm from the small intestine of dog showing scolex with hooklets and suckers and entire strobila

Life Cycle

The worm passes its life cycle in two hosts.

Definitive Hosts

Dog, wolf, fox, jackal. The adult worm lives in the small intestine of these animals who discharge a large number of eggs in their feces. The dog is the optimum definitive host.

Intermediate Hosts

Sheep, pig, cattle, horse, goat, man. The larval stage is passed in these animals and man giving rise to hydatid cyst. The sheep appears to be the optimum intermediate host.

Life Cycle

The eggs are discharged with the stools of definitive host (dog). These are swallowed by intermediate hosts (sheep and other domestic animals) and also by man (particularly children) due to intimate handling of infected dog. In the duodenum, the embryos are hatched out. After 8 hours of ingestion, the embryos bore their way out of the intestinal wall and enter the radicles of the portal vein. The embryos are carried to the liver (1st filter). Some of the embryos pass through the hepatic capillaries and enter pulmonary circulation to filter out of the lungs (2nd filter). A few embryos pass through the pulmonary capillaries enter the blood stream and lodge in various organs. They are mainly found in liver and lungs. Wherever, the embryo settles it forms a hydatid cyst, in which the larvae is transformed into a hollow bladder (hydatids means a drop of water). From the inner side of the cyst, brood capsules with a number of scolices are developed. A hydatid cyst developing from a single egg (oncosphere) may contain thousands of scolices. Usually when the infection occurs in man, it is a dead end. The natural cycle is maintained by dog and sheep because dog ingests these fertile hydatids which grow into adult worms (Figs 39.8 and 39.9).

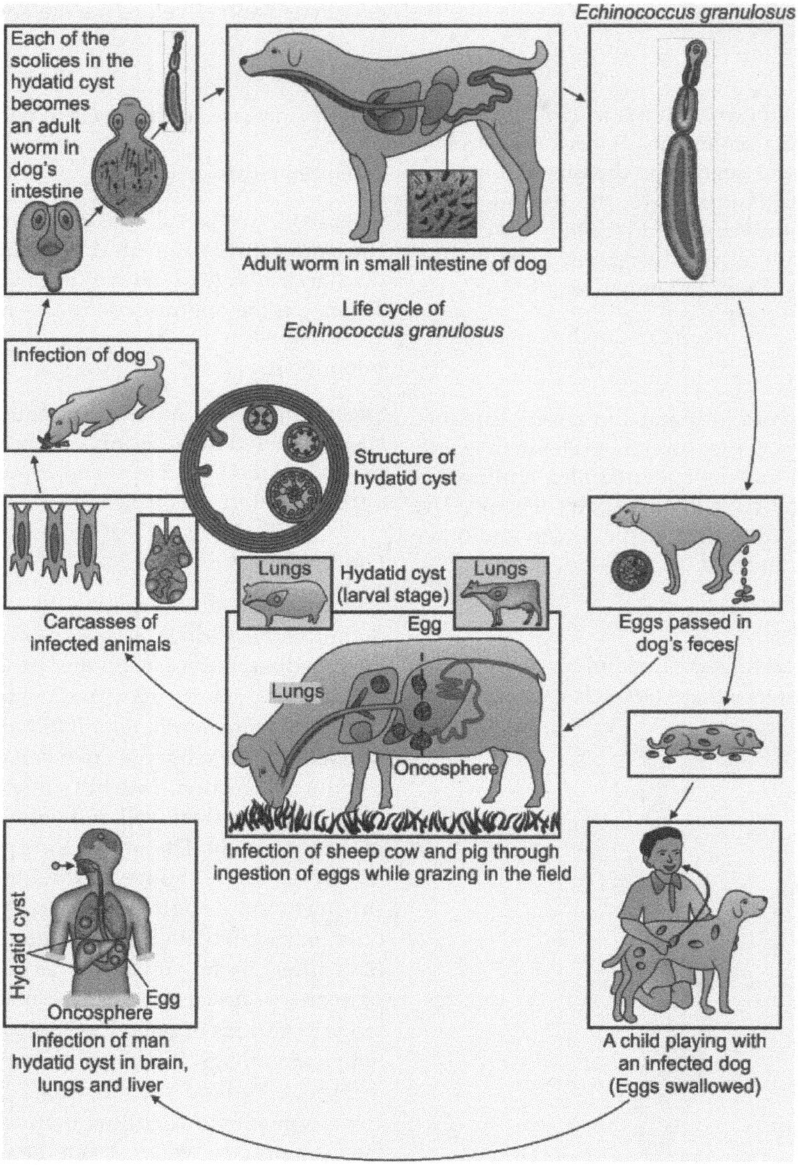

Fig. 39.8: Shows the life cycle of *Echinococcus granulosus*

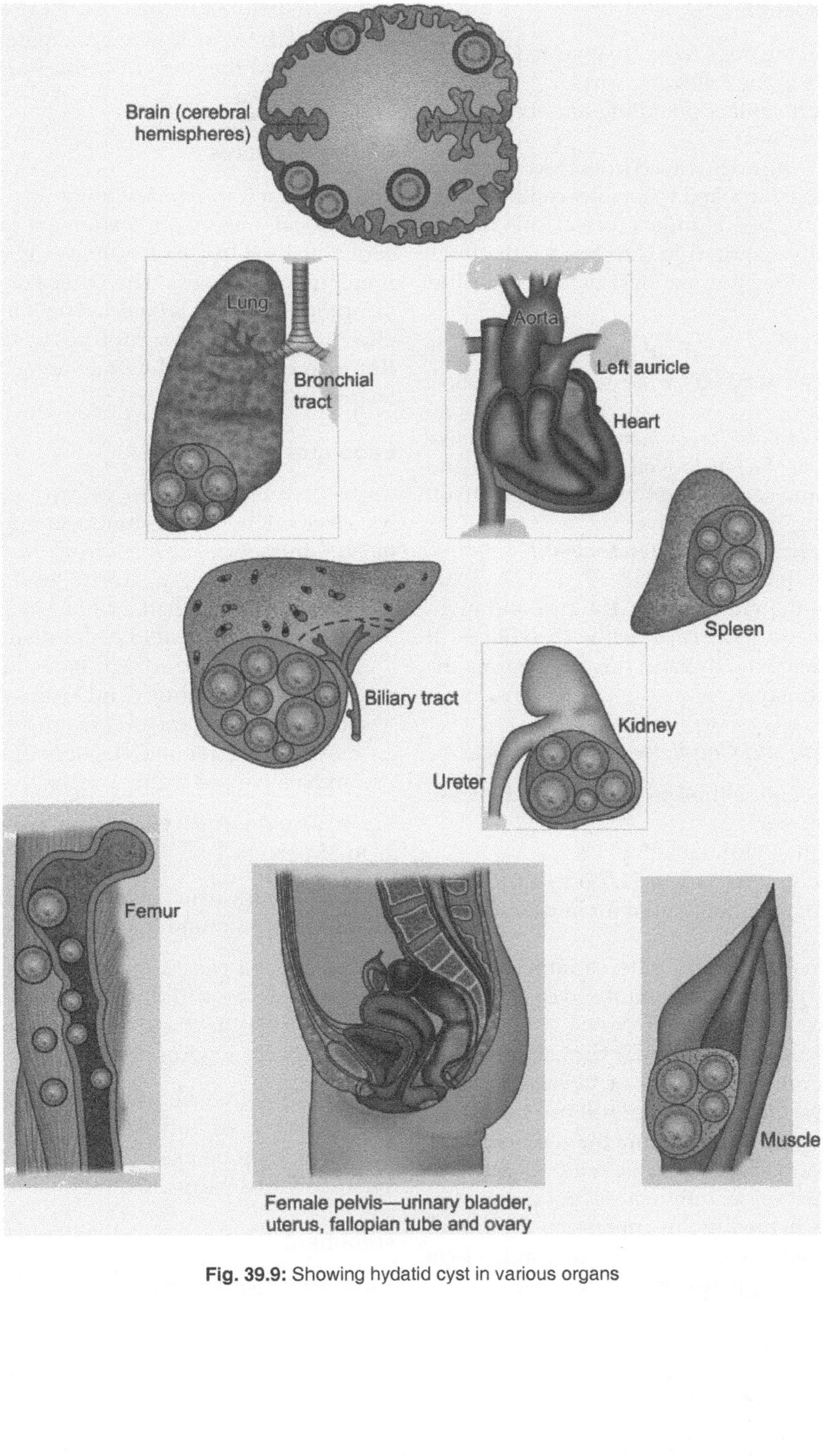

Fig. 39.9: Showing hydatid cyst in various organs

Mode of Infection

The eggs in the dogs feces are ingested by man. This occurs in the following ways:
1. By direct contact (handling and fondling of infected dogs).
2. By allowing dogs to feed from the same plate.
3. By taking uncooked vegetables contaminated with infected canine faeces. Infection is generally acquired in childhood though the disease does not manifest before adult life.

Hydatid Cyst

The cyst wall secreted by the embryo consists of two layers:
1. Outer cuticular layer (**ectocyst**). It looks like the white of a hardboiled egg. It is elastic and when incised or ruptured curls on itself exposing the inner layer.
2. Inner germinal layer **(endocyst).**
   - It is thin and cellular.
   - It is the vital layer of the cyst and gives rise to brood capsules with scolices. It secretes the hydatid fluid and forms the outer layer.

Composition and Character of Hydatid Fluid

1. Clear colorless fluid to pale yellow in color.
2. Highly toxic.
3. Reaction slightly acidic pH 6.7.
4. Specific gravity is low (1.005 to 1.010).
5. It is antigenic, being used for immunological tests.
6. Contains sodium chloride, sodium sulphate, sodium phosphate, sodium and calcium salts of succinic acid.
7. **Hydatid sand**: A granular deposit, settles at the bottom. It consists of liberated brood capsules, free scolices, and loose hooklets.

Brood capsules sprout from the germinal layer of the hydatid cyst. The scolices numbering 5 to 20 or more develop within these brood capsules. A fully developed scolex represents the future head of the adult worm with suckers and a circle of hooklets invaginated inside the scolex.

The hydatid cyst grows very slowly. At the end of the 1st year it is approximately 4 cm in diameter and the brood capsules and scolices begin to appear.

Clinical Features

The chief clinical manifestations are dependent upon local signs and if the cyst is situated superficially it causes a visible swelling. In the majority of cases, the disease remains symptomless and it is detected only by pressure effects or when the cyst ruptures or suppurates. Rupture of a hydatid cyst is associated with anaphylactic symptoms.

Laboratory Diagnosis

Casoni reaction: This is an immediate hypersensitivity skin test introduced by Casoni in 1911. Intradermal injection of:
- Two mL of fresh sterile hydatid fluid produces within half-an-hour in all positive cases a large wheal (5 cm in diameter) with multiple pseudopodia, it fades in an hour.
- Sterile normal saline (2 mL) is injected in the other arm for control. Hydatid fluid from human cases (removed by operation) or from animals is used as an antigen.

Blood examination shows eosinophilia of 20 to 25 percent.

Serological tests carried out with hydatid antigen fluid have been found to be positive.

Exploratory cyst puncture An accurate diagnosis may be made by withdrawing a few mL of the hydatid fluid and examining it under the microscope for scolices or hooklets.

Radiological Often helpful in the diagnosis of hydatid cyst of lungs and liver. Hepatic photoscan may be useful in locating the site of hydatid cyst of the liver.

Treatment

There is no specific drug.

Prophylaxis

This consists of the following:

1. Prevention of infection of dogs and deworming of dogs.
2. Cleaning of hands before eating.
3. Avoiding contamination of fingers while examining dog feces.

Nemathelminthes

NEMATODA

General Characters

1. The nematodes are **unsegmented, elongated** and **cylindrical,** both **ends are often pointed.**
2. They can be 5 mm in size as in *T. spiralis* and *S. stercoralis* or very large, (*D. medinensis*) upto 1 meter.
3. The body is covered with a tough cuticle.
4. The worm has a body cavity in which the various organs such as the digestive and genital systems float. Excretory and nervous systems are very primitive.
5. The alimentary canal is complete.
6. The nematodes are all **diecious helminths,** i.e. the sexes are separate. **The male is generally smaller than the female and the posterior end is curved or coiled ventrally.**

Life Cycle

Man is the optimum host for all nematode parasites. They pass their life cycle in one host except superfamilies *Filarioidea* and *Dracunculoidea* where 2 hosts are required. **In *Filarioidea,* the second host is an insect vector** in which the larval development takes place. **In Dracunculoidea, the second host is cyclops.**

- Most nematodes localise in the intestinal tract and start developing. The eggs are expelled out of the body and undergo developmental changes before they can enter a new host.

Classification of Nematodes

A. **According to Habitat of Adult worms**

Intestinal

Small intestine — Cecum and vermiform appendix

- *Ascaris lumbricoides (Roundworm)*
- *Ancylostoma duodenale (Hookworm)*
- *Necator americanus (American hookworm)*
- *Strongyloides stercoralis*
- *Trichinella spiralis*
- *Capillaria philippinensis*

Somatic (Inside the tissues and organs)

Lymphatic system

- *Wuchereria bancrofti*
- *Brugia malayi*

Subcutaneous tissues

- Loa loa (African eye worm)
- Onchocerca volvulus
- *Dracunculus medinensis* (Guinea worm)

Lungs

- Strongyloides stercoralis

Mesentery

- *Dipetalonema perstans*
- *Mansonella ozzardi*

Conjunctiva

- *Loa loa*
- Out of these we shall only study some as representatives of the whole species.

B. **Systematic classification (Table 39.3).**

C. Classification based on the stool examination findings (Table 39.4).

Mode of Infection of Nematode Parasites

1. By ingestion of:
   a. **Embryonated eggs** contaminating food and drink, as in *A. lumbricoides, E. vermicularis* and *T. trichiura.*
   b. Growing embryos in an intermediate host (infected cyclops), as in *D. medinensis.*

Table 39.3: Classification of Intestinal Nematodes (optional)

Subclass	*Order*	*Superfamily*	*Genus*	*Species*
Aphasmidia (No caudal chemoreceptors)	Enoplida	Trichinelloidea	*Trichinella*	*T. spiralis*
			Trichuris	*T. trichiura*
			Capillaria	*C. philippinensis*
		Rhabditoidea	*Strongyloides*	*S. stercoralis*
		Strongyloidea	*Ancylostoma*	*A. duodenale*
	Rhabditida		*Necator*	*N. americanus*
		Metastrongyloidea	*Angiostrongylus*	*A. cantonensis*
		Oxyuroidea	*Enterobius*	*E. vermicularis*
Phasmidia (Having caudal chemoreceptors)		Ascaridoidea	*Ascaris*	*A. lumbricoides*
			Wuchereria	*W. bancrofti*
			Brugia	*B. malayi*
			Onchocerca	*O. volvulus*
			Dipetalonema	*D. perstans*
	Spirurida	Filarioidea		*D. streptocerca*
			Mansonella	*M. ozzardi*
			Dirofilaria	*D. conjunctivae*
				D. immitis
			Loa	*L. loa*
		Dracunculoidea	*Dracunculus*	*D. medinensis*
		Spiruroidea	*Gnathostoma*	*G. spinigerum*

Table 39.4: Classification of Intestinal Nematodes on the basis of stool examination findings Intestinal Nematodes

- Larvae in Stool — *S. stercoralis*
- Eggs in stool — Colored (bile-stained)
  - *A. lumbricoides*
  - *T. trichiura*

  — Colourless (not bile-stained)
  - Hookworms (*A. duodenale*)
  - *N. americanus*
  - *E. vermicularis* (Rarely)
- Eggs on perianal skin — Colorless (not bile-stained)
  - *E. vermicularis*

c. Encysted embryos in infected pig's flesh, as in *T. spiralis*.

2. By penetration of the skin: The filariform larvae boring through the skin, as in *A. duodenale*, *N. americanus* and *S. stercoralis*.
3. By blood-sucking insects, as in the parasites belonging to the superfamily Filarioidea.
4. By inhalation of infected dust containing embryonated eggs, as in *A. lumbricoides* and *E. vermicularis*.

INDIVIDUAL PARASITES: *TRICHURIS TRICHIURA*

Common name—Whipworm.

Geographical Distribution

Worldwide. Commoner in warm-moist regions.

Habitat

The adult worms, lives in the large intestine of man, the caecum and vermiform appendix.

Morphology

Adult Worm

In shape and general appearance, the worm resembles a whip, the anterior three-fifth is very thin and hair like, the posterior part is stout and resembles the handle of the whip. The worm lives in the large intestine (caecum), the anterior portion is embedded in the mucous membrane. The adult worm may live in the human bowel for many years. The male is slightly smaller than the female and the posterior part is shaped like a comma or an arc (Fig. 39.10A).

Eggs

The important features of a Trichuris egg are as follows:

1. Size—50 μm in length by 25 μm in breadth.
2. Color—brown (bile-stained) has a double shell, the outer one is bile-stained.
3. Barrel-shaped with a mucus plug at each pole.
4. Contains an unsegmented ovum when the egg leaves the human host.
5. Floats in a saturated solution of common salt.

The eggs when freshly passed are not infective to man (Fig. 39.10B).

Life Cycle

No intermediate host is required as the worm passes its life cycle in one host. The eggs come out of the human host with the feces and the development proceeds slowly in water or damp earth depending upon the environmental conditions. In warmer climate the **rhabditiform** larvae develops quickly within the egg (in a matter of 3 to 4 weeks). The embryonated eggs are infective to man.

Man gets infected when the embryonated eggs are swallowed with food or water. The egg shell is dissolved with digestive juices and the larvae come out from one of the poles. The liberated larvae pass down into the **caecum**, their site of localisation. They grow directly into adult worms and embed their anterior parts in the mucosa of the intestine. The worms become sexually mature within a month from the time of ingestion of the eggs and the gravid female begins to lay eggs. The cycle is then repeated (Fig. 39.11).

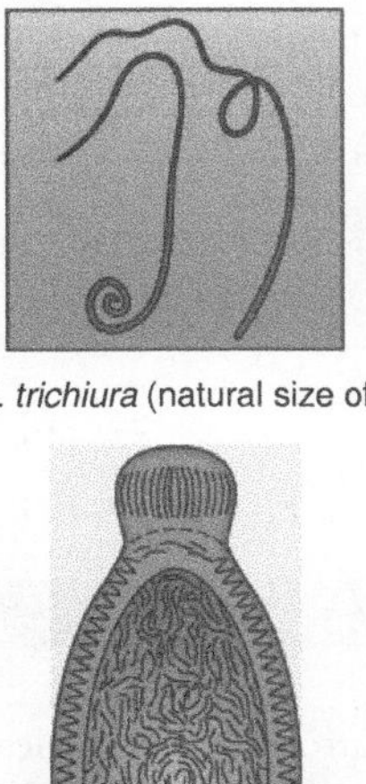

Fig. 39.10A: *T. trichiura* (natural size of adult worms)

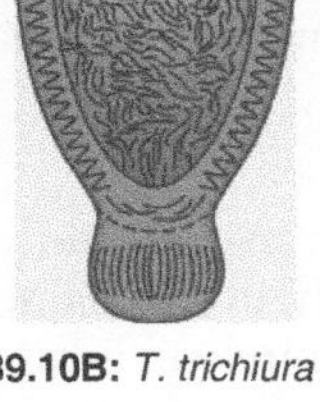

Fig. 39.10B: *T. trichiura eggs*

Clinical Features

Infection with *T. trichiura* is known as trichuriasis. Usually the worms do not produce pathogenic effects. The worms staying in the vermiform appendix may give rise to symptoms of acute appendicitis. In heavy infections, the patient complains of abdominal pain, mucus diarrhea often with blood streaked stool and loss of weight.

Laboratory Diagnosis

This is seen by the finding of characteristic eggs by a direct microscopical examination of a saline emulsion of stool. Adult worms may occasionally be present.

Treatment

Drugs are Thiabendazole, Mebendazole.

Prophylaxis

1. Proper disposal of feces.
2. Prevention of the consumption of uncooked vegetables and fruits.

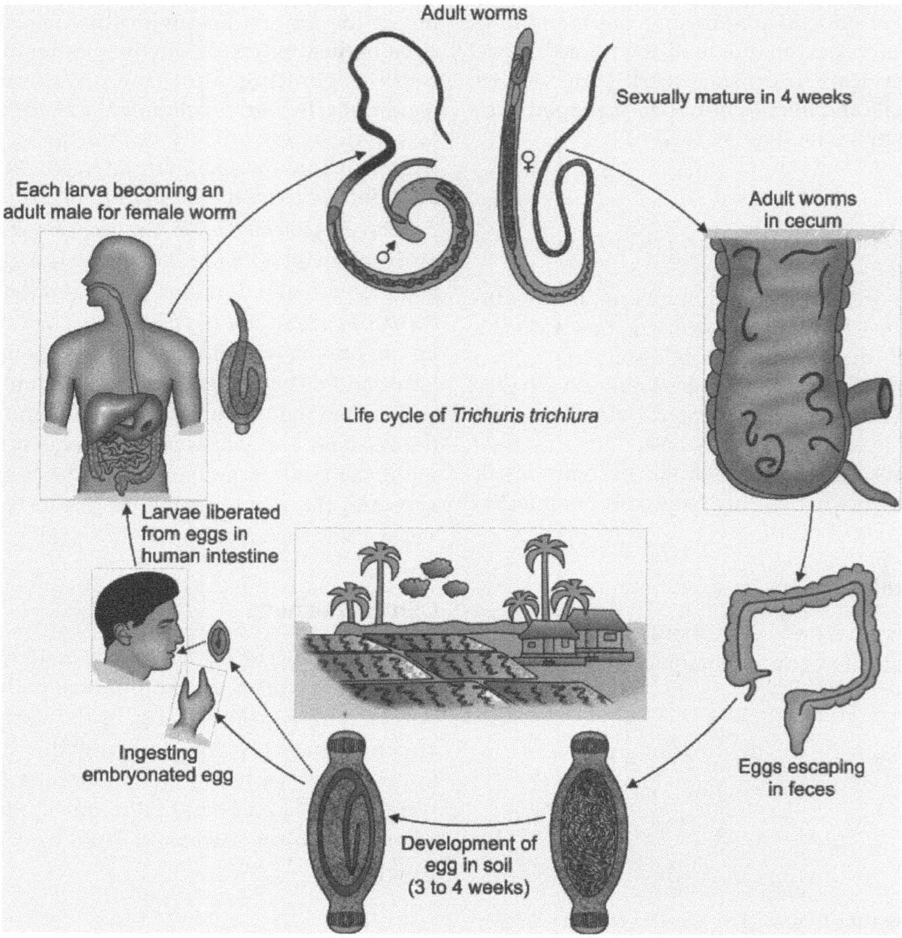

Fig. 39.11: Life cycle of *Trichuris trichiura*

ANCYLOSTOMA DUODENALE

Common name (The Old World Hookworm)

Geographical Distribution

It is widely distributed in all tropical and sub-tropical countries extending from parallel 36°N to parallel 30°S occurring in places wherever humidity and temperature are favorable for development of larvae in the soil. It is found in Europe, North Africa, India (Punjab and UP), Srilanka, Central and North China, Pacific Islands and Southern states of America.

Habitat

The adult worm lives in the small intestine of man, particularly in the jejunum, less often in duodenum and rarely in ileum.

Morphoglogy

Adult Worm

It is small, greyish-white cylindrical worm. When freshly passed, the worm has a reddish brown color due to ingested blood in its intestinal tract. The anterior end of the worm is bent slightly dorsally hence the name hook worm. The female is longer than the male (male 8 mm, female 12.5 mm).

The adult worm can live for 3 to 4 years in the human intestine.

Eggs

The eggs are passed out with the feces and the important features of the egg are:

1. Oval or elliptical in shape measuring 65 μm × 40 μm.
2. Colorless (not bile-stained).
3. Surrounded by a transparent hyaline shell membrane.
4. Contains a segmented ovum usually with 4 blastomeres. Has a clear space between the egg shell and the segmented ovum.
5. Floats in a saturated solution of common salt.

The eggs are first laid in an unsegmented stage and during their passage through the bowel segmentation proceeds up to the 4-celled stage. The eggs when passed out with the feces are not infective to man (Fig. 39.12).

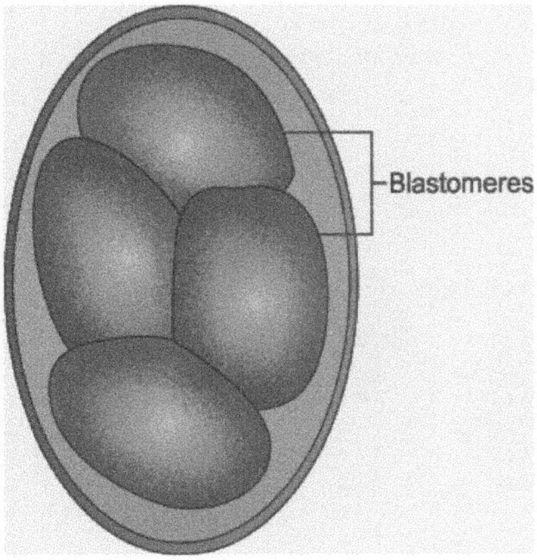

Fig. 39.12: Eggs of *A. duodenale*, showing four blastomeres

Life Cycle

No intermediate host is required and like other helminths, multiplication of worms does not occur inside the human body. Man is the only definitive host for *A. duodenale*. The following are the various stages of the life cycle (Fig. 39.13).

Stage 1 ***Passage of eggs from the infected host***
The eggs containing segmented ova with 4 blastomeres are passed out in the feces of the human host.

Stage 2 ***Development in the soil***
From each egg, a **rhabditiform larva** (250 μm in length), hatches out in the soil in about 48 hours. After about 10 days of development and two moultings it changes into a **filariform** larvae (500 to 600 μm) in length, which is the infective stage of the parasite. The time taken for the development to occur from eggs to filariform larvae is 8 to 10 days.

Stage 3 ***Entrance into a new host***
The filariform larvae are infective to man. The larvae cast off their sheaths and gain entrance to the body by penetrating the skin.

Stage 4 ***Migration***
This stage of migration is very interesting because the passage extends from the subcutaneous tissues to the intestine. From subcutaneous tissues, they pass through the lymph vascular system into venous circulation and are carried via the right heart into pulmonary capillaries, where they break through the capillary walls and enter into the alveolar spaces. Then they migrate onto the bronchi, trachea and larynx and slip over the epiglottis to the back of the pharynx and are ultimately swallowed. On entering the esophagus, a third moulting takes place. This time taken for migration is about 10 days.

Stage 5 ***Localization and laying of eggs***
The growing larvae settle down in the small intestine, undergo a fourth

moulting and develop into adolescent worms. In 3 to 4 weeks time, they become sexually mature and the fertilised females begin to lay eggs in the feces. The cycle is thus repeated. **The interval between the time of skin infection and the first appearance of eggs in the feces is about 6 weeks.**

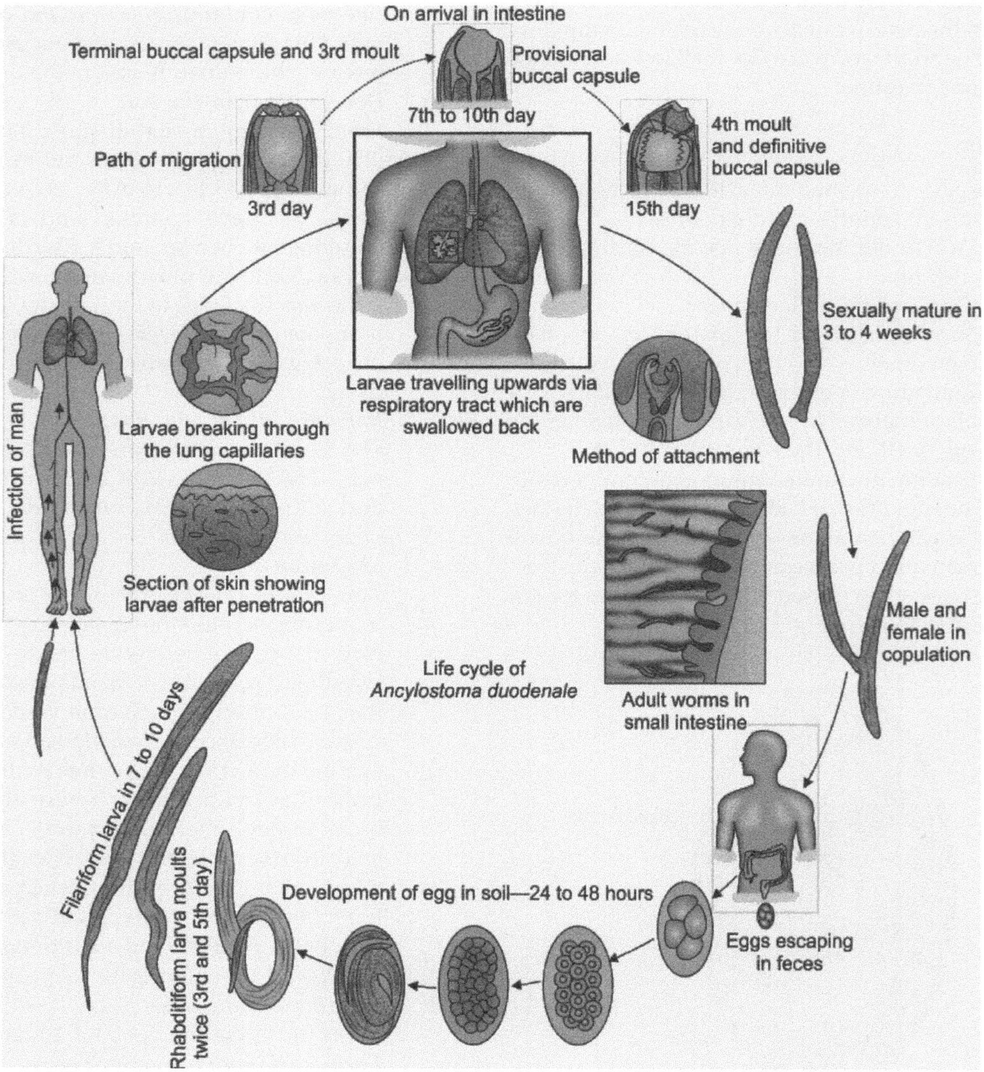

Fig. 39.13: Life cycle of *A. duodenale*

Mode of Infection

This occurs when man walks bare foot on fecally contaminated soil. The **filariform larvae** penetrate directly through the skin with which they come in contact. Usually it is the thin skin between toes or on the inner side of the soles.

Pathogenic Effects

These may be considered under two heads:

1. ***Those produced by the larval forms*** while entering the skin of the host and during migration through the lungs.
2. ***Those produced by the adult worms in*** the small intestine.

Pathogenic Effects Caused by Ancylostoma Larvae

a. *Lesions in the skin*
   1. Ancylostome dermatitis
   2. Creeping eruption

   Ancylostome dermatitis: It is a skin irritation which occurs at the site of entry.

   Creeping eruption is a condition in which the filariform larvae wander about through the skin in an aimless manner for several weeks or months producing a reddish itchy papule along the path traversed by the larvae (termed larva migrans). This is particularly seen with those species of parasites (*A. braziliense* and *A. caninum*) which are not adapted to man and therefore having penetrated the skin layers cannot proceed to normal development in the small bowel. The migration proceeds for many months before the larva dies.
b. *Lesions in the lungs*: Bronchitis and bronchopneumonia may occur when the larvae break through the pulmonary capillaries and enter alveolar spaces. A marked eosinophilia occurs at this stage.

Pathogenic Effects Caused by Adult Worms

The adult worms inhabit the small intestine (jejunum) of man and attach themselves to the mucous membrane by means of their powerful buccal teeth. In course of time, a severe progressive anemia of microcytic hypochromic **type develops.**

Cause of Anemia: The worm, a habitual blood sucker is primarily responsible but it appears that some other factors also operate

i. *Chronic blood loss*: This occurs by the withdrawal of blood by the parasites for their food and chronic hemorrhages from the punctured sites. Each worm is capable of drawing 0.3 to 0.2 mL of blood and when many parasites draw a lot of blood over a long period, it causes anemia. There is a loss of about 1 percent of hemoglobin for 12 worms.
ii. *Nutritional defects*: If there is deficiency of the available iron and other hematopoietic substances in the diet, it makes the anemia worse. If there is deficiency of folic acid and vitamin B_{12}, a macrocytic anemia occurs and iron, vitamin B_{12} and folic acid deficiency together results in a dimorphic anemia.

Symptoms of Anemia: Gastrointestinal disturbances. There is pain in the epigastric region resembling duodenal ulcer pain. Occasionally the patient may have an abnormal apetite showing an altered taste. He may have an abnormal appetite for things such as earth mud or lime (pica). Bowels are generally constipated.

Signs of Anemia: The skin assumes a light yellow color. The face appears puffy with the swelling of lower eyelids and edema of feet and ankles. The general appearance of the patient is a pale plumpy individual with protuberant abdomen and dry hair. Growth in children may be stunted. The mucous membrane of the eyes, lips and tongue show extreme pallor (Fig. 39.14).

Laboratory Diagnosis

Direct Method

Examination of stool: A macroscopic examination of the stool is necessary to find out the adult worms. A microscopic examination of stool may easily demonstrate the presence of characteristic hookworm eggs. The eggs are quite typical.

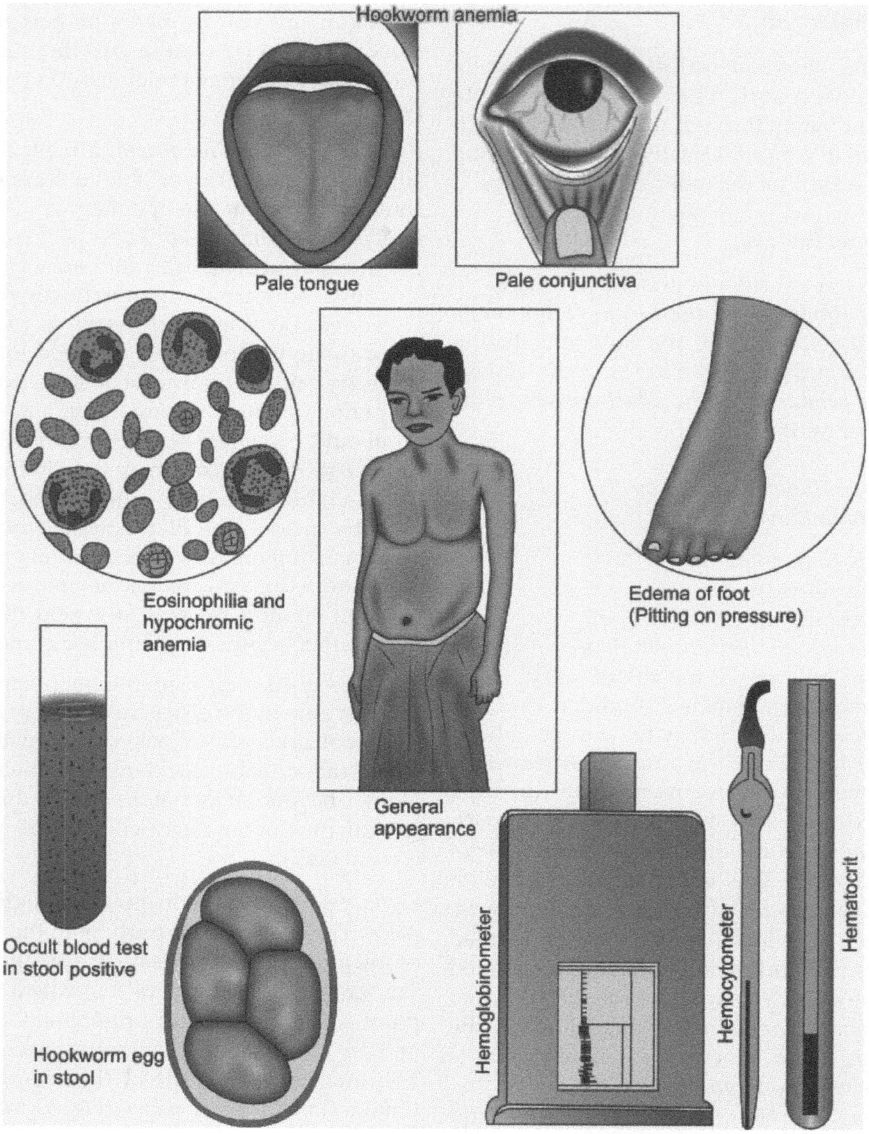

Fig. 39.14: Clinical and laboratory diagnosis of hookworm anemia

Study of duodenal contents: The material obtained by duodenal intubation may show either eggs or adult worms.

Indirect Methods

Examination of blood: This is carried out to ascertain the nature of anemia and presence of eosinophilia.

In a majority of cases of hookworm anemia, test for occult blood in the stool gives a positive reaction. Charcot-Leyden crystals are often found in stool.

Treatment

For the treatment of hookworm infection, the following steps are taken:

a. Expulsion of worms by anthelminthic drugs.
b. Treatment of anemia.

Prophylaxis

1. Attack on adult parasite—by means of treatment.
2. Attack on larvae—by proper control of sewage.
3. Personal protection—Wearing of boots and gloves.

Species Diagnosis

Another species of hookworm is *Necator americanus* which is called the American hookworm or the New World hookworm.

This is common in Sri Lanka and India (except in Punjab and UP). Although first discovered in America, it is more likely of African origin.

The life cycle, general morphology, pathogenicity, diagnosis and treatment are the same as described for *A. duodenale*.

Specific Diagnosis

A species diagnosis of hookworm anaemia whether due to *A. duodenale* or *N. americanus* can be only made by studying the morphology of adult worms or the mature infective filariform larvae (Table 39.5).

Table 39.5: Differentiating features between the two species *A. duodenale* and *N. americanus*

	A. duodenale	*N. americanus*
Adult worms		
Size	Adult worms large and thicker	Adult worms smaller and more slender
Anterior end	Bends in the same direction as the body curvature	Bends in the opposite direction to the body curvature
Buccal capsule	6 teeth–4 hook-like teeth on the ventral surface and 2 knob-like on dorsal surface	4 chitinous plates–2 on ventral surface, 2 on dorsal surface
Posterior end of female	A spine is present	There is no spine
Pathogenicity	More pathogenic—blood loss is higher in A. duodenale because i. It is a larger worm ii. It is armed with teeth iii. It is more migratory, leaving more bleeding points	Less pathogenic
Larva (Filariform Larvae)		
Buccal	Shorter	Larger
Cavity	Lumen larger	Lumen shorter
Shape of the head	Slightly conical	Rounded

ASCARIS LUMBRICOIDES

Common name—Roundworm

Geographical Distribution

It is worldwide in its distribution but it is especially present in the tropics—China, India and South East Asia. It occurs in persons with unhygienic habits.

Habitat

The adult worm lives in the lumen of the small intestine (jejunum).

Morphology

Adult Worms

It resembles an ordinary earthworm and it is the **largest intestinal nematode parasitizing man.** When fresh from the intestine, it is light brown or pink in color, but it gradually changes to white. In shape it is rounded and tapers at both ends, the anterior end being thinner than the posterior. The mouth is at the anterior end and has three finely toothed lips, one dorsal, and two ventral. The digestive and reproductive organs float inside the body cavity containing an irritating fluid. Allergic manifestations are due to the fluid. The life span of the adult worm in the human host is less than one year (Fig. 39.15).

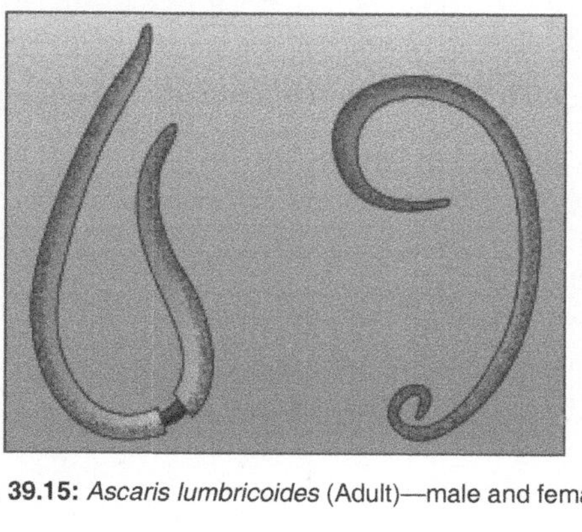

Fig. 39.15: *Ascaris lumbricoides* (Adult)—male and female

The male is 15 to 25 cm in length whereas the female is longer and stouter than the male and measures 25 to 40 cm in length. The female is tapering and the male is coiled. The eggs liberated by a fertilized female pass out of the human host with the feces.

Eggs

The characteristics of a *fertilized egg* is are follows (Fig. 39.16):

i. Round or oval in shape (60 to 75 µm in length by 40 to 50 µm in breadth).
ii. Always bile stained and brownish (golden brown) in color.
iii. Surrounded by a thick smooth translucent shell with an outer aluminous coat which is thrown into rugosities. This outer coat is sometimes lost (*decorticated egg*).
iv. Contains a very large conspicuous unsegmented ovum (the nucleus is concealed by a large amount of coarse yolk granules), there is a clear crescentic area at each pole.
v. Floats in a saturated solution of common salt.

The female even if not fertilized is capable of liberating eggs. The characteristics of the *unfertilized eggs* are as follows:

i. Narrower, longer (80 µm × 55 µm) and more elliptical.
ii. Brownish in color (bile-stained).
iii. Has a thinner shell with an irregular coating of albumin.
iv. Contains a small atrophied ovum with a mass of disorganized, highly refractile granules of various sizes.
v. Does not float in salt solution (heaviest of all helminthic eggs).

Both fertilized and unfertilized eggs are found in a sample of stool but if a specimen shows only unfertilised eggs, it signifies that the host is harbouring the female ascaris or that mating has not occurred.

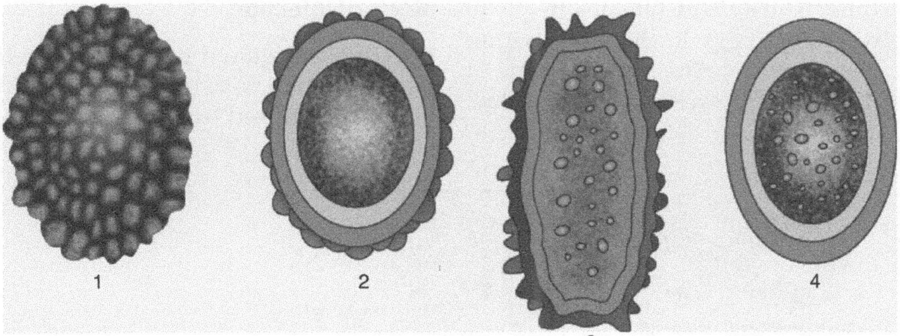

Fig. 39.16: The fertilized and unfertilized eggs of *A. lumbricoides* (1)) Surface view of *A. lumbricoides* egg, (2) Median view of *A. lumbricoides* fertilized egg, (3) Unfertilized *A. lumbricoides* egg, (4) Decorticated *A. lumbricoides* egg *(For color version see Plate 4)*

Life Cycle

The worm passes its life cycle in one host. No intermediate host is required. Continuation of the species is maintained by transference from one individual to another. Man is the only known definitive host of *Ascaris lumbricoides* (Fig. 39.17).

The various stages in the life cycle are:

Stage I ***Eggs in the feces***
The fertilized eggs containing the unsegmented ovum are passed in the feces. They are not infective to man when freshly passed.

Stage II ***Development in the soil***
A rhabditiform larva is developed from the unsegmented ovum within the egg shell in 10 to 40 days time depending on the conditions. The ripe egg is infective to man. Before hatching the larva undergoes a moulting and becomes 2nd stage larva from 1st stage larva.

Stage III ***Infection by ingestion and liberation of larvae***
When ingested with food, drink or raw vegetables, the embryonated eggs pass down to the duodenum where digestive juices weaken the egg shell and stimulate the enclosed larvae into activity. The egg shell splits and the rhabditiform larvae are liberated in the upper part of the small intestine.

Stage IV ***Migration through the lungs***
The larvae liberated in the small intestine do not directly develop into mature worms. They penetrate the mucous membrane of the small intestine and are carried by the portal circulation to the liver, where they live for a period of 3 to 4 days. Then they pass out of the liver, enter the right heart and then the pulmonary circulation. In the lungs they grow much bigger and increase in length from 0.2 mm to 2.0 mm. Here they moult twice. They break the capillary wall and reach lung alveoli. This takes about 10 to 15 days.

Stage V ***Reentry into stomach and the small intestine***
From the lung alveoli the larvae crawl up the bronchi and trachea and helped by the current of ciliated epithelium of the respiratory tract, they are propelled into the larynx and pharynx and are swallowed. The larvae pass down the esophagus to the stomach and localize in the upper part of the small intestine, their normal habitat. Another moulting takes place here.

Stage VI ***Sexual maturity and egg liberation***
The larvae on reaching their habitat grow into adult worms and become sexually mature in about 6 to 10 weeks

time. The gravid females begin to discharge eggs in the stool within about two months from the time of infection. The cycle is again repeated.

Mode of Infection

Infection is acquired by swallowing ripe eggs (embryonated) with raw vegetables cultivated on a soil fertilized by infected human excreta.

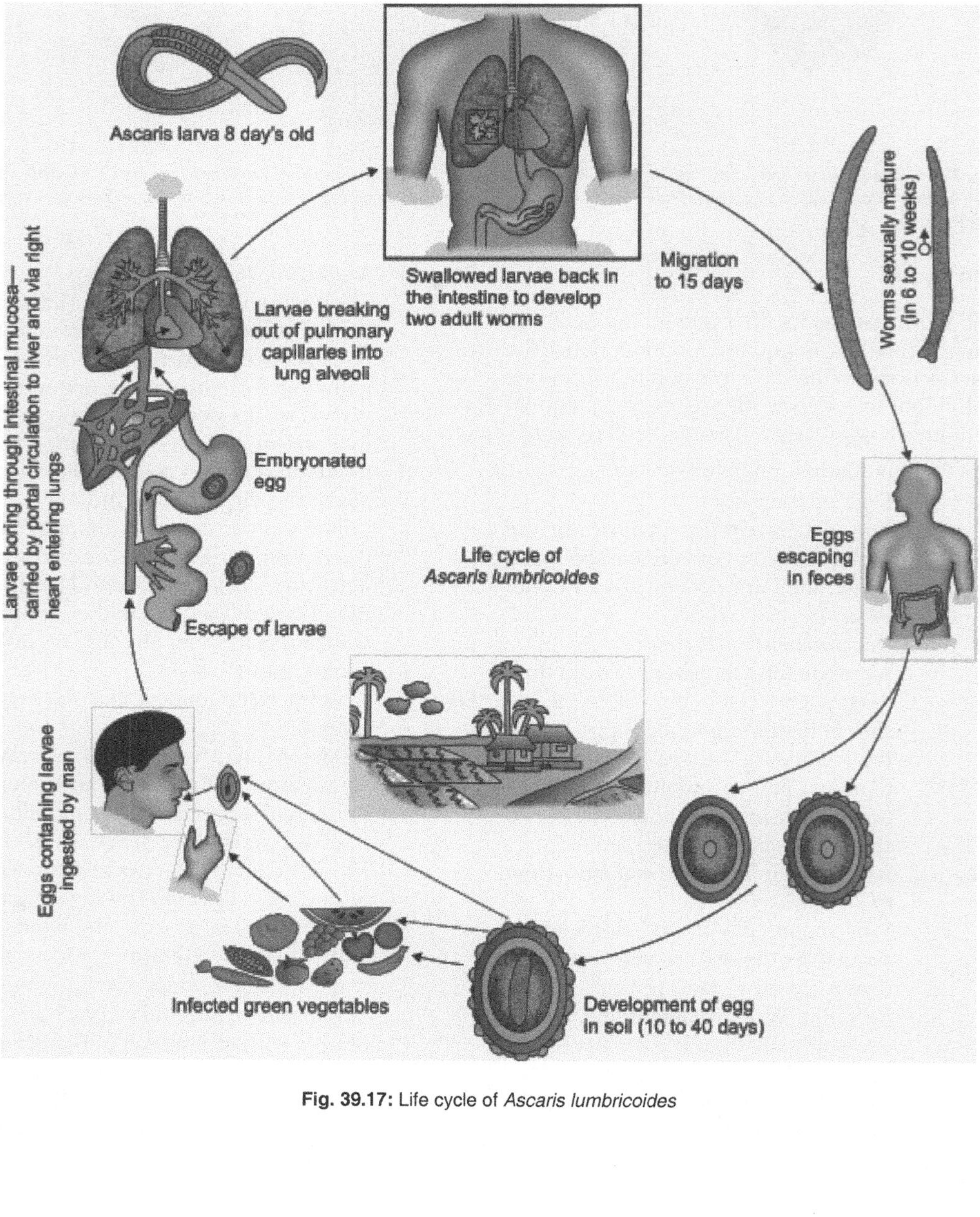

Fig. 39.17: Life cycle of *Ascaris lumbricoides*

Water supplies may be contaminated with infected human excreta.

Clinical Features

Infection of *Ascaris lumbricoides* in man is called ascariasis. The symptoms are:
1. Those produced by the migrating larvae.
2. Those produced by adult worms.

Symptoms due to Migrating Larvae

In heavy infections, typical symptoms of pneumonia such as fever, cough and dyspnea may appear because of the presence of larvae in the lungs. This is called Ascaris pneumonia **or** Loeffler's syndrome. **Sputum is often blood tinged and contains Ascaris larvae. Urticarial rash and eosinophilia (20%) are seen in such cases.**

If the ascaris larvae pass beyond pulmonary capillaries and reach the general circulation, they may reach various organs where there may be different clinical symptoms.

Symptoms due to Adult Worms

Incubation period is usually two months. This is the time taken from exposure to development of clinical symptoms. The symptoms are mostly related to the gastrointestinal tract. The adult worm produces pathogenic effects in these two ways:
1. *Spoliative action* By robbing the host of its nutrition. It takes up a lot of protein and vitamin because the protein content of the worm is high and contributes to protein-energy malnutrition. Ascaris infection may cause vitamin A deficiency.
2. *Toxic action* The body fluid of Ascaris (Ascoron) when absorbed is toxic and gives rise to fever. Other allergic reactions seen are urticaria, edema of the face, conjunctivitis and irritation of the upper respiratory tract.
3. *Mechanical effects* The presence of *Ascaris lumbricoides* has led to the development of intussusception. An **intussusception** (a blockage of the intestine) is a medical condition in which a part of the small intestine has invaginated into another section of intestine, similar to the way in which the parts of a collapsible telescope slide into one another.
   It may also penetrate through the ulcers of the alimentary canal, causing perforation. A large number of Ascaris worms together in the intestine produce intestinal obstruction.
4. *Ectopic Ascariasis*: This means that the Ascaris worms enter places where they are not supposed to enter, for example, they may pass through the esophagus at night, coming out through the mouth or nose. Sometimes they may enter the respiratory passages causing suffocation. When they enter the biliary passage they causes obstructive jaundice and acute hemorrhagic pancreatitis.

Laboratory Diagnosis

Direct Evidences

Finding of adult worms
- i. *In the stool or vomit* The worm may pass out spontaneously or a specific anthelminthic may lead to its expulsion.
- ii. *X-ray diagnosis* The presence of *Ascaris lumbricoides* has been demonstrated by barium emulsion which being ingested by the worm within 4 to 6 hours casts an opaque shadow (string-like shadow).

Finding of eggs
- i. *In the stool*: A simple saline emulsion of the stool sample can be studied to see the presence of Ascaris eggs.
- ii. *In the bile*: Microscopical examination of the bile obtained by duodenal intubation may show Ascaris eggs.

Indirect Evidences

Blood examination: Eosinophilia is present only at the early stages of invasion.

Dermal reaction (allergic): Scratch test with powdered ascaris antigen has often been found to be positive.

Serological diagnosis: This is done especially in cases of allergic pneumonitis.

Treatment

For Ascaris the drug of choice is a piperazine salt.

Prophylaxis

The measures should consist of:
i. Proper disposal of human feces.
ii. Treatment of parasitized individuals.
iii. Education of children in schools.

ENTEROBIUS VERMICULARIS

Common names—Threadworm, Pinworm, Seat worm.

Geographical Distribution

It is found all over the world.

Habitat

Adult worms (gravid females) live in the caecum and vermiform appendix of man on the surface of the mucosa and may sometimes enter the submucosa also.

Morphology

Adult Worms

It is small, white in color, spindle-shaped and looks like a short piece of thread.

Male: It measures 2 to 4 mm in length and 0.1 to 0.2 mm across. The posterior third of the body is curved. It usually dies after fertilizing the female (Fig. 39.18).

Female: It measures 8 to 12 mm in length and 0.3 to 0.5 mm across its thickest part. It is straight posterior and ends in a long tapering and pointed tail which is 1/3rd of the length of the worm. The gravid female dies after laying the eggs within 2 to 3 weeks.

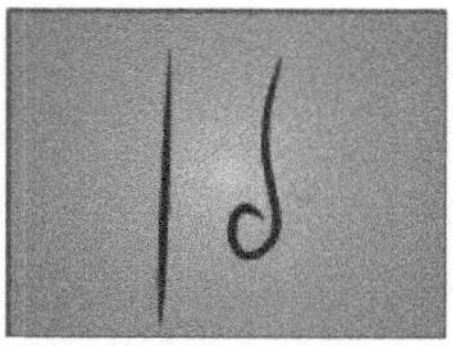

Fig. 39.18: The male and female worm of *E. vermicularis*

Eggs

The general characteristics of the egg are as follows (Fig. 39.19):
1. Colorless (not bile-stained).
2. Asymmetrical in shape, being plano convex that is flattened on one side (ventral) and convex (dorsal) on the other.
3. Measures 50 × 60 μm in length × 30 μm in breadth.
4. Surrounded by a transparent shell.
5. Contains a coiled tadpole like larvae.
6. Floats in a saturated solution of common salt.

Life Cycle

No intermediate host is required. The eggs, laid on the perianal skin contain a tadpole like larvae. These complete their development in 24 to 36 hours time in the presence of oxygen. Infection occurs by ingestion of these eggs. The egg shells

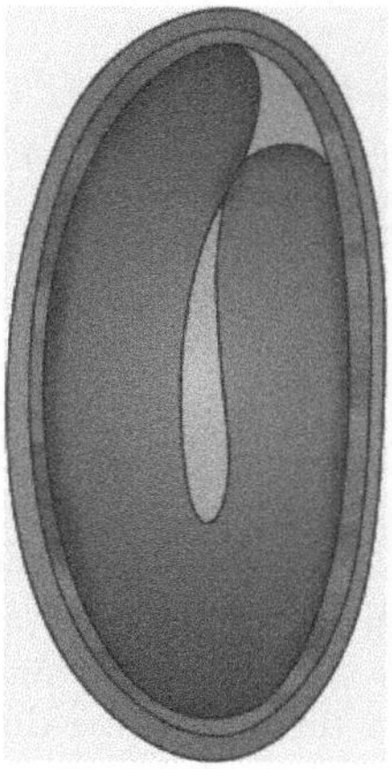

Fig. 39.19: Eggs of *E. vermicularis*

are dissolved by digestive juices and the larvae escape in the small intestine where they develop into young worms. After the worms become sexually mature, the male fertilizes and the female dies. The gravid female then migrates from the small intestine down to the caecum and the colon and vermiform appendix and remains there till the eggs develop. The fertilized female then goes down the rectum and out of the anus during the night after the patient has gone to sleep, to deposit eggs on the perianal skin. The cycle is then repeated. The whole cycle is completed in 2 to 4 weeks time (Fig. 39.20).

Mode of Infection

Children are the ones most commonly infected.

1. *Autoinfection*: The movement of the worms at the time of laying eggs causes intense itching. The patient scratches the affected part and

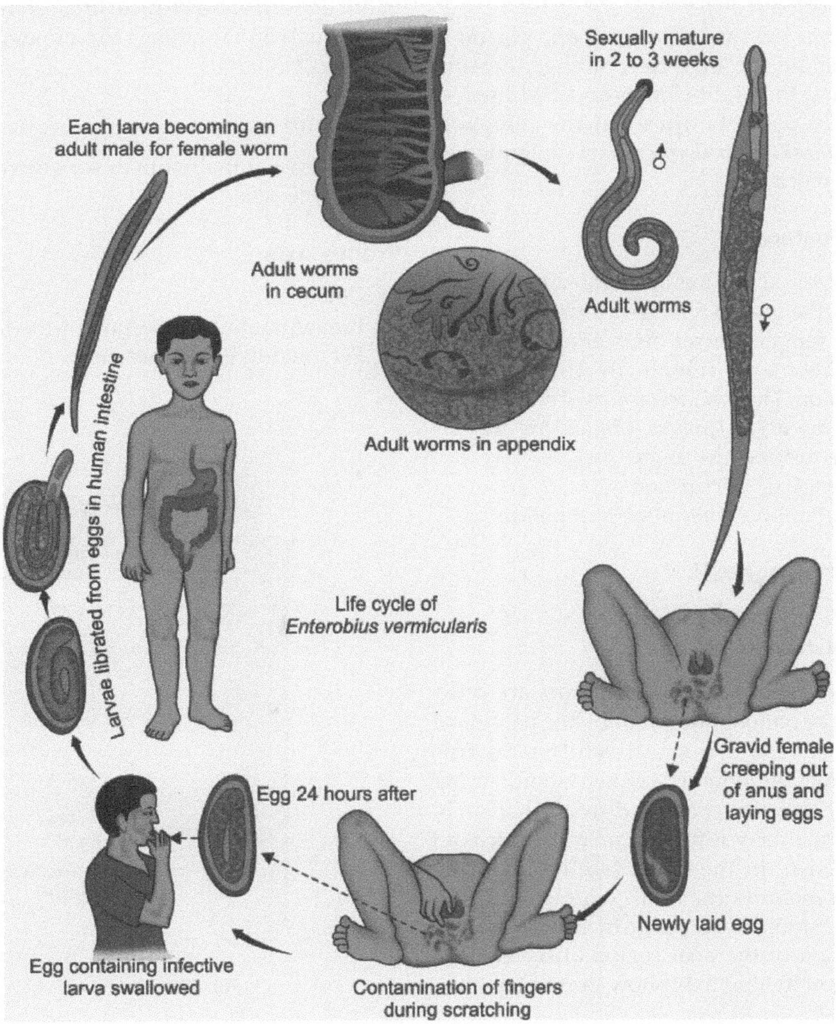

Fig. 39.20: Life cycle of *E. vermicularis*

thereby picks up the eggs containing the infective larvae on his fingers. These eggs are transferred to food and swallowed by the patient himself or the infection may occur directly from anus to mouth, as occurs in children.

2. *Retroinfection*: This is the process in which the eggs laid on the perianal skin immediately hatch into infective stage larvae and migrate through the anus to develop into young forms in the colon.
3. Transmission can occur from one person to another by the ingestion of eggs. Persons handling the night clothes and bed linen of infected patients often get the infection. Transmission can also occur by contaminated food or drink.

Clinical Features

The main clinical features are because of irritation caused by the gravid females around anus. The migrating female worms often enter the female genital tract and female urethra causing inflammation. The manifestations of enterobiasis or infection with *Enterobius vermicularis* are:

- Itching around the anus
- Frequency of micturition
- Inflammation of vermiform appendix.

Laboratory Diagnosis

1. ***Detection of adult worm.***
2. ***Demonstration of eggs.***

Detection of adult worms: The worms are often found by the patient himself or by the parents of children. These are small whitish worms discovered in the stool. The patient should bring such stool samples preserved in alcohol or 10 percent formaldehyde for examination which can be obtained from the lab before he takes the sample. Sometimes the adult worms are easily seen in the stool after a purge or enema.

Inspection of the anal region at the time of beginning of itching may show gravid females.

Demonstration of eggs: Microscopical examination of stool for eggs of *E. vermicularis* can be done by a direct smear examination, or by concentration method. Eggs can be demonstrated in the scrapings from the perianal skin by a NIH swab. It is advisable to take the swab immediately after the patient wakes up in the morning. It has a cellophane paper attached to a rubber rod and tied with a rubber band which can be opened on the slide by releasing the rubber band. Eggs can also be recovered from under the finger nails and washings from under garments (Fig. 39.21).

Treatment

The specific anthelminthics for enterobiasis are piperazine salts.

Prophylaxis

This includes:

1. Prevention of re-infection of the individual.
2. Personal hygiene measures.

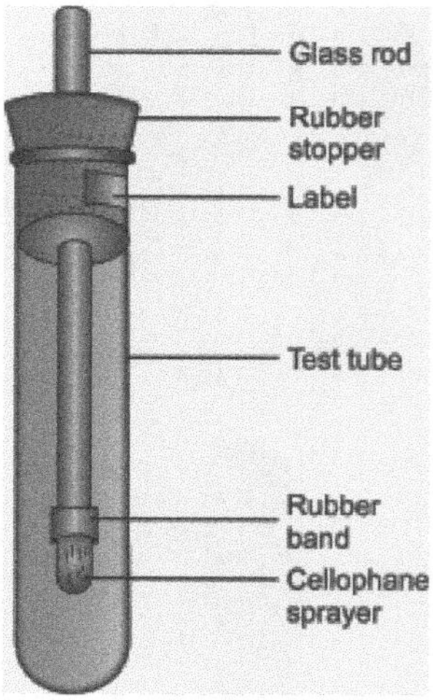

Fig. 39.21: NIH swab

SUPERFAMILY FILARIOIDEA

INTRODUCTION

This superfamily includes nematodes which inhabit the blood vessels, lymphatics, connective tissues and the cavities of man and animals. The adult worms are slender and thread like and usually measure 2 to 10 cm in length. The females are much longer than the males. The females are **viviparous** giving birth to larvae known as **microfilaria.**

The life cycle is passed in two hosts—man and a blood-sucking insect. Microfilaria complete their development in the insect host giving rise to the infective form. Infection is transmitted to man by the bite of the insect. Species diagnosis is made from a study of larval forms, adult worms are rarely obtained.

Depending on the differential characters of microfilariae, they are divided into many types. We shall be studying two types found in the blood in India.

- *Mf. bancrofti* (Mf. = Microfilaria).
- *Mf. malayi* (Flow chart 39.1 and Fig. 39.22).

WUCHERERIA BANCROFTI

Geographical Distribution

The parasite is found in tropics and subtropics (India, West Indies, Southern China, Japan, Pacific Islands, West and Central Africa and South America). In India it is found in Rajasthan, Punjab, UP and Delhi.

Habitat

Adult worms are found in the lymphatic vessels and lymph nodes of man only.

Morphology

Adult Worms

These are long hair-like, transparent nematodes creamy white in color. They are filiform in shape and both ends are tapering, the head end terminating in a slightly rounded swelling. The male measures 2.5 to 4.0 cm whereas the female measures 8 to 10 cm. The females are **ovo-viviparous** (laying eggs with well-developed embryos). The life span of the adult worms is about 5 to 10 years. Females are more in number than males (Fig. 39.23).

Microfilariae

From the lymph nodes, the microfilariae find their way through the main lymphatic trunks into the circulating blood. They are very active in their habits. When unstained, they appear as colorless and transparent bodies with blunt heads and pointed tails. It has a hyaline sheath which is much larger than the body so that the larvae can move forwards and backwards within it. Inside this sheath are nuclei which extend from the head to the tail end (Fig. 39.24).

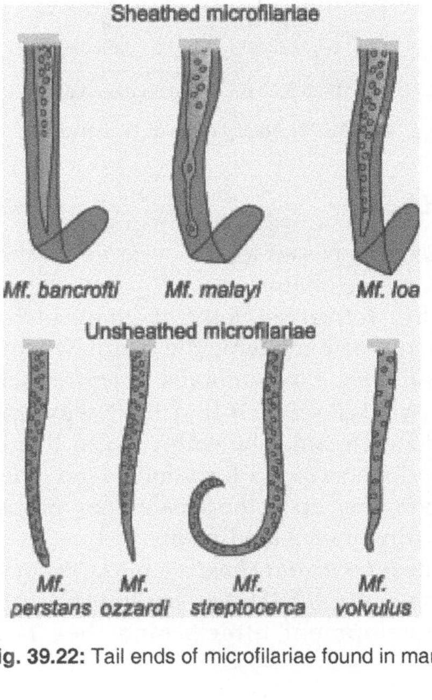

Fig. 39.22: Tail ends of microfilariae found in man

Flow chart 39.1: Differential characters of Microfilariae

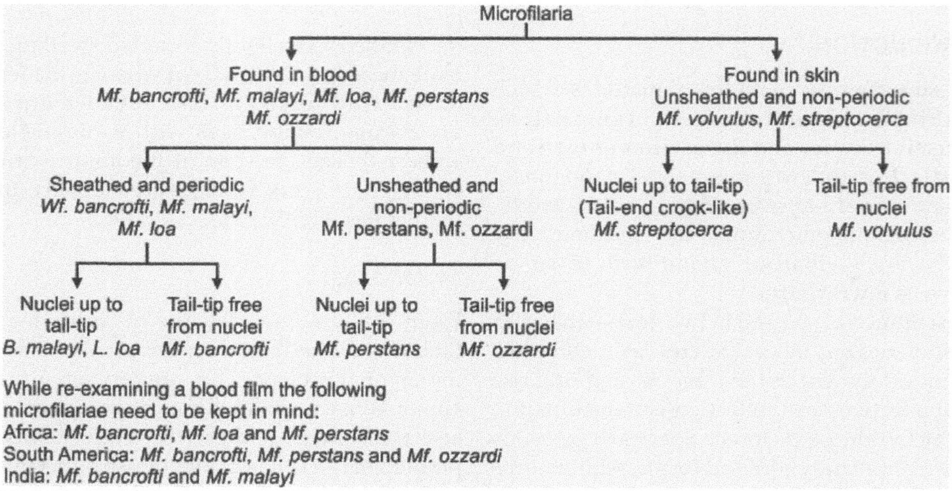

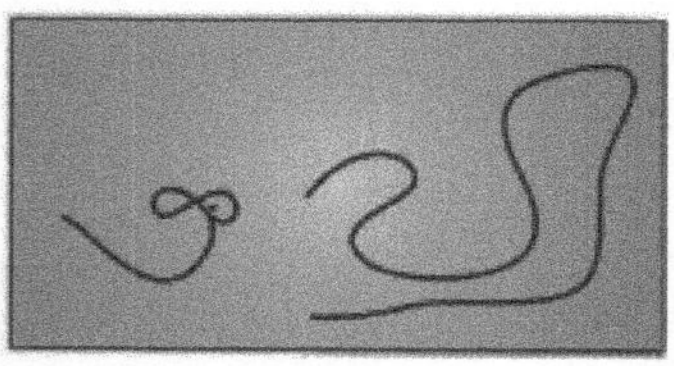

Fig. 39.23: Adult worms of *W. bancrofti*

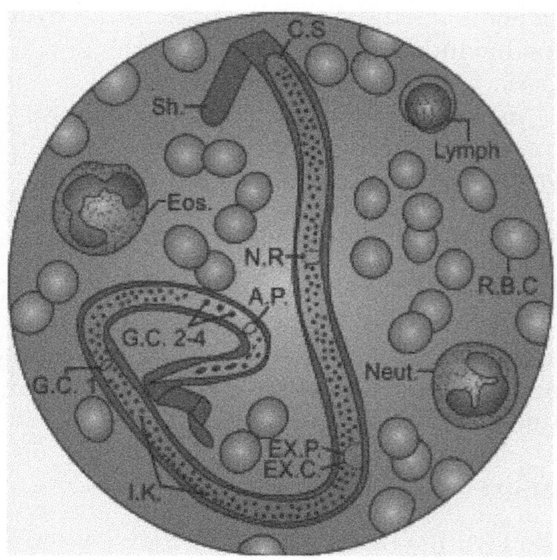

Fig. 39.24: Morphology of *Microfilaria bancrofti*

Life Cycle

W. bancrofti passes its life cycle in two hosts—man and mosquito.

1. The ***definitive host*** is man in whose lymphatic system, the adult worms are harbored. Live embryos (microfilariae) are discharged which find their way into the blood stream. The embryos can live in the peripheral blood for a long time. They are then taken up by the female culex mosquitoes during their blood meal.
2. The ***intermediate host*** is a mosquito in which the microfilariae undergo further development after which they become infective to man. A large number of species of mosquito belonging to genus *Culex, Aedes* and *Anopheles* act as intermediate hosts for *W. bancrofti*.

Stages in the Development of Microfilaria in the Mosquito

1. Sheathed microfilariae ingested by the mosquito during its blood meal, penetrate the gut and migrate to the thoracic muscles. Here they rest and begin to grow.
2. In the next few stages they pass from first stage larvae to second stage and then third stage larva. After the third stage larvae are developed they enter the proboscis sheath of the mosquito on about the 14th day.

Entrance into Man and Development into Adult Worms

When the infected mosquito bites a human being, the third stage larvae are not directly injected into blood stream like the malarial parasites but are deposited on the skin near the site of puncture. Later the larvae enter through the puncture wound or penetrate through the skin on their own.

The third stage larvae penetrate the skin, reach the lymphatic channels, settle down at some place (inguinal, scrotal or abdominal lymphatics) and begin to grow into adult forms. After 5 to 18 months they become sexually mature. The male fertilizes the female and the gravid females give birth to larvae. Microfilaria are again emitted which pass through the thoracic duct or right lymphatic duct to the venous system and pulmonary capillaries and then to the peripheral circulation.

Clinical Features

Infection with *W. bancrofti* is called filariasis. **Adult worms living or dead produce the pathogenic effects. The living microfilariae circulating in the blood are not known to produce any pathogenic effect except in occult filariasis**. The adult worm causes an inflammatory reaction of the lymphatic system called **lymphangitis** which forms the basic lesion in classical filariasis. Lesions in occult filariasis are caused by microfilariae and are found not only in lymph nodes but also in lungs, liver and spleen.

The lesions produced in ***classical filariasis*** are:

1. Inflammation of the lymph glands and vessels—***lymphangiitis with lymphadenitis***.
2. Dilatation of lymphatics.
3. Lymphangiovarix (small blood vessels rupture into dilated lymphatics).
4. Hyperplasia of the skin and connective tissue.
5. Secondary bacterial infection.

Lymphangitis

This means inflammation of the lymphatics. It is caused by an inflammatory response of the worm. The parts usually involved are the lymphatics of the testicle and epididymis, the lymphatics of the spermatic cord (funiculitis) abdominal lymphatics—(retroperitoneal lymphangitis) and the lymphatics of the upper and lower extremities. The favourite site for the adult worm of *W. bancrofti* is the epididymis. The visible lymphatic trunks appear as red congested streaks on the skin. On palpation they are found to be painful and appear as cord-shaped swellings.

Lymphadenitis

Inflammation of the regional lymph nodes. They are usually found in the groin and sometimes in the axilla. They appear as soft, more or less lobulated masses. The skin over the swelling is not adherent and unless acutely inflamed, the swelling is not painful and tender.

Hydrocele

This means swelling of the scrotum due to inflammation of the lymphatics of the testis and epididymis. **Recurrent attacks of wuchererial orchitis and epididymitis predispose to the occurrence of hydrocele. The fluid usually contains the microfilariae but the microfilariae die in the hydrocele fluid.**

Elephantiasis

The affected part becomes very enlarged producing a tumor-like solidity. **This is the end**

result of wuchererial infection and follows years of continuous infection.

Chyluria

Escape of chyle through the urine due to rupture of varicose chyle vessels through the mucous membrane of the urinary tract is called chyluria. In short the clinical manifestations of classical filariasis may be written as follows:

A. ***Asymptomatic filariasis*** These are cases of light infections.
B. ***Symptomatic filariasis*** These can be roughly divided into:
   - ***Inflammatory Phase***—Lymphangitis and lymphadenitis.
   - ***Obstructive Phase***—Characterized by enlarged lymph nodes, and elephantiasis of various parts. These occur in sites where inflammatory reaction has occurred. The obstructive phase may take 20 years to develop.

Diagnosis

The procedures adopted are as follows:

Direct Evidences

This includes a search for microfilariae and adult worms. The *microfilariae are found* in the peripheral blood, chylous urine, exudate of lymphvarix and in the hydrocele fluid. The microfilariae are not found in the following conditions:

1. In case of elephantiasis due to lymphatic obstruction.
2. After an attack of lymphangitis due to death of the adult worm.
3. During early allergic manifestations.
4. In occult filariasis.

The adult worms can be looked for in the biopsied lymph node or as the calcified worm by X-ray.

Indirect Evidences

Allergic tests

- Blood examination—shows eosinophilia of 5 to 15 percent.
- Intradermal skin test—an immediate hypersensitivity reaction.

Immunological test

- Complement fixation test—a sensitive test for occult filariasis.

Occult filariasis (Meyers Kouwenaar syndrome): This is a condition in which there is massive eosinophilia (30 to 80%), absolute eosinophil count > 3000/mm^3, generalized lymph node enlargement, hepatosplenomegaly, pulmonary symptoms and absence of microfilaraemia. The adult worm produces the microfilaria continuously but they do not reach the peripheral blood because they are destroyed in the tissues. It is an unusual host reaction to filarial antigen resulting in the development of an eosinophil granuloma in which a large number of eosinophils aggregate around a microfilaria.

We come to know about its filarial origin by:

1. Filarial complement fixing antibody in high titer.
2. Clinical, hematological and serological manifestations respond readily to DEC (Diethyl carbamazine) (Table 39.6).

Table 39.6: Differences between classical and occult filariasis

	Classical filariasis	*Occult filariasis*
Basic pathology	Acute inflammation followed by an epitheloid granuloma surrounding the adult worm	An eosinophilic granuloma (allergic or hypersensitivity reaction)
Organs involved	Lymphatic system (lymphatic vessels and lymph nodes)	Lymphatic system—lungs, liver and spleen
Microfilaria	Present in blood	Present in affected tissue but not in blood
Therapeutic response	No response to any drug	Responds to microfilaricidal drug—diethyl carbamazine
Serological test	Complement fixation test not so sensitive	Complement fixation test highly sensitive

Tropical pulmonary eosinophilia: (Eosinophilic lung, Weingarten's syndrome). This is a manifestation of occult filariasis and is characterized by low fever, loss of weight, cough and scanty sputum, dyspnoea and splenomegaly. Chest X-ray shows increased markings or diffuse miliary mottling.

Microfilaria may be demonstrated in tissues by lung biopsy.

Brugia Malayi

This worm is basically similar to *W. bancrofti* with some minor differences:

1. The geographical distribution is in Indonesia, Thailand, Vietnam, Malaysia, Burma, Southern China, Korea, Japan and Sri Lanka. In India it is reported from Kerala, Orissa, Madhya Pradesh and Assam.
2. The microfilaria of *B. malayi* and *W. bancrofti* differ in some minor respects.
3. The life cycle is the same as *W. bancrofti*. The intermediate hosts in India are various species of Mansonia, and one species of Anopheles.
4. In Malayan filariasis there is absence of chyluria and rarity of scrotal swellings.

DRACUNCULUS MEDINENSIS

Common names—Guinea worm

Geographical Distribution

It is found in India, Pakistan, Burma, Saudi Arabia, Iraq, Iran, eastern regions of USSR, Africa, West Indies and South America. In India the parasite is found in Punjab, Rajasthan, Madhya Pradesh, Gujarat, Maharashtra and South India.

Habitat

The adult females are found in the subcutaneous tissues especially of the legs, arms and back.

Morphology

Adult Worms

Male: The male worm has not been recovered from man. As always the male is much smaller than the female.

Female: This is a slender long worm measuring 60 cm to 1 m in length with a diameter of 1.5 to 1.7 mm. The body is cylindrical, smooth and milk white in color. The posterior extremity is tapering and is bent to form a hook. The worm is viviparous which means it discharges embryos. The body fluid is toxic and causes a blister if it escapes into the tissues.

The life span of the female is about one year and that of the male 6 months.

Embryos

These are coiled bodies with rounded heads and long thin tails. After the embryos are discharged in water, further development proceeds in the body of a minute fresh water crustacean of the genus *Cyclops*. Unless they are taken up by cyclops, they can live only for a very short period.

Life Cycle

The worm passes its life cycle in two hosts—man and cyclops (Fig. 39.25).

1. ***Definitive host***: Man harbours the adult parasite in the subcutaneous tissue.
2. ***Intermediate host***: Cyclops in which the embryos undergo developmental changes before they become infective to man.

Let us start the life cycle by entrance into man. The cyclops containing the infective larvae is swallowed by man with raw drinking water. On reaching the stomach, the cyclops is digested by the gastric juice and the larvae are liberated. They come out of the gut wall and enter the connective tissue where they grow to sexual maturity.

The larvae in man become adult males and females. The males die after fertilizing the

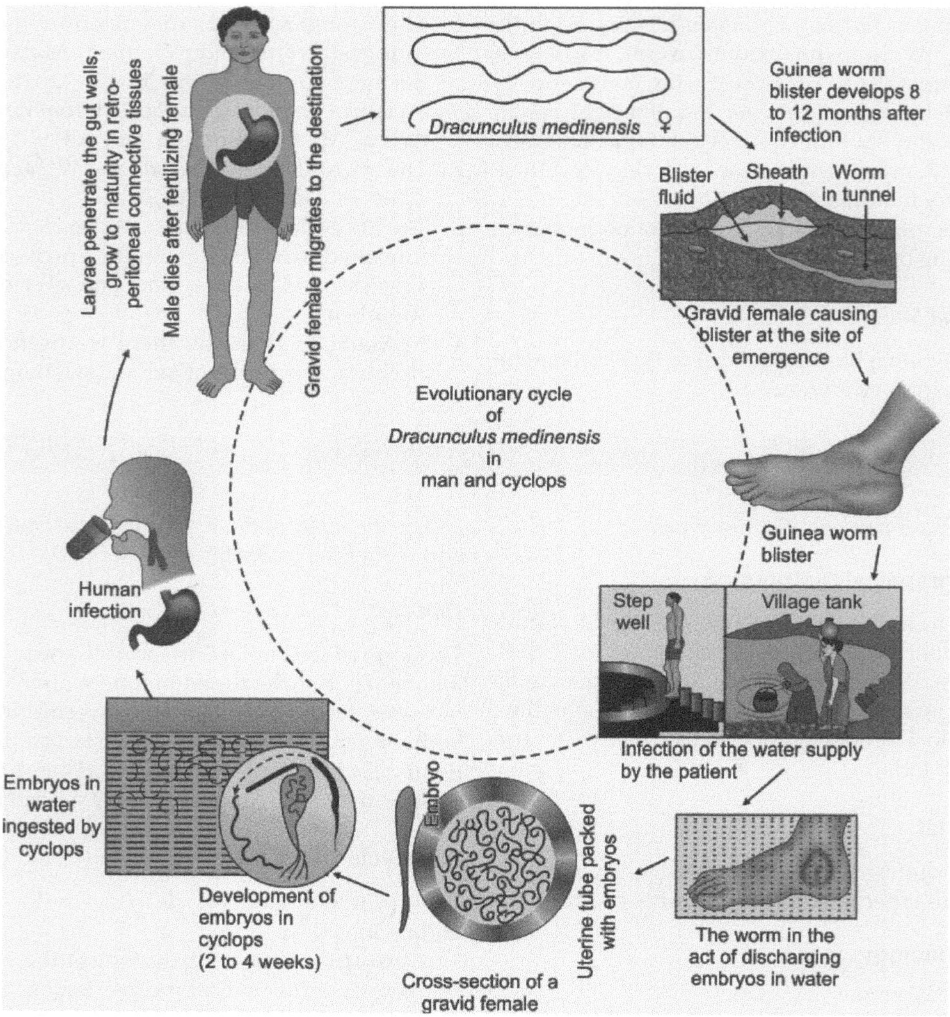

Fig. 39.25: Evolutionary cycle of *Dracunculus medinensis* in man and cyclops

females and disappear within 6 months of infection. The union between males and females occurs in the deeper connective tissues and it takes 6 months for the gravid female to select its site for discharging embryos in water. It selects those places which are likely to come in contact with water. On reaching the skin surface it secretes a toxin producing a blister which ruptures and forms an ulcer. Through this a milky fluid is secreted which contains a number of coiled embryos ejected from the uterus. The embryos reach water which are then taken up by a cyclops. Each cyclops can ingest as many as 15 to 20 guinea worm embryos. The cyclops usually die at the end of 42 days but with a heavy infection they do not live for more than 15 days.

The cycle is thus repeated.

Clinical Features

Infection with *D. medinensis* in man is called guinea worm disease or **dracunculosis**. The symptoms are due to the blister formation and liberation of a toxic substance causing allergic manifestations.

Blister Formation

The lesion appears whenever the female worm makes an attempt to come to the surface of the body where it can readily discharge its embryos. In majority of cases, the female worm chooses some part of the legs or arms, trunk, buttock, scrotum, head or neck. The gravid female goes to her destination where it pierces the skin. The head of the worm tries to come to the surface resulting in itching or burning sensation in that area. An irritant secreted by the worm produces a small red spot which gets converted to a small bleb or blister. The fluid in the blister is sterile and yellow in color, it contains many monocytes, eosinophils and neutrophil granulocytes. When the blister ruptures we can see a small hole through which the head of the worm protrudes. The central hole leads to a tunnel in the subcutaneous tissue where the female worm lies.

Laboratory Diagnosis

We can either detect the adult worm or detect the embryos.

1. *Detection of adult worm*: This is possible when the female worm appears at the surface of the skin.
2. *Detection of embryos*: The affected part through which the head of the worm is protruding must be bathed in water to encourage the discharge of embryos from uterus. The milky fluid containing many embryos can be pipetted off and examined under the microscope.

Intradermal Tests

Injection of dracunculus antigen intradermally causes a wheal to appear in the course of 24 hours.

X-ray Examination

Worms in deeper tissues after death become calcified or absorbed. The position of calcified worms may be seen. Blood examination shows eosinophilia.

Treatment

Ambilhar is a drug which is used for the treatment. One method of extracting the worm is to encourage the parasite to discharge it's embryos by careful douching with cold water. As soon as the female worm shows herself, the end is tied with a fine silk to a match stick or a similar object. Then it is rolled out by gentle traction in about 15 to 20 days.

Prophylaxis

1. Prevention of pollution of drinking water by infected individual.
2. Chemical treatment of water supply for eradication of cyclops.
3. Drinking water should be strained, filtered or boiled.

Section 6

Mycology

Mycology

Introduction

In the recent years, Medical Mycology has become a discipline in its own right. With the control of bacterial infections, more of fungal infections are being exposed. Opportunistic fungal infections are increasing in immunocompromised patients. The role of fungi in causing allergic asthma and hypersensitivity reactions is also being studied.

This section provides the basics of mycology and the correct diagnostic methods to be used in the laboratory for the diagnosis of fungal infections. As the diagnostic techniques differ from the ones used in bacterial diseases, it becomes important to learn and master the methods used for fungal diagnosis.

CHAPTER

40

Medical Mycology

LESSON PLAN

- Definition and Introduction
- Structure of a Fungus
- Classification of Fungi
- Mycoses (Fungus Infections)
- Superficial Mycoses
- Deep Mycoses
- Opportunistic Mycoses
- Laboratory Diagnosis of Fungal Infections
  - Laboratory Diagnosis of Superficial Fungal Infections
  - Laboratory Diagnosis of Deep Fungal Infections

DEFINITION AND INTRODUCTION

Medical mycology is the branch of microbiology which deals with the study of fungi.

Fungi, as we know are **eukaryotic protists** that are different in many ways from bacteria and other prokaryotes.

- Fungi have rigid cell walls containing chitin, mannan and other polysaccharides
- Their cytoplasmic membrane contains sterols.
- They have true nuclei with nuclear membrane and paired chromosomes
- They divide asexually, sexually or by both processes
- They may be unicellular or multicellular
- They show various degrees of specialization.

Why Have Fungal Infections Become More Important?

With the control of bacterial infections in the developed countries, fungal infections have now emerged more important. Most of the fungi are soil saprophytes and human infections are mainly **opportunistic** that is, they occur when body defenses are low. Modern advances in treatment such as antibiotics, steroids and immunosuppressive agents have led to a decrease in immunity and lowering of normal protective bacterial flora. These reasons have led to an increase in the fungal infections.

STRUCTURE OF A FUNGUS

- The simplest type of fungus is the unicellular budding **yeast**.
- Elongation of the cell produces a tubular thread-like structure called the **hypha**.
- A tangled mass of hypha constitutes the **mycelium**.
- Fungi which form mycelia are called **moulds or filamentous fungi**.
- Hyphae may have partitions which are called ***septa***. Accordingly they are called septate or non-septate.
- The septa when present have pores through which the free flow of cytoplasmic material can take place.

CLASSIFICATION OF FUNGI

Depending on the structure of the cell, fungi can be divided into four classes:
1. Yeasts
2. Yeast like fungi
3. Moulds
4. Dimorphic fungi.

Yeasts are unicellular fungi which occur as spherical or elliptical cells and reproduce by simple budding. On culture they form smooth creamy colonies. The only pathogenic yeast is *Cryptococcus neoformans*.

Yeast like fungi grow as yeast and also as elongated cells resembling hyphae. The latter form a pseudomycelium. *Candida albicans* is pathogenic yeast like fungus.

Moulds or filamentous fungi form true mycelia and reproduce by the formation of different types of spores. Dermatophytes are examples of pathogenic moulds.

Dimorphic fungi These can occur as filaments or as yeasts depending on the conditions of growth. In host tissues or cultures at 37°C they occur as yeasts while in the soil and in cultures at 22°C they appear as moulds. Most fungi causing systemic infections are dimorphic fungi.

MYCOSES (FUNGUS INFECTIONS)

Human fungus infections are of three types:
- Superficial
- Systemic (deep-seated)
- Opportunistic infections.

Superficial infections are caused by fungi that invade only superficial keratinized tissue (skin, hair, nails).

The characteristics of fungi causing superficial infections are:
- They cause a mild but chronic disease
- They are more common than the other types
- These fungi are specialized saprophytes with the capacity to digest keratin
- They include the various types of tinea or ringworm affecting skin, hair and nails.

Systemic (deep-seated) infections are caused by soil saprophytes. Infection is accidental. Systemic mycoses can be asymptomatic or turn into a fatal disease.

Opportunistic fungal infections occur in patients with debilitating diseases such as cancer or diabetes or when the immunity is low, e.g. treatment with immunosuppressive drugs, steroids, X-rays or broad spectrum antibiotics. These infections are caused by fungi that are normally avirulent such as *Mucor, Penicillium or Aspergillus*.

SUPERFICIAL MYCOSES

Superficial mycoses are of two types:
- Surface infections
- Cutaneous infections.

Surface Infections

The fungi live on the dead layers of the skin and its appendages (nail, hair). They have no contact with the living tissue and hence there is no inflammatory response. The only changes produced are cosmetic defects.

1. ***Tinea versicolor (Pityriasis versicolor)*** This is a chronic asymptomatic involvement of the stratum corneum in which there are discrete patches of depigmentation of the skin. The areas involved are chest, abdomen, upper limbs and back. The causative agent is a fungus called *Malassezia furfura* (*Pityro sporum or biculare*). The disease is more common in tropics, and in young adults. Diagnosis is done by examining skin scrapings, which show yeast like cells and short-branched filaments (Fig. 40.1). This fungus can be seen on normal skin also and in this way, it is considered to be an opportunistic infection
2. ***Tinea nigra*** is a localized infection of the stratum corneum especially the palms producing black or brownish macular lesions. It is caused by *Cladosporium mansonii*.
3. ***Piedra*** is a fungus infection of the hair characterized by the appearance of firm irregular nodules along the hair shaft.

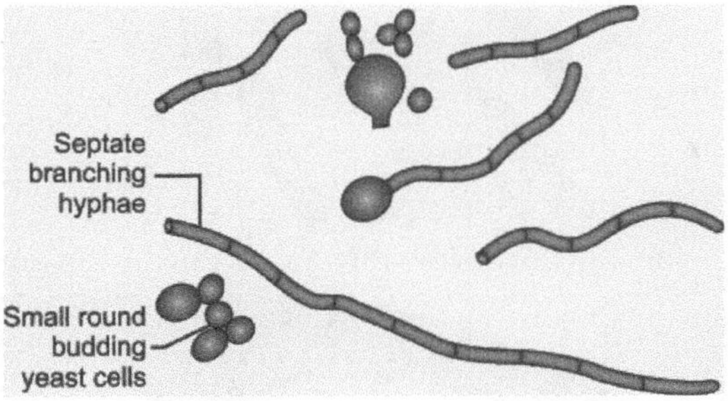

Fig. 40.1: *Pityrosporum orbiculare* in stratum corneum clusters of small round budding yeast cells are interspersed among septate branching hyphae. Skin scraping, KOH preparation

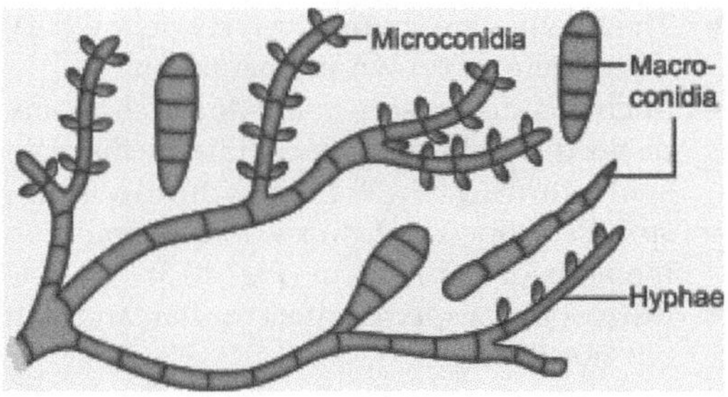

Fig. 40.2: *Trichophyton rubrum*: Culture mount showing microconidia along sides of hyphae and long cylindrical macroconidia

Cutaneous Infection

The most important cutaneous infection is **dermatophytosis** caused by a group of related fungi called ***dermatophytes***. Infection is in the cornified layer of the skin and its appendages, but a variety of inflammatory and allergic responses are induced in the host by the presence of fungi and their metabolic products. Another type of cutaneous infection is caused by *Candida albicans*. Though candida infection is mostly seen in skin and mucosa it can cause systemic disease involving every organ. Candida infection therefore represents a bridge connecting superficial and deep mycoses.

Dermatophytoses

Definition: Dermatophytoses are diseases caused by a group of related fungi called dermatophytes. It is the most common cutaneous infection.

Dermatophytes: These are filamentous fungi that infect only superficial keratinized tissues—skin hair and nails. The clinical conditions which they cause are called dermatophytoses also known as tinea or ringworm infection. All dermatophytes have a saprophytic existence and infect man accidentally.

They are classified into three genera:

a. *Trichophyton*
b. *Microsporum*
c. *Epidermophyton*

Around 40 species of dermatophytes are known.

- All dermatophytes grow on Sabauraud's dextrose agar medium forming characteristic colonies.
- If we make a Lactophenol cotton blue preparation of the culture we see septate hyphae and 2 types of asexual spores—microconidia and macroconidia.
- Differentiation into 3 genera is based on the nature of macroconidia.

Trichophyton

Colonies are powdery, velvety or waxy with different pigmentation characteristic of different species. Microconidia are abundant and are arranged in clusters along the hyphae or borne on conidiophores.

Macroconidia are scanty. They are elongated with blunt ends.

Macroconidia have special shapes in different species and are of importance in species identification. Trichophytons infect skin, hair and nails. Some of the species are:

- *T. rubrum*
- *T. mentagrophytes*
- *T. tonsurans*

T. rubrum is the most common species infecting man. It often causes chronic treatment resistant lesions (Fig. 40.2).

Microsporum

- The colonies are cottony, velvety or powdery with white to brown pigmentation
- Microconidia are scanty and do not show any distinctive feature. Macroconidia are the main spore form. They are large multicellular, spindle-shaped structures, borne singly on the ends of the hyphae (Fig. 40.3)
- Microsporum species infect the hair and skin but not the nails.

Epidermophyton

- The colonies are powdery and greenish yellow in color
- Microconidia are absent
- Macroconidia are multicellular, pear-shaped and typically arranged in clusters (Fig. 40.3)
- Epidermophyton attacks the skin and the nails but not the hair
- The genus contains only one species—*E. floccosum.*

See Table 40.1 for the common characteristics of dermatophytes.

Pathogenicity

Dermatophytes grow only on the keratinized layers of the skin. They do not penetrate into the living tissues. The fungal products give rise to local inflammation or a hypersensitivity reaction.

Clinically the ringworm can be classified depending on the site involved. **Tinea corporis** is the ringworm of the smooth or non-hairy skin of the body.

Tinea cruris is involvement of the groin and perineum.

Tinea barbae or barber's itch is the involvement of the bearded areas of the face and neck.

Tinea pedis or athlete's foot is the ringworm of the foot.

Tinea capitis—It is the ringworm of the scalp.

Favus is a chronic type of ringworm in which dense crusts (scutula) develop in the hair follicles which lead to alopecia and scarring. Scalp infections sometimes produce severe boggy lesions with marked inflammatory reaction called **kerion** (Tables 40.2 and 40.3).

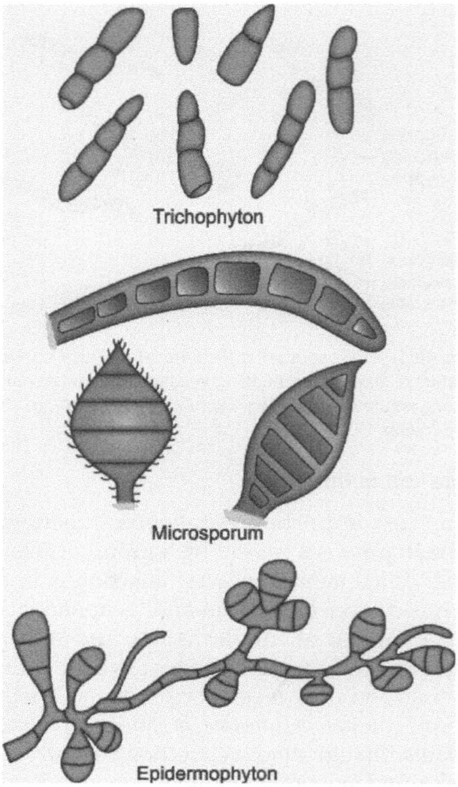

Fig. 40.3: Macroconidia of dermatophytes. Cylindrical in trichophyton, fusiform in microsporum and club-shaped in Epidermophyton

Epidemiology

Dermatophytosis occurs throughout the world but certain types of disease and some species of fungi show a particular distribution. Example—Tinea pedis is common in temperate cliimates and not tropics.

Laboratory Diagnosis of Dermatophyte Infection

The routine method of diagnosis is by the examination of KOH mounts. Scrapings are taken

Table 40.1: Some characteristics of common dermatophytes

Species	*Colony*	*Morphology*
T. rubrum	Velvety, red pigment on reverse	Few, long, pencil-shaped macroconidia
T. mentagrophytes	White to tan, cottony or powdery. Pigment variable	Clusters of microconidia. Cigar-shaped macroconidia with terminal tail-filaments
T. tonsurans	Cream or yellow, with central furrows	Abundant microconidia. Thick-walled, irregular macroconidia
T. schoenleinii	Smooth, waxy, brownish	Hyphal swellings, chlamydospores, favic chandelier
T. violaceum	Very slow growing. Waxy, violet to purple pigment	Distorted hyphae, Conidia rare
M. audouinii	Velvety, brownish, slow growing	Thick-walled chlamydospores, conidia rare and irregular
M. canis	Cottony, orange pigment on reverse	Abundant, thick-walled, spindle-shaped macroconidia with upto 15 septa
M. gypseum	Powdery, buff-coloured	Abundant, thin-walled macroconidia with 4-6 septa
E. floccosum	Yellowish green, powdery	Club-shaped macroconidia in clusters

Table 40.2: Clinical types of dermatophytoses and their common causative agents

Disease	*Common causative agents*
Tinea capitis	*Microsporum* any species, *Trichophyton* most species
Favus	*T. schoenleinii, T. violaceum, M. gypseum*
Tinea barbae	*T. rubrum, T. mentagrophytes, T. verrucosum*
Tinea corporis	*T. rubrum and any other dermatophyte*
T. cruris	*E. floccosum, T. rubrum*
T. pedis	*T. rubrum, E. floccosum*
Ectothrix hair infection	*Microsporum species, T. rubrum, T. mentagrophytes*
Endothrix hair infection	*T. schoenleinii, T. tonsurans, T. violaceum*

Table 40.3: Some clinical features of dermatophyte infection

Skin disease	*Location of lesions*	*Clinical appearance*	*Fungi most Frequently responsible*
Tinea corporis (ringworm)	Non-hairy, smooth skin	Circular patches with advancing red, vesiculated border and central scaling. Pruritic	*Microsporum canis Trichophyton mentagrophytes*
Tinea pedis (athlete's foot)	Interdigital spaces on feet of persons wearing shoes	Acute: itching, red vesicular. Chronic: itching, scaling, fissures	*Trichophyton rubrum, T. mentagrophytes, Epidermophyton floccosum*
Tinea cruris (jock itch)	Groin	Erythematous scaling lesion in intertriginous area. Pruritic	*T. rubrum, T. mentagrophytes. E. floccosum*
Tinea capitis	Scalp hair, endothrix: fungus inside hair shaft. Ectothrix: fungus on surface of hair	Circular bald patches with short hair stubs or broken hair within hair follicles. Kerion rare. *Microsporum*-infected hairs fluoresce	*M. canis, Trichophyton tonsurans*
Tinea barbae	Beard hair	Edematous, erythematous lesion	*T. rubrum, T. mentagrophytes*
Tinea unguium (onychomycosis)	Nail	Nails thickened or crumbling distally discolored, lusterless. Usually associated with Tinea pedis	*T. rubrum, T. mentagrophytes E. floccosum*
Dermatophytid (id reaction)	Usually sides and flexor aspects of fingers, palm. Any site on body	Pruritic vesicular to bullous lesions. Most commonly associated with Tinea pedis.	No fungi present in lesion. May become secondarily infected with bacteria

from the edges of ringworm lesions. The specimen is mixed with a drop of 10 percent KOH and after placing a coverslip, the preparation is gently heated to bring about clearing. Microscopy shows branched septate hyphae (Fig. 40.4).

Infected hair can be seen through examination through UV light (Wood's lamp). Infected hair is fluorescent. Two types of hair infection can be seen in wet mounts **ectothrix** in which arthrospores are seen as a sheath surrounding the hair and **endothrix** in which the spores are inside the hair shaft (Fig. 40.5). Demonstration of fungus in nails is difficult and can be done after immersion in KOH for a day or two.

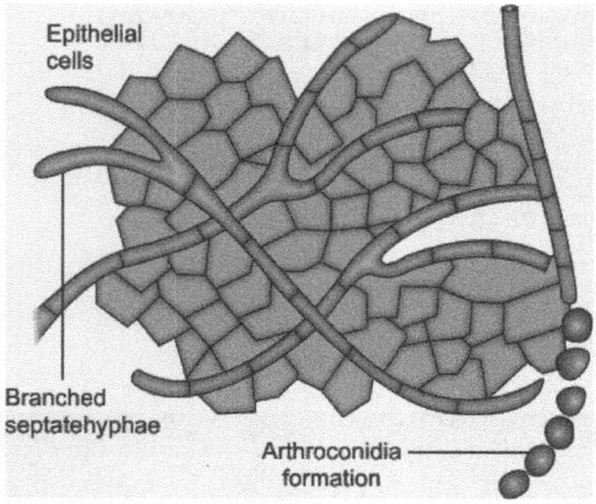

Fig. 40.4: Dermatophyte hyphae in skin scraping, KOH mount. Partly digested epithelial cells in background. Branched hyphae. Arthroconidia formation

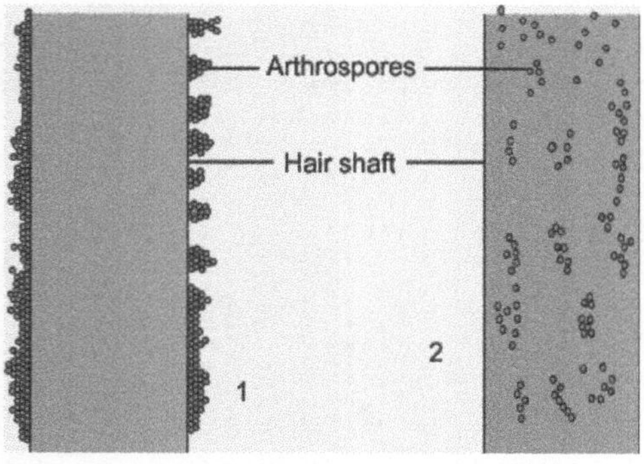

Fig. 40.5: Ectothrix and endothrix types of hair infection. (1) Ectothrix type with fungal arthrospores surrounding hair, (2) Endothrix type—showing arthrospores insde hair shaft

Species identification is done by culture on SDA (Sabouraud's Dextrose Agar) and incubated at room temperature. Growth is slow and colonies appear only in one to 3 weeks.

See ahead for detailed discussion on laboratory diagnosis of superficial infections.

Candidosis

It is also called moniliasis and is an infection of the skin, mucosa and sometimes of internal organs.

It is caused by yeast like fungus *Candida albicans* and sometimes by other candida species.

Candida albicans is an ovoid or spherical budding cell which produces pseudomycelia both in culture and in tissues. It produces two kinds of spores—blastospores which are thin-walled and seen in exudates and chlamydospores which are thick-walled and seen in cultures (Figs 40.6 and 40.7).

Candida species are normally found on the skin and the mucosa, as a part of normal flora. So candidosis is an **opportunist endogenous infection** and the commonest predisposing factor is diabetes.

There are many sites in the body where candidosis can develop:

1. *Cutaneous candidosis*: It may be intertriginous between folds or paronychial. Paronychia is a lesion around the nail and is seen in those in whom there is frequent contact with water. The lesions in the former are erythematous

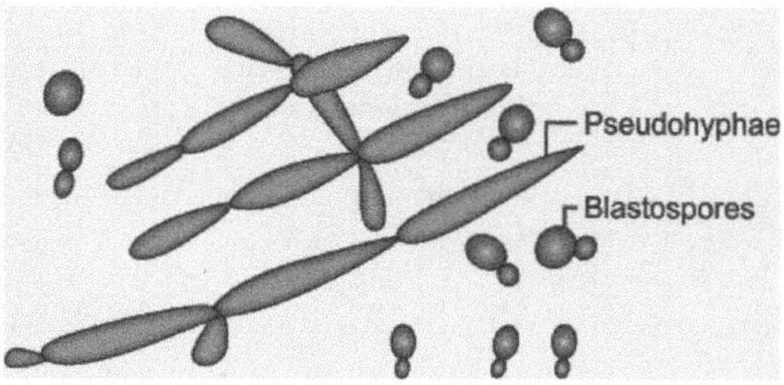

Fig. 40.6: Blastospores (blastoconidia) and pseudohyphae in exudates

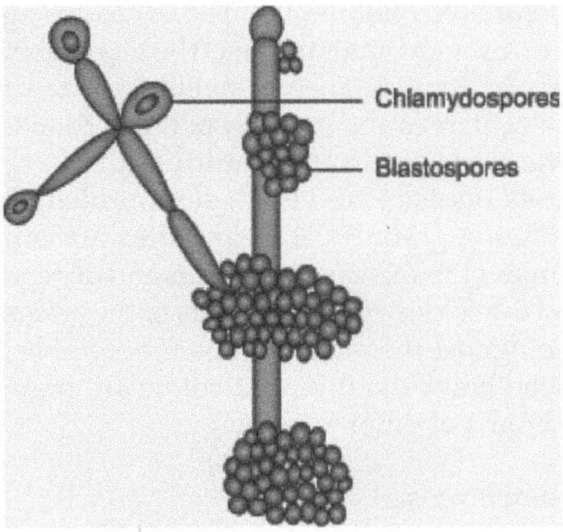

Fig. 40.7: Blastoconidia, pseudohyphae and chlamydoconidia (chlamydospores) in culture at 20°C

or moist lesions with sharply demarcated borders. The sites affected are those where skin is moist with perspiration, e.g. groin, perineum, axillae and inframammary folds.

2. *Mucosal*: The common mucosal lesions are vaginitis and oral thrush. There is an curdy white discharge in vaginitis and can be found in pregnancy.
   Oral thrush is found in bottle-fed infants, the aged and the debilitated. Creamy white patches appear on the tongue or buccal mucosa leaving a red oozing surface on removal.
3. *Intestinal*: This is seen after eating oral antibiotics for long periods. It presents as diarrhea not responding to treatment
4. *Others*: Bronchopulmonary candidosis is seen as a rare complication of preexisting pulmonary or systemic disease. Candida granuloma and chronic mucocutaneous candidiasis are serious manifestations in immunodeficiencies.

Diagnosis

It can be established by microscopy and culture. Wet films or Gram's stained smears from lesions or exudates show budding gram-positive cells. As candida is a normal skin contaminant, only

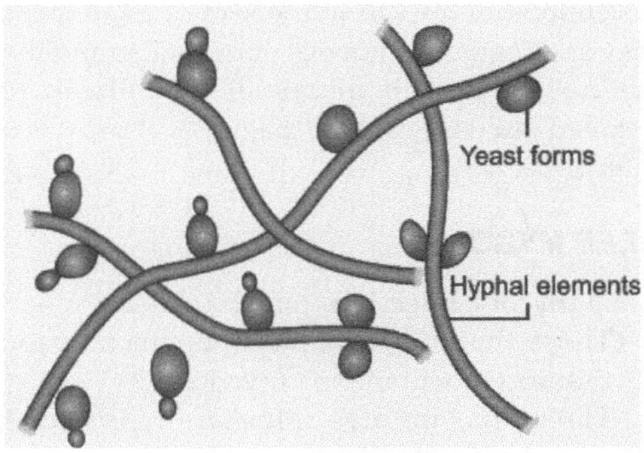

Fig. 40.8: *Candida albicans* in a stained specimen of sputum. The presence of hyphal elements in addition to yeast forms indicates colonization of tissue by the organism

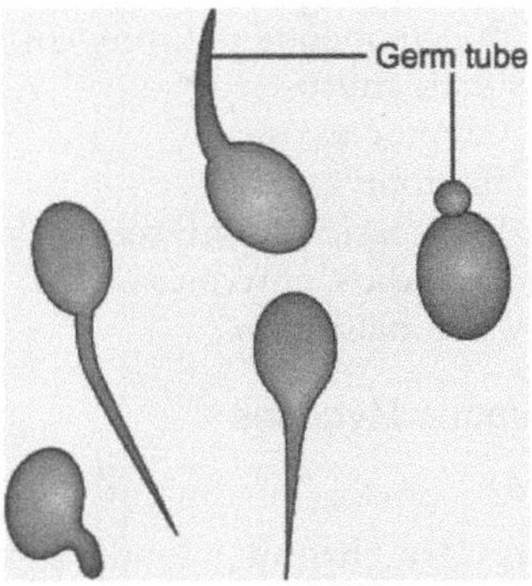

Fig. 40.9: Young cultures of *Candida* form germ tubes when placed in serum for 3 hours at 37°C

their presence in great numbers indicates infection. Also demonstration of mycelial forms indicates colonisation and tissue invasion (Fig. 40.8). Culture can be done on Sabouraud's dextrose agar or on any other ordinary media. Colonies are creamy, white smooth and with a yeasty odor.

Candida albicans can be identified from other candida species by growth characteristics and sugar assimilation tests. A rapid method of identifying *Candida albicans* is based on its ability to form germ tubes within 2 hours when incubated in human serum at 37°C (**Reynolds-Braude phenomenon**) (Fig. 40.9).

Antibodies appear in the sera of patients but they are frequent in normal persons also and they are not helpful in diagnosis. See ahead for detailed discussion on lab diagnosis of superficial infections.

DEEP MYCOSES

Deep mycotic infections may be classified as:

- Those that affect mainly the subcutaneous tissues (subcutaneous mycoses)
- Those that involve internal organs (deep seated or systemic mycoses).
  - A. Subcutaneous mycoses:
    1. Mycotic mycetoma
    2. Chromoblastomycosis
    3. Sporotrichosis
    4. Rhinosporidiosis
    5. Subcutaneous phycomycosis
  - B. Systemic mycoses:
    1. Cryptococcosis
    2. Blastomycosis
    3. Paracoccidioidomycosis
    4. Coccidioidomycosis
    5. Histoplasmosis.

Subcutaneous Mycoses

Mycetoma

Mycetomas are chronic, slowly progressive infections of the subcutaneous tissue usually of the foot. The disease was originally reported by Gill from Madura, South India. So it is called **Madura foot.** It is mainly seen in the tropics. It is common in Tamil Nadu but rare in Kerala. It is caused by a number of Nocardia, filamentous fungi and Actinomycetes. The causative agent enters through minor trauma. The disease begins as a small subcutaneous swelling of the foot which enlarges and goes deeper. It is connected to the surface through multiple discharging sinuses discharging viscid, seropurulent fluid containing granules. The **granules are micro-colonies** of the aetiological agents and depending upon the colour and consistency of the grains we can diagnose the causative agent. See Table 40.4 which shows the different colour of grains in mycetoma of different etiology.

Chromomycosis

The term chromomycosis includes a group of clinical manifestations caused by various pigmented fungi. The causative agents are soil inhabiting fungi. They get entrance through the skin by traumatic implantation and develop into a warty cauliflower. The disease is common among barefooted agricultural workers. Diagnosis is established by culture or by KOH mounts. Tissue sections show a typical morphology (Fig. 40.10).

Sporotrichosis

Sporotrichosis is caused by the fungus *Sporothrix schenckii* and is characterized by the development on the skin, in subcutaneous tissues and in lymph nodes of nodules which soften and break down to form ulcers. The fungus is a saprophyte found widely on plants, thorn and timber. Infection is acquired through thorn pricks or other minor injuries. Diagnosis is made by culture and

Table 40.4: Color of grains in mycetoma of various aetiology

Color of grain		
White of yellow	*Brown to black*	*Red*
Nocardia asteroides	*Madurella mycetomi*	*Actinomadura pelletieri*
Nocardia brasiliensis	*Madurella grisea*	
Actinomadura madurae	*Phialophora jeanselmei*	
Streptomyces somaliensis		
Allescheria boydii		

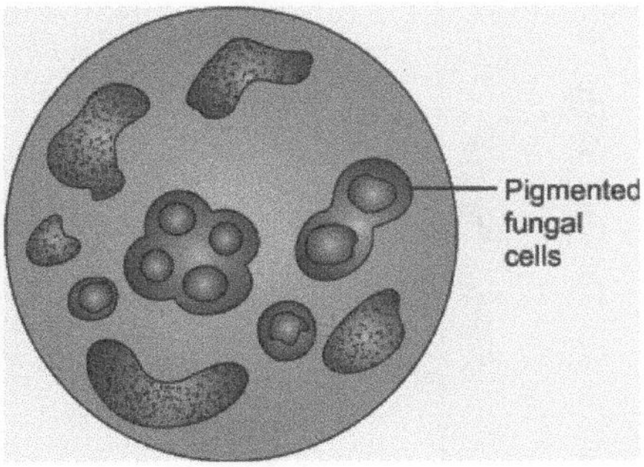

Fig. 40.10: Chromomycosis. Pigmented fungal cells seen in a giant cell

histology. Serology can also be done. Figure 40.11 shows the morphology of a culture mount of *Sporothrix schenckii.*

Rhinosporidiosis

Rhinosporidiosis is a chronic granulomatous disease characterized by the development of friable polyps usually confined to the nose, mouth or eye, but rarely on the genitalia or other mucous membranes. Large majority of cases are from India or Sri Lanka. The disease is generally confined to mucous membranes. Hematogenous dissemination has also been seen. Diagnosis is made histologically. It has not been cultivated (Fig. 40.12).

Subcutaneous Phycomycosis

This is a painless subcutaneous nodule which enlarges to involve a whole limb or large areas of the body. This condition is seen in many Asian and African countries. The causative agent is **Basidiobolus haptosporus** found in decaying vegetation.

Systemic Mycoses

Cryptococcosis

Cryptococcosis is a sub acute or chronic infection caused by the yeast *Cryptococcus neoformans.* It is a round or ovoid budding cell 4 to 20 μm in diameter with a prominent polysaccharide capsule. It is a soil saprophyte and is found in the feces of pigeons and other birds.

Infection is usually acquired by inhalation but may sometimes be through skin and mucosa. Most infections are asymptomatic.

The various areas of infection by cryptococcus could be:

1. Pulmonary
2. Visceral
3. Cutaneous
4. Meningeal

Cryptococcal meningitis is the most serious type of infection.

Diagnosis is done by demonstration of **capsulated budding yeast** cells in the lesions and by culture (Fig. 40.13). The capsules stand out in India ink preparations. The fungus grows on

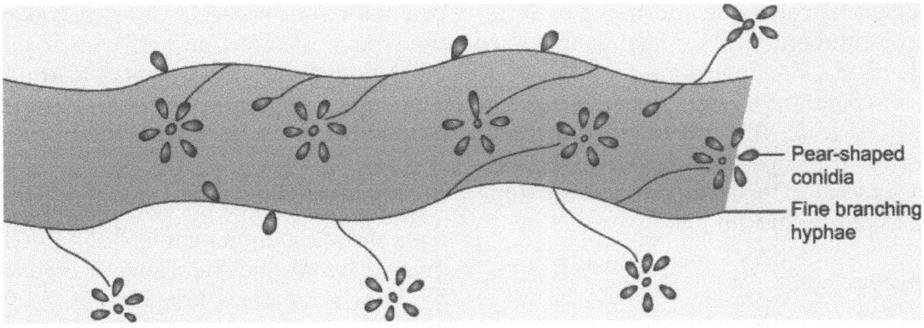

Fig. 40.11: *Sporothrix (sporotrichum) schenckii*: Culture mount showing fine branching hyphae and pear-shaped conidia borne in rosette like clusters at tips of lateral branches and singly along sides of hyphae

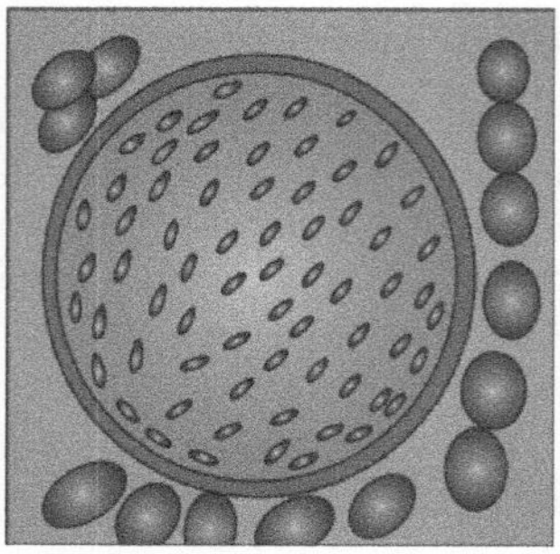

Fig. 40.12: *Rhinosporidium*: Mature sporangium (centrally located) in the stroma of a lesion

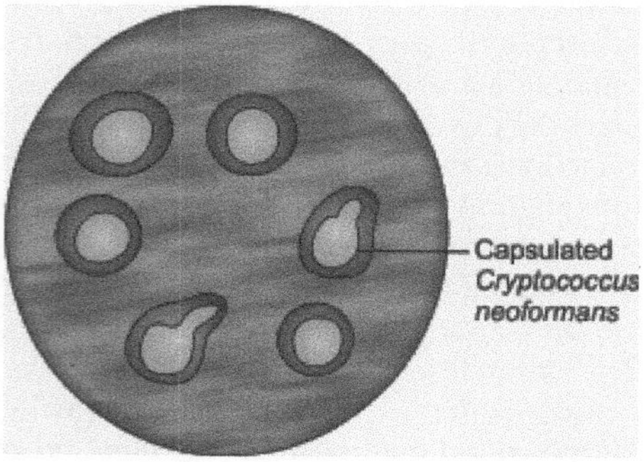

Fig. 40.13: *Cryptococcus neoformans*, India ink preparation of spinal fluid

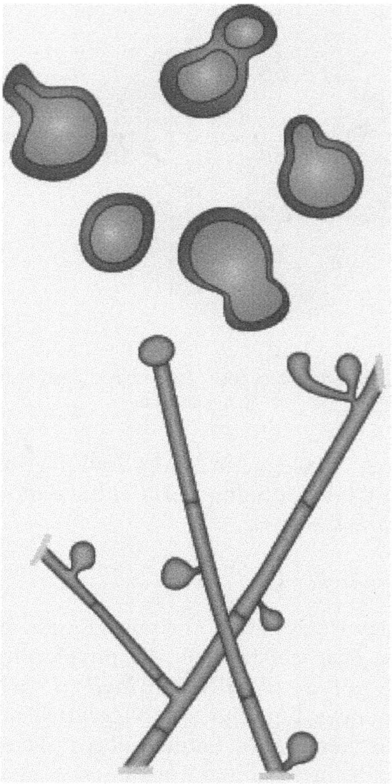

Fig. 40.14: *Blastomyces dermatidis* (a) In tissue or culture at 37°C, (b) In culture at 20°C on Sabouraud's agar

SDA forming smooth mucoid cream colored colonies. The ability to grow at 37°C and hydrolyze urea differentiates *C. neoformans* from non-pathogenic cryptococci.

Pathogenicity can be demonstrated by intracerebral or intraperitoneal inoculation into mice which develop a fatal infection.

Four serological types of cryptococcal capsular polysaccharide A, B, C, D have been seen. Demonstration of capsular antigen by precipitation can sometimes be useful to diagnose some cases of cryptococcal meningitis.

Blastomycosis

This is a chronic infection caused by fungus *Blastomyces dermatidis* and shows the formation of suppurative and granulomatous lesions in any part of the body especially lungs and skin. Soil is the source of infection and it is acquired by inhalation. As the infection is in North America it is known as North American blastomycosis (Fig. 40.14).

Paracoccidioidomycosis

It is a chronic granulomatous disease of the skin, mucosa, lymph nodes and internal organs caused by *Paracoccidioides brasiliensis*. Ulcerative granulo-mas of the buccal and nasal mucosa are an important part of this disease (Fig. 40.15).

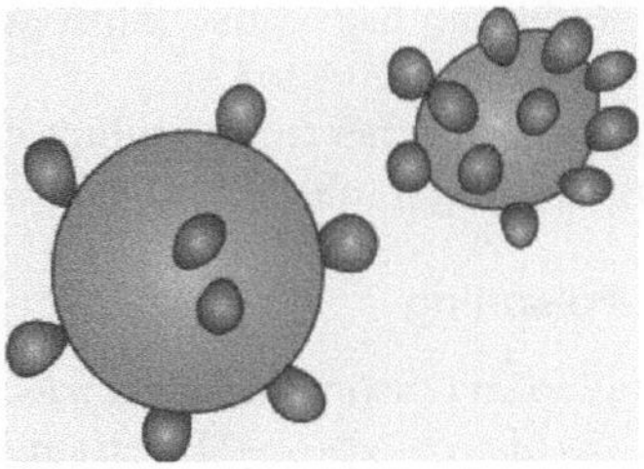

Fig. 40.15: *Paracoccidioides brasiliensis.* In tissue or culture at 37°C; Multiple budding

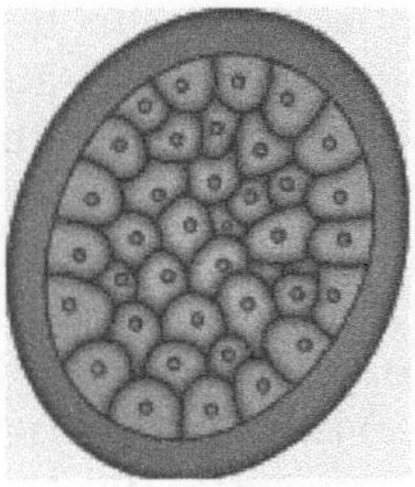

Fig. 40.16: *Coccidioides immitis*; tissue phase showing spherule with numerous endospores

Coccidioidomycosis

This is an infection caused by the fungus *Coccidioides immitis*. Infection is acquired by inhalation of dust containing arthrospores of the fungus. In most cases, respiratory infection is asymptomatic but some people develop a self-limited influenza-like fever (Fig. 40.16).

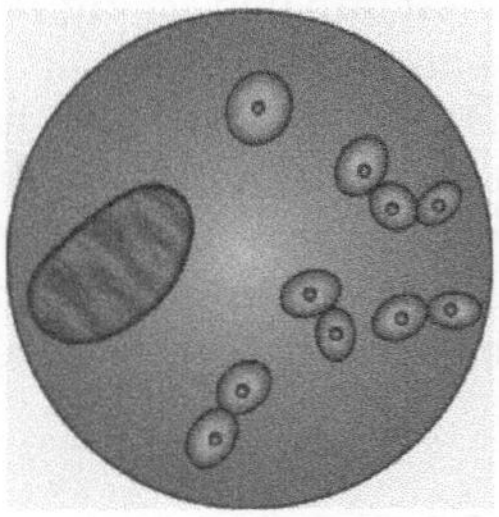

Fig. 40.17: *Histoplasma capsulatum* (Macrophage containing blastoconidia)

Histoplasmosis

Histoplasmosis is an intracellular infection of the reticuloendothelial system caused by fungus *Histoplasma capsulatum* (Figs 40.17 and 40.18).

The disease is worldwide in distribution but is common in USA where it is endemic. The fungus is present in the soil, rotting trees and bird feces. The large majority of infections are asymptomatic. Some infected persons develop pulmonary disease which resembles tuberculosis. The reticuloendothelial system is involved along with lymphadenopathy and hepatosplenomegaly, etc.

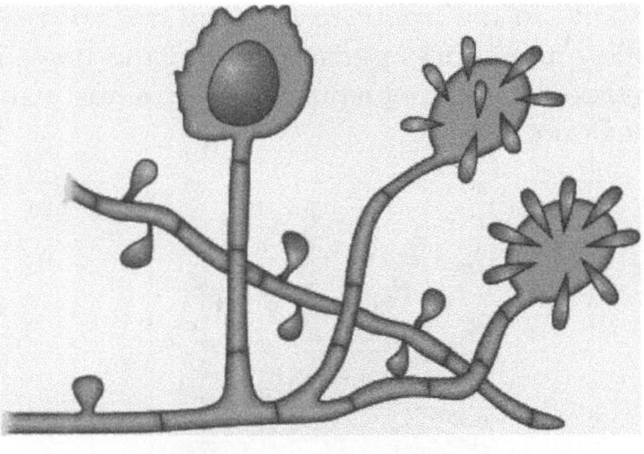

Fig. 40.18: *Histoplasma capsulatum.* Macro- and microconidia in culture at 20°C

OPPORTUNISTIC MYCOSES

These fungi are present in the atmosphere and can grow as contaminants on culture media. However, if a person is debilitated, it can cause serious infection.

Aspergillosis

Aspergillus is the fungus that grows on damp bread. The commonest species to cause human disease is *Aspergillus fumigatus*. Systemic aspergillosis occurs as the following types:

1. Pulmonary aspergillosis
   a. Aspergillus asthma
   b. Bronchopulmonary aspergillosis
   c. Aspergilloma
   d. Invasive aspergillosis
2. Disseminated aspergillosis.

Aspergillus asthma can occur in atopic individuals following sensitisation to inhaled aspergillus spores. **In bronchopulmonary aspergillosis**, the fungus grows within the lumen of bronchioles which may be occluded by the fungus plugs. The fungus can be demonstrated in sputum. Colonizing aspergillosis usually develops in preexisting pulmonary cavities such as tuberculosis or cystic disease. The fungus grows into large balls (**Aspergilloma**). **In invasive aspergillosis** the fungus invades the lung tissue. **Disseminated aspergillosis** involves brain, kidney and other organs.

Diagnosis is made by microscopic examination and by culture. The fungus grows rapidly on culture media (Fig. 40.19).

As aspergilli are common contaminants their demonstration in exudates should be interpreted with care.

Mucormycosis

It is an invasive disease caused by species of Rhizopus, and Mucor. The primary infection is usually in the upper respiratory tract or nose where the spores germinate and the mycelia invade the adjacent sinuses—orbit, sinuses and the brain.

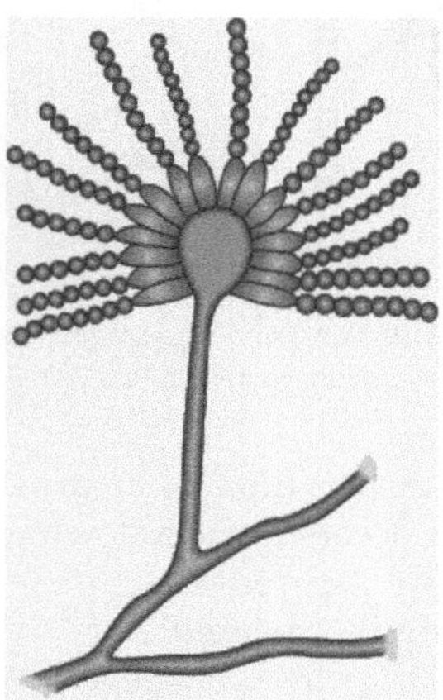

Fig. 40.19: *Aspergillus* morphology on a lactophenol cotton blue preparation on the culture medium. It shows un branched nonseptate conidiophores terminating in a globose vesicle bearing phialids from which arises chains conidia

This fungus can also cause infections of the ear and eye (Figs 40.20A to C).

Penicillium is another fungus which can cause opportunistic fungal infection.

Mycotic Poisoning

Many fungi form poisonous substances. Mycotic poisoning is of two types—**Mycetism** in which the fungus as whole causes toxic effects and **mycotoxicosis** in which fungal toxins contaminate food articles Example of mycetism is mushroom poisoning and example of mycotoxicosis is aflatoxin produced by *Aspergillus flavus*.

LABORATORY DIAGNOSIS OF FUNGAL INFECTIONS

The methods of lab diagnosis of fungal infections differ from that of bacterial infections.

1. We utilize more direct methods and less of serology because there is antigenic cross reactivity between the fungi of different genera and also because patients suffering from systemic fungal disease are immunologically unresponsive as a result of toxic therapy.
2. Fungi are much less in number as compared to bacteria in clinical samples. Therefore, many samples of affected tissue needs to be taken.
3. The culture media used for isolation of fungi are acidic and have high concentration of sugar such as glucose.

Laboratory Diagnosis of Superficial Fungal Infections

The samples to be collected in dermatophyte infection should be in adequate amounts.

Sample Collection

Skin scrapings: A curved disposable blade is used for taking samples by scraping across the inflamed margin of the lesion into apparently healthy tissue. The epidermal scales are collected from the outer active edge of lesion in a sterile

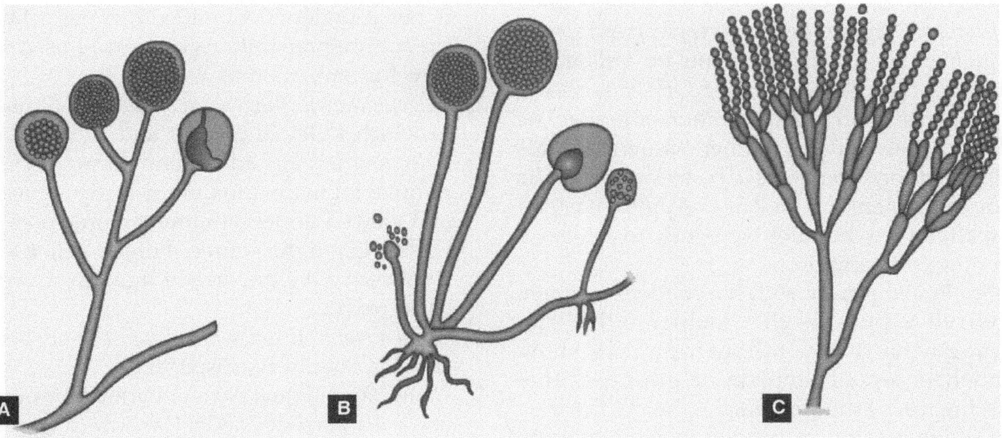

Figs 40.20A to C: Common contaminant fungi, culture mount, (A) *Mucor* showing nonseptate mycelium without rhizoids (root-like structures). Sporangiophores which may be branched, terminate in large globose sporangia containing numerous spores. (B) *Rhizopus* showing nonseptate mycelium with rhizoids. Unbranched sporangiophores arise opposite rhizoids. (C) *Penicillium* showing the 'penicillus' or brush, consisting of chains of spores extending from the ends of short branches of conidiophores

Petri-dish or black paper. If vesicles are present, the tops should be removed with fine scissors and sent for examination.

Skin strippings: This is the alternative method for collection of skin specimens. Water proof transparent vinyl adhesive tape is applied firmly to the affected area and peeled off. The tape now bearing a thin layer of skin is applied to a sterile glass microscope slide for transport to the lab. It is good for culture of dermatophytes and yeast.

Nail: Friable material or discolored areas should be removed from under the nail or nail clippings may be taken from the distal border with scissors or nail clippers. In case of paronychia in which a yeast infection is suspected, exudate is expressed from the paronychial folds by probing with a flat excavator and collecting with a swab previously moistened with sterile saline.

Hair: Infected hair should be removed by plucking with an epilating sterile forceps. It should not be cut as it fails to remove the area most likely to harbor the fungus that is the base of the hair shaft around the follicle. The affected hair strands may fluoresce under a Woods lamp.

Transport

1. The transport of skin, hair and nail specimens for fungal studies should be done by wrapping them in black paper or in an envelope. In such conditions, ringworm fungi remain viable for weeks or even months.
2. The samples should not be packed in air tight containers because we want them to dry out to prevent overgrowth of saprophytic bacteria and fungi. Neither should the samples be refrigerated as viability of the samples is affected.
3. Tape stripping which is stuck to a microscopic slide should be placed in a protective box for transport.
4. For collection of skin scrapings, two slides can be taken, one used to scrape the skin and another one kept at the bottom to collect the scrapings. Both the slides are sent in an envelope.

Direct Examination

Unstained: Prepare specimens for microscopy by reducing skin to thin fragments on a slide and adding a drop of 10 percent KOH. This allows rapid penetration and maceration of tissue. The alkali digests cells and other tissue materials enabling fungal elements to be seen clearly. The slide can be gently heated also. Apply cover slip and after a few minutes tap gently to achieve a very thin preparation.

See in low power with the condenser down. Observe hyphae as fine filaments that run through the tissue. Microscopy may show branched septate hyphae or gram-positive budding cells as in Candida.

Demonstration of fungus in nails may be difficult and may be possible only after keeping the clippings in KOH for a day or two.

Two types of hair infection may be seen in wet mounts—ectothrix in which the arthrospores are seen as a sheath surrounding the hair and endothrix in which spores are seen inside the hair shaft. If we want to get more information in hair infections, we can obtain that under **Wood's light**—a source of filtered UV light with maximum emission at 366 nm. Some fungi produce a **greenish fluorescence** at the base of hair shaft. Those areas of hair shaft that fluoresce have visible crusted areas which are selected and closely examined for arthrospores.

Stains:

1. Lactophenol cotton blue stain

Phenol crystals	20 g
Lactic acid	20 mL
Glycerol	40 mL
Distilled water	20 mL

   Cotton blue/methyl blue = 0.075 g
   - Glycerol helps in mounting and prevents drying
   - Lactic acid preserves the fungal structure
   - Phenol crystals kill the fungus
   - Cotton blue stains it.

   Place a drop of dye on the slide. Tease out culture fragments. Add a cover slip avoiding bubbles and exert gentle pressure. Remove excess stain. Wait for a few minutes. May heat it. See it under 10 x or 40 x. It is used more for culture preparations but can be used for direct examination as well.
2. *Calcoflour white fluorescent stains* may be used in which KOH 20 percent and *Calcoflour white* is added and allowed a few minutes for maceration. A cover slip is placed and viewed under a fluorescent microscope with a UV light source. Fungal cell walls fluoresce a bright green against a dark background.
3. *Gram's stain*: If gram-positive cells are seen candida should be suspected.
4. *Other stains*: Equal parts of Parker blue black ink + 10 percent NaOH. We can diagnose *Pityriasis versicolor* by staining with Parker blue black ink. They show many short curved hyphae with groups of spherical cells giving a **banana and grape arrangement**.

Culture

1. We want a culture media for fungi that is inhibitory to bacteria and in certain cases non-pathogenic fungi as well.
2. There are many reasons why we do not want to heat the culture media for fungi to a high temperature.
   a. Agar is hydrolysed by heat at low pH and high temp.
   b. The culture medium for fungus has high concentration of sugar and heating tends to char sugar.

   So autoclaving is done at 115°C.

- The culture medium which we use is SDA or *Sabouraud's Dextrose Agar*

  This has

  Glucose ⇒ 20 g

  Peptone = 10 g

  Agar = 15 gm

  Water = 1 liter

  Steam and adjust pH to 5.4.

  Autoclave at 115°C for 15 mins.

  Dispense 20 mL into plates or 5 mL into tubes.

  We can prepare one plain medium and one

with antibiotics namely penicillin, streptomycin cycloheximide, natamycin or chloramphenicol. These antibiotics are to avoid contamination with bacteria.

- *Malt Peptone Agar*
  This is an alternative culture medium.
  It has:
  Malt extract-40 g
  Peptone = 5 g
  Agar = 15 g
  Water = 1 liter
- Other culture mediums are:
  1. *Dermatophyte test medium*
  2. *Rice agar*
  3. *Niger seed agar for cryptococcus*
     Incubation for fungi is done at 28 to 30°C for 4 weeks.

Method of Fungal Culture

Skin and nails should be reduced in size to pieces approximately 1 mm across. Hair roots should be selected where crushed fluorescent material exists. The inocula should be gently implanted into agar on each plate at well-spaced intervals.

All dermatophytes have an optimum temperature for growth in culture of 28° to 30°C. We should incubate cultures in parallel. One at 22°C and one at 37°C. The one at 37°C should be discarded after one week if there is no growth of yeast or other fungi. The one at 22°C should be incubated for 3 to 4 weeks.

The cultures should be examined at 4 to 5 days intervals. Growth of a dermatophyte occurs in seven to ten days and colonies appear as light colored. Colonies that are blue black or dark green should be regarded as non-dermatophyte. The following characteristics should be noted:

1. Rate of growth of the colony.
2. Texture and color of the colony.
3. Underside of the colony and pigmentation on the reverse.

Trichophyton: Colonies are powdery or velvety or waxy with red pigment on the reverse.

Microsporum: The colonies are cottony, velvety or powdery with white/brown pigment.

Epidermophyton: Powdery-greenish yellow in color.

Just like we make a Gram's stain in bacteriology, a lacto phenol cotton blue preparation is made in mycology. The conventional method of making this preparation for microscopy is by using needles to take a representative sample of the colony. The sample is then teased out and a drop of lactophenol cotton blue stain is placed on it. After placing a cover slip, this preparation is studied under the microscope.

No Growth From Positive Material

Failure to isolate a fungus from a specimen of skin or hair in which hyphae were seen in a microscopy sample can be attributed to:

1. Insufficient sample
2. Improperly collected sample
3. Prior treatment of lesion with an agent having antifungal activity
4. Incorrect storage such as refrigeration or holding the material in a container that retains moisture.

Serology and Animal Inoculation

There are not helpful for diagnosis.

Laboratory Diagnosis of Deep Fungal Infections

The diagnosis of deep fungal infections has been discussed earlier. Here we will deal with the detailed diagnosis of two of them, namely infections by *Cryptococcus* and *Candida*.

Cryptococcus

- *Samples* to be collected
  - Spinal fluid
  - Exudates
  - Sputum
  - Urine
  - Serum
- *Microscopy* Specimens are examined in a wet mount directly. India ink preparation makes the capsules stand out. India ink preparation

of centrifuged CSF reveals encapsulated yeast in 50 percent cases.

- *Culture* Growth is rapid at 20 to 30°C. Creamy colonies are seen. Sputum culture is positive in only 10 percent.
- *Biochemistry* Sugar assimilation tests are done.
- *Animal pathogenicity tests* can be demonstrated by intracerebral or intraperitoneal inoculation into mice which produces a fatal infection. Capsulated cells can be demonstrated in brain of infected mice.
- *Serology* Four serological types of cryptococcal capsular polysaccharide A, B, C, D have been identified.

Tests for both antigen and antibody can be done on CSF and serum. Latex slide agglutination is normally done to detect antigen or antibody.

Serology is positive in only 1/3rd of patients.

Candida

Samples:

- Swabs and scrapings from surface lesions.
- Sputum.
- Exudates.

Microscopy: Gram-stained smears of samples show pseudohyphae and budding cells.

Culture: The culture on Sabouraud's dextrose agar shows soft creamy colonies, with a yeasty odour. If a lactophenol cotton blue preparation is made from culture, hyphae will be observed. *Candida albicans* can be distinguished from other species of *Candida* by:

1. Germ tube test.
2. Sugar fermentation tests.
3. Formation of chlamydospores on corn meal agar at 20°C.

Germ tube test: Touch a single colony of candida with a loop or a pasteur pipette. Emulsify it in 0.5ml of horse or other serum in a small test tube. Incubate at 37°C in a water bath for 2-4 hours. Germ tubes are formed if the species is *Candida albicans*. Germ tubes are extensions of typical yeast cells which gives a drumstick appearance.

Sugar fermentation tests of glucose, maltose sucrose and trehalose are positive in *Candida albicans*.

Serology: In systemic candidiasis, a rise in titre of antibodies to candida may be detected by various tests.

Skin Test: It is universally positive because most people have been exposed to the antigen.

Section 7

Applied Microbiology

- Normal Microbial Flora of the Human Body
- Vaccines

Applied Microbiology

Introduction

Applied Microbiology deals with the application of the principles and techniques of microbiology to associated fields. Here, we have picked up two topics. The first one deals with the study of the normal microbial flora of the human body which helps us in differentiating between pathogenic and non-pathogenic bacteria and arriving at a correct diagnosis.

The other chapter discusses the vaccines given routinely for prevention of diseases. This chapter is extremely important as it helps us to apply the principles of immunology and bacteriology to the prevention and control of microbial spread.

CHAPTER

41

Normal Microbial Flora of the Human Body

LESSON PLAN

- Introduction
- Advantages of Normal Flora
- Disadvantages of Normal Flora
- Normal Flora of the Skin
- Normal Flora of the Mouth and Upper Respiratory Tract
- Normal Flora of the Conjunctiva
- Normal Flora of the Nose, Nasopharynx and Sinuses
- Normal Flora of the Intestinal Tract
- Normal Flora of the Genitourinary Tract
- Bacteria in Blood and Tissues
- Opportunist Pathogenicity

INTRODUCTION

The normal microbial flora means the population of microorganisms which are present in or on the body of normal healthy people. They are divided into residents and transients. Residents consist of a constant type of microorganisms. They vary in different age groups or geographical areas and if disturbed, quickly come back. Transients are non-pathogenic or potentially pathogenic microorganisms that inhabit the skin or mucous membranes for some time and are derived from environment. They are of no significance as long as the resident normal flora is intact, but if resident flora is disturbed, transient microorganisms may colonize, proliferate and produce disease.

ADVANTAGES OF NORMAL FLORA

1. The resident population prevents permanent colonization of the body by other organisms which may be pathogenic. So they are protective and form a part of the natural immunity of the host.
2. The micro flora of the intestinal tract synthesizes vitamin K and several group B vitamins.
3. Some bacteria of the normal flora produce antibiotic substances (colicins) which have a harmful effect on pathogens.
4. Some bacteria of the normal flora release endotoxins which help the defense mechanism of the body.
5. The bacterial flora stimulates the production of surface antibody IgA, which prevents pathogenic organisms from invasion into deeper tissues.

DISADVANTAGES OF NORMAL FLORA

1. They can become pathogenic when host defenses are lowered, or they are introduced in large numbers in unusual sites, e.g. streptococci of the viridans group are the most common resident organisms of the upper respiratory tract. If large numbers of them are introduced into the blood stream following tooth extraction or tonsillectomy

they may settle down on deformed heart valves and cause endocarditis.
2. They cause confusion in diagnosis because of their presence and their resemblance to some pathogens.
3. Penicillinase producing organisms of normal flora can aggravate bacterial resis-tance, interfering with therapy.
4. Streptococci of mouth can cause dental caries.

In environments which are full of pathogens as hospitals, a shift in the normal flora of the individuals can occur, e.g. an increase in carriage of antibiotic resistant staphylococci.

NORMAL FLORA OF THE SKIN

- Human skin is constantly bombarded by organisms present in the environment. It is also contaminated by one's own secretions and excretions depending on personal hygiene
- Flora depends on
  - Area of the body
  - Clothing
  - Occupation
  - Environment
- Usual organisms
  - Diphtheroids
  - Staphylococci (aerobic and anaerobic)
  - Gram-positive aerobic spore bearers
  - *Streptococcus viridans*
  - *Streptococcus faecalis.*

Gram-negative bacilli—*E. coli*, *Proteus* and other intestinal organisms.

- Mycobacteria (non-pathogenic)
- *Candida albicans*
- *Cryptococcus*
- *Pityrosporum ovale*
- Pathogenic hemolytic streptococci and staphylococci
- Penicillin resistant staphylococci are seen in individuals in hospitals.

Hair: *Staphylococcus aureus* is present on the hair.

NORMAL FLORA OF THE MOUTH AND UPPER RESPIRATORY TRACT

The mouth contains many microorganisms:

- Micrococci
- Gram-positive aerobic spore bearers
- Coliforms
- Proteus
- Lactobacilli.

The gum pockets between the teeth and crypts of tonsils have a wide spectrum of anaerobic flora:

- Anaerobic micrococci
- Anaerobic streptococci
- Vibrios
- Fusiform species
- *Corynebacterium* species
- *Mycoplasmas*
- *Neisseria*
- *Candida.*

Within 12 hours after birth, alpha hemolytic streptococci are found in the upper respiratory tract and become the dominant organism of the oropharynx and remain so for life. Few bacteria are found in normal bronchi. Smaller bronchi and alveoli are normally sterile. *Haemophilus* species and *Branhamella catarrhalis* may also be seen.

NORMAL FLORA OF THE CONJUNCTIVA

- The conjunctiva is relatively free from organisms due to flushing action of tears
- The predominant organisms of the eye are diphtheroids (*Corynebacterium xerosis*), *Moraxella* species, staphylococci and non-hemolytic streptococci.

NORMAL FLORA OF THE NOSE, NASOPHARYNX AND SINUSES

The floor of the nose harbors corynebacteria, staphylococci and streptococci.

The nasopharynx of the infant is sterile at birth. Two to three days after birth, it gets common commensal flora and the pathogenic flora carried by the mother and the attendants.

Nasopharynx can be considered the natural habitat of the common pathogenic bacteria which cause infections of the nose, throat, bronchi and lungs.

NORMAL FLORA OF THE INTESTINAL TRACT

Within 4 to 24 hours of birth an intestinal flora is established.

- In breastfed children, the intestine contains lactobacilli, enterococci, colon bacilli and staphylococci. *L. bifidus* constitutes 99 percent of total organisms in the feces.
- In bottle-fed children, colon bacilli, enterococci, gram-positive aerobic and anaerobic bacilli exist. Instead of *L. bifidus, L. acidophilus* is found.

Effect of Diet

Diet has a marked influence on the relative composition of the intestinal and fecal flora.

In normal adult, the microorganisms on the surface of the esophageal wall are those swallowed with saliva and food.

Because of the low pH of the stomach, it is virtually sterile except soon after eating. In patients with carcinoma of the stomach or achlorhydria or pyloric obstruction there is proliferation of gram-positive cocci and bacilli.

The number of bacteria increases progressively beyond the duodenum to the colon, being lesser in the small intestine than large intestine.

In the duodenum and upper ileum, lactobacilli and enterococci predominate but in the lower ileum and caecum, the flora resembles the fecal flora.

In the adult normal colon the resident bacterial flora are mostly (96 to 99%) anaerobes:

- Anaerobic streptococci
- Anaerobic lactobacilli
- Clostridia
- Bacteroides

The remaining bacteria are aerobes.

(One to four % aerobes)—Enterococci, coliforms, and small numbers of proteus, pseudomonas, lactobacilli, *Mycoplasma*, *Candida* and others.

NORMAL FLORA OF GENITOURINARY TRACT

- *Mycobacterium smegmatis*, a harmless commensal is found in the smegma of the genitalia of both males and females.
- Male urethra has aerobic and anaerobic bacteria. They are lactobacilli, *Gardnerella vaginalis*, a haemolytic streptococci, *bacteroides species*, *Chlamydia trachomatis* and *Ureaplasma urealyticum*
- Female urethra is either sterile or contains a few gram-positive cocci.

Vagina

At birth—It is sterile.

After 24 hours—It is invaded by micrococci, enterococci and diphtheroids.

In 2 to 3 days—Because of presence of maternal estrogen, glycogen deposition occurs which leads to the growth of lactobacillus (**Döderlein's bacillus**) which produces acid from glycogen. After the passively transferred oestrin has been eliminated in the urine, glycogen disappears and pH of the vagina becomes alkaline. This brings about a change in the flora to micrococci, alpha and non-hemolytic streptococci, coliforms and diphtheroids.

At puberty, glycogen reappears and the pH changes to acid due to the metabolic activity of Döderlein's bacilli, *E. coli* and yeasts. This change probably helps in prevention of colonisation by possible harmful microorganisms. During pregnancy, there is an increase in *Staphylococcus albus*, Döderlein's bacilli and yeasts. Occasionally other members of the intestinal flora may be present. After menopause the flora resembles that found before puberty. The normal vaginal flora includes clostridia, listeria, anaerobic streptococci, mycoplasma, *Gardnerella vaginalis*, neisseriae and non-pathogenic treponema species.

BACTERIA IN BLOOD AND TISSUES

Commensals from the normal flora of the mouth, nasopharynx and intestinal tract may get into blood and tissues. They are usually quickly eliminated by normal defense mechanisms of the body.

Unless the organisms of doubtful pathogenity are isolated more than once in serial blood cultures they have little significance.

OPPORTUNIST PATHOGENICITY

Opportunist pathogenicity occurs when the host defences are impaired and microbes which do not cause disease in normal hosts become pathogenic. The normal flora is a good source of such organisms. They occur in large numbers adjacent to tissues, well placed to invade and infect if the host defenses become impaired. For example, when patients become neutropenic through disease or anticancer chemotherapy, they are frequently infected by their own gut, skin or respiratory flora unless precautions are taken. The opportunistic bacteria can also come from the hospital and natural environments and sometimes from other people's skin or nasopharynx of hospital staff.

CHAPTER

42

Vaccines

LESSON PLAN

INTRODUCTION

As we have studied earlier, immunity or the resistance to infection is of two types—Innate and acquired. Innate immunity is the immunity that we have due to our genetic make up. Acquired immunity is the resistance which the individual acquires during his life. Acquired immunity is of two types—Active and Passive. Active immunity is the resistance developed by an individual as a result of an antigenic stimulus. Active immunity may be natural or artificial. Natural active immunity results from either a clinical or in apparent infection with a microorganism. Artificial active immunity is the resistance induced by vaccines.

WHAT ARE VACCINES?

Vaccines are preparations of live or killed microorganisms or their products used for immunization.

CLASSIFICATION

Vaccines are of two types—Live and Killed.

LIVE VACCINES

Live vaccines initiate an infection that is similar to natural infection though it is much milder. The immunity lasts for several years but booster doses may be necessary. Live vaccines may be administered orally or parenterally.

KILLED VACCINES

Killed vaccines are generally less immunogenic than live vaccines and the protection lasts only for a short period. They have to be administered repeatedly, generally at least two doses bein grequired for the production of immunity. The first is known as the primary dose and the subsequent doses as booster doses.

IMMUNOPROPHYLAXIS

Prophylaxis means protection. The application of immunization methods for the prevention of diseases is called immunoprophylaxis.

Active immunoprophylaxis can be considered under two headings.

1. Routine immunization of children which forms a part of basic healthcare of communities.
2. Immunization of individuals or selected groups exposed to risk of particular infections.

Routine immunisation schedules have been developed for different countries based on the prevalence of infectious diseases and their pubic health importance. The expanded programme on immunisation recommended by the World Health Organization for the developing countries is directed against tuberculosis, diphtheria, pertussis, tetanus, poliomyelitis and measles.

A schedule of immunisation is shown in the Table 42.1. We shall now study a few vaccines.

BCG

BCG stands for Bacillus Calmette-Guérin named after two scientists, Calmette and Guérin. This is given for protection against tuberculosis.

Although BCG vaccine has been in use for about 60 years its efficiency is still doubtful. Several trials show protection rates from nil to 80 percent. It is beheved that BCG may be useful in infants and children particularly against the more serious types of infection, meningitis and miliary tuberculosis. It is, therefore, recommended that the vaccine is to be administered to the infant soon after birth, before the mother and baby are discharged from the hospital. Booster doses are not given because in the developing countries natural infections with tubercle bacilli maintain immunity. In countries where tuberculosis is rare immunity following a single dose of BCG becomes less and a booster dose is given at school entry.

Complications are few and there may be local ulceration, enlargement and suppuration of the draining lymph nodes and keloid formation.

It has been seen that BCG gives some protection against leprosy and leukemia. The vaccine is manufactured at BCG Laboratory at the King's Institute Guindy, Chennai and Serum Iinstitute of India, Pune.

DPT

Diphtheria, pertussis and tetanus are important childhood infections which can be prevented by immunization.

DPT vaccine contains the toxoids of diphtheria and tetanus and a killed suspension of pertussis bacilli. The pertussis vaccine acts as an adjuvant for the toxoids. The primary course of DPT immunisation consists of 3 subcutaneous injections with an interval of 4 to 8 weeks between the 1st and 2nd and 8 to 12 weeks between the 2nd and 3rd. This gives better antibody response than giving the vaccine at monthly intervals. We should start the DPT vaccine at 2 months because there is little maternal immunity against pertussis which can be a very severe illness in young babies. Before two months, immunization is not effective due to immaturity of the immune system. Diphtheria is rare in children under 6 months of age as they are protected by maternal antibodies then. Tetanus in the newborn can be prevented by immunizing pregnant women with tetanus toxoid. A booster dose of DPT istetanus toxoid. A booster dose of DPT is recommended at 18 months of age.

Diphtheria and pertussis do not occur after 5 years but tetanus can occur at any age. Therefore, a booster of tetanus toxoid is advisable at school entry. This should give life long protection. Adverse reactions to DPT vaccine are rare and consist of local inflammation, fever and convulsions.

Poliomyelitis

Two effective vaccines are available against poliomyelitis—the oral vaccine and the inactivated parenteral vaccine. Oral polio vaccine is ideally suited for mass immunization.

Table 42.1: Schedule of immunization

Sl No.	*Age*	*Disease*	*Vaccination*	*Remarks*
		Recommended Immunization Schedule Followed In India		
1	At Birth	Hepatitis B	HEP B Vaccine -I	
2	At Birth	Polio	Oral PV 0 Dose	
3	Birth To 6 weeks	Tuberculosis	BCG	
4	4–6 weeks	Hepatitis B	HEP B Vaccine -II	
		Diphtheria		
		Pertusis	DPT-I	
5	6 weeks	Tetanus	OPV -I	
		Polio		
		Diphtheria	DPT-II	*Delhi Govt
		Pertusis	OPV-II	Recommendation
6	10 weeks	Tetanus	HEP B Vaccine III*	
		Polio		
		Hepatitis B		
		Diphtheria		
		Pertusi	DPT-III	*Delhi Govt
7	14 weeks	Diphtheria	OPV- III	Recommendation
		Stetanus	HEP B Vaccine IV*	
		Polio		
8	24 weeks	Hepatitis B	HEP B Vaccine III*	*IAP Recommendation
9	9–12 months	Polio Measles	OPV-IV Measles	
		Mumps		
10	15–18 months	Measeles	MMR*	
		Rubella		
		Diphtheria	DPT –Booster I	*Recommended By
11	18 months	Pertusis	OPV –V	Delhi Govt & Iap Only
		Tetanus		
		Polio		
12	24 months	Typhoid	Typhoid*	*IAP Recommendation
		Diphtheria		
		Pertusis		
13	4–5 Years	Tetanus	DPT Booster–II	
		Polio	OPV -VI	
		Other Available Vaccines		
14	6 weeks	H Influenza B	HiB	*IAP Recommendation
15	10 weeks	H Influenza B	HiB	
16	14 weeks	H Influenza B	HiB	*IAP Recommendation
17	18 months	H Influenza B	HiB	*IAP Recommendation
18	24 months	Hepatitis A	H A Vaccine-I	Suggested Vaccination
19	30 months	Hepatitis A	H A Vaccine -II	Suggested Vaccination
20	12 months	Chickenpox	Varicella Vaccine	Suggested Vaccination
21	24 months	Meningococcal A&C	Meningococcal Vaccine	Suggested Vaccination
22	12 months	Pneumococcal	Pneumococcal Vaccine	In Special Circumstances
23	12 months	Influenza	Influenza Vaccine	In Special Circumstances
		On Going Vaccinations		
24	10 Years	Tetanus	TT	Every Five Years
25	5 Years	Typhoid	Typhoid	Every Three Years
26	5 Years	Meningococcal A&C	Meningococcal Vaccine	Every Three Years
27	NID's† and SNID's‡	Polio Eradication	Pulse Polio	As Per Govt Directives

* IAP—Indian Academy of Pediatrics
† NID's—National Immunization Days
‡ SNID's—Sub-National Immunization Days

A three dosage schedule was widely used in the tropics but seroconversion rates in India and many other tropical countries were poor. Many reasons have been proposed for this poor response:

1. Improper storage.
2. Interference by other enteroviruses in the gut.
3. Neutralization by antibodies in breast.
4. Presence of inhibitors in gastrointestinal secretions.

To circumvent this problem a high potency vaccine is used. Precautions to be observed for a good vaccine response are:

- Avoiding breastfeeding for some hours before and after administration of vaccine
- Increasing the number of doses to five
- Simultaneous vaccination of all infants and children in one locality.

For the present, the best course is to give five doses of oral polio vaccine as suggested in the schedule.

Measles

Measles is the commonest exanthematous disease of childhood. Live attenuated measles vaccines has been found to be effective. The earlier vaccines gave rise to fever but the later vaccines do not cause any serious side-effects.

The vaccine is given as a single dose of S/C injection in children 9 to 12 months old. Younger children have some maternal antibodies and vaccination in them may prove ineffective. Booster injections are not necessary.

Mumps

The live vaccine is available in advanced countries. This may be given alone or in combination with measles and rubella vaccine. It is however not needed in developing countries where mumps is a minor illness.

Rubella

The vaccination is given to pregnant women in whom there is a danger of infection leading to fetal malformations.

Now MMR vaccine has been introduced as a combined vaccination for the three diseases (Measles, Mumps, Rubella) above.

Smallpox

Small pox eradication programme was initiated by Who in 1957 and global eradication of small pox was achieved by 1980 . Therfore the vaccine is No longer indicated. It's production has been discontinued in India. Large stocks of vaccine are maintained by the WHO to be used in the unlikely event of smallpox reappearing.

Typhoid Vaccine

The monovalent typhoid vaccine was introduced by Wright in 1897. During the 1st World War when British troops had to serve in Europe, Africa and Asia, where typhoid and paratyphoid fevers were common, the typhoid vaccine was supplemented with killed paratyphoid A and B bacilli in the hope that polyvalent TAB vaccine would protect against typhoid and paratyphoid fevers. Immunity lasts from 6 months to some years.

These days the various types of typhoid vaccine available are:

1. Acetone killed and dried vaccine
2. Heat-killed phenolized vaccine

Because paratyphoid B does not occur in India, this component of TAB vaccine has been deleted. The vaccine manufactured at present contains only typhoid and paratyphoid A bacilli. It is at present not used routinely in the general population but only in special groups such as armed forces, nurses and other hospital workers in whom it is given annually.

Mass immunization is sometimes practised when:

1. There occurs a large outbreak of enteric fever in an area.
2. Household contacts of patients with enteric fever.

Two doses of typhoid vaccine are given S/C at an interval of one month to children of about two years.

A booster at school entry may be helpful.

A more effective oral typhoid vaccine prepared from Ty 21 a mutant strain proved very effective in a clinical trial in Egypt. Its administration is cumbersome, requiring prior neutralisation of gastric acidity.

Cholera

- ***Killed parenteral cholera*** vaccine is used
- It provides limited protection for upto 6 months only
- Trials in Calcutta and Indonesia with aluminium phosphate adjuvant vaccine has given better results. This gives protection for about 2 years especially in young children. But the vaccine has not been manufactured for routine use as yet.

At present cholera vaccine is misused because whenever there is an outbreak of gastroenteritis this vaccine is given. Many of these outbreaks may not be cholera at all.

Influenza

Inactivated influenza virus vaccines are used in Britain annually before the onset of winter in special groups such as the elderly with chronic bronchitis. This helps reduce morbidity and mortality in them. In the tropics where annual winter epidemics of influenza are not a feature, routine immunization is not called for influenza. Immunization becomes necessary when a pandemic spread is anticipated.

Other Vaccines

1. **Polyvalent pneumococcal polysaccharide** vaccine containing common serotypes is used in the USA in selected vulnerable groups.
2. **Meningococcal vaccines** containing the protective polysaccharide antigens have been used against epidemic meningococcal meningitis.
3. **Killed *Pseudomonas aeruginosa*** vaccines have been used in severely burnt patients.
4. **A live chickenpox vaccine** developed in Japan is recommended in leukaemic and other high-risk children.
5. **The 17D yellow fever vaccine** is manufactured at the Central Research Institute, Kasauli. As yellow fever does not occur in India, the vaccine is used only for persons travelling to endemic areas.
6. An effective vaccine has been developed in Japan for **Japanese encephalitis**. As the disease has now become a serious problem vaccination has become necessary. The vaccine is being manufactured at the CRI, Kasauli.
7. **An inactivated vaccine for KFD (Kyasanur Forest disease)** has been developed in India. The vaccine has not been manufactured in bulk nor mass immunization attempted.
8. **Rabies vaccine**—Neural vaccines are Sample or BPL vaccines. These carry the risk of neuroparalytic complications. The human diploid cell vaccine is safe and effective but expensive.
9. **Hepatitis vaccines**—Vaccines exist for Hepatitis A and Hepatitis B. They are recombinant DNA vaccines and are given intramuscularly. Hepatitis A is given in two injections, a month apart. Hepatitis B is given in 3 injections at 0, 1 month and 6 months. A booster dose is given every 5 years.

Autovaccines

For chronic infections, autovaccines are found to be useful. The infecting strain of the bacterium is grown and graded doses of a suspension of the bacteria killed by heat and phenol are given. Staphylococci and streptococci are the bacteria commonly used for autovaccine preparation.

PASSIVE IMMUNIZATION

The antitoxic sera in common use are:

- antidiphtheritic
- antitetanus
- antigas gangrene.

Active immunization is used in case of diphtheria and antidiphtheritic serum is not used these days. Antitetanus serum however is used extensively in treatment. However, it should be used only for tetanus prone wounds. As active immunisation against gas gangrene is not available, antigas gangrene serum still has a place in crush injury. Antisera have been used in the prophylaxis and treatment of many viral diseases. Convalescent sera or specific immune globulin has been used for protection of contacts against smallpox, chickenpox, measles and hepatitis. Human gammaglobulin preparations contain antibodies against all common viral infections and have been used as broad spectrum antiviral immunoprophylactics.

VACCINATION REQUIREMENTS

Most countries insist on Yellow Fever vaccination and a few still require cholera vaccination.

READER SUGGESTIONS SHEET

Please help us to improve the quality of our publications by completing and returning this sheet to us.

Title/Author: **Microbiology Theory for MLT** *by Namita Jaggi*

Your Name and Address:

Phone and Fax:

E-mail Address:

How did you hear about this book? [please tick appropriate box(es)]

- ☐ Direct mail from publisher
- ☐ Conference
- ☐ Bookshop
- ☐ Book review
- ☐ Lecturer recommendation
- ☐ Friends
- ☐ Other (please specify)
- ☐ Website

Type of purchase: ☐ Direct purchase ☐ Bookshop ☐ Friends

Do you have any brief comments on the book?

Please return this sheet to the name and address given below.

JAYPEE BROTHERS MEDICAL PUBLISHERS (P) LTD
4838/24, Ansari Road, Daryaganj
New Delhi 110 002, India

Index

Page numbers followed by *f* refer to figure and *t* refer to table